Jane W. Ball, RN, CPNP, DrPH
Executive Director
Trauma System Consultant
American College of Surgeons
Gaithersburg, Maryland

Ruth C. Bindler, RNC, PhD
Professor
Washington State University
College of Nursing
Spokane, Washington

Kay J. Cowen, RNC, MSN
Clinical Associate Professor
UNCG School of Nursing
Greensboro, NC

Pearson
New York   Boston   San Franscisco   London   Toronto
Sydney   Tokyo   Mexico City   Paris   Cape Town
Hong Kong   Montreal

Library of Congress Cataloging-in-Publication Data

Ball, Jane.
   Clinical handbook for pediatric nursing / Jane W. Ball, Ruth C. Bindler, Kay J. Cowen. — 2nd ed.
      p. ; cm.
   Rev. ed. of: Clinical handbook for pediatric nursing / Jane W. Ball, Ruth C. Bindler. c2006.
   Includes bibliographical references and index.
   ISBN-13: 978-0-13-500506-4
   ISBN-10: 0-13-500506-X
   1. Pediatric nursing—Handbooks, manuals, etc.   I. Bindler, Ruth McGillis.   II. Cowen, Kay J.
   III. Title.
   [DNLM: 1. Pediatric Nursing—methods—Handbooks. 2. Child Development—Handbooks.
   3. Nursing Assessment—Handbooks.   WY 49 B187c 2010]
   RJ245.B345 2010
   618.92'00231—dc22

                                                                                    2009006261

Publisher: Julie Levin Alexander
Assistant to Publisher: Regina Bruno
Editor-in-Chief: Maura Connor
Assistant to the Editor-in-Chief: Marion Gottlieb
Executive Acquisitions Editor: Pamela Fuller
Assistant to the Executive Acquisitions
   Editor: Sarah Wrocklage
Director of Marketing: Karen Allman
Senior Marketing Manager: Francisco del Castillo
Marketing Specialist: Michael Sirinides
Managing Editor, Production: Patrick Walsh

Production Editor: Erin Melloy, S4Carlisle
Production Liaison: Anne Garcia
Manufacturing Manager: Ilene Sanford
Senior Design Coordinator: Maria
   Guglielmo-Walsh
Tile Art: Courtesy of Rydal Elementary
   School, Abington, PA
Tile Art Photographer: Michal Heron
Composition: S4Carlisle Publishing Services
Printer/Binder: Bind-Rite Graphics, Robbinsville
Cover Printer: Bind-Rite Graphics, Robbinsville

Notice: Care has been taken to confirm the accuracy of information presented in this book. The authors, edi-tors, and the publisher, however, cannot accept any responsibility for errors or omissions or for conse-quences from application of the information in this book and make no warranty, express or implied, with respect to its contents.

The authors and publisher have exerted every effort to ensure that drug selections and dosages set forth in this text are in accord with current recommendations and practice at time of publication. However, in view of ongoing research, changes in government regulations, and the constant flow of information relating to drug therapy and reactions, the reader is urged to check the package inserts of all drugs for any change in indications or dosage and for added warning and precautions. This is particularly important when the recom-mended agent is a new and/or infrequently employed drug.

Pearson Education Ltd., London
Pearson Education Singapore, Pte. Ltd.
Pearson Education Canada, Inc.
Pearson Education—Japan
Pearson Education Australia PTY, Limited

Pearson Education North Asia, Ltd., Hong Kong
Pearson Educación de Mexico, S.A. de C.V.
Pearson Education Malaysia, Pte. Ltd.
Pearson Education Upper Saddle River, New Jersey

www.pearsonhighered.com

10 9 8 7 6 5 4 3 2 1
ISBN-13: 978-0-13-500506-4
ISBN-10:   0-13-500506-X

Contents

PREFACE

As a nursing student or practicing nurse, you face challenging client situations that test your knowledge base, your ability to prioritize, and your familiarity with certain clinical skills. The *Clinical Handbook for Pediatric Nursing, 2e,* has been created to help you in situations like these. The handbook provides general information on growth and development, vital signs, assessment, and more, with information specific to the care of children in the community or hospital. Included are principles of pediatric medications, pain management, immunization schedules, and an overview of clinical and nursing management for conditions organized by body systems. Each content area includes key information about clinical therapy, as well as how to use the nursing process to plan appropriate nursing management. Critical nursing assessments and interventions are identified, and specific examples are given regarding documentation of care.

As a valuable resource, the *Clinical Skills Manual for Pediatric Nursing, Fourth Edition,* can be consulted for detailed instructions on how to perform the techniques and procedures referred to in this book.

Although the handbook provides condensed information about each subject area, critical aspects of nursing practice have been included. It is our hope that this book will enhance pediatric nursing practice, provide a quick overview in the clinical setting, and help nurses provide safe, competent care to all children.

We would also like to acknowledge and thank the following reviewers for their helpful feedback and participation:

Vicky H. Becherer, MSN, RN
Pediatric Clinical Instructor
University of Missouri–St. Louis
St. Louis, Missouri

Tracy B. Chamblee, MS, RN, CNS
Clinical Nurse Specialist
Golisano Children's Hospital
University of Rochester Medical Center
Associate Professor
St. John Fisher College
Rochester, New York

Virginia M. White, RN, BSN, MN, APRN-BC
ARNP—Nursing Faculty Adjunct
Olympic College
Bremerton, Washington

Michele Wolff, RN, MSN
Professor of Nursing
Saddleback College
Mission Viejo, California

1 NORMAL VITAL SIGNS

Table 1–1 Normal Respiratory Rate Ranges for Each Age Group

Age	Respiratory Rate per Min
Newborn	30–55
1 year	20–40
3 years	20–30
6 years	16–22
10 years	16–20
17 years	12–18

Table 1–2 Heart Rate Ranges and Average Heart Rates for Each Age Group

Age	Heart Rate Range (Beats/Min)	Average Heart Rate (Beats/Min)
Newborns	100–170	120 when stabilized
Infants to 2 years	80–130	110
2–6 years	70–120	100
6–10 years	70–110	90
10–16 years	60–100	85

Table 1–3 Blood Pressure Levels for Boys by Age and Height Percentile*

Age (Year)	BP Percentile	Systolic BP (mm Hg) Percentile of Height							Diastolic BP (mm Hg) Percentile of Height						
		5th	10th	25th	50th	75th	90th	95th	5th	10th	25th	50th	75th	90th	95th
1	50th	80	81	83	85	87	88	89	34	35	36	37	38	39	39
	90th	94	95	97	99	100	102	103	49	50	51	52	53	53	54
	95th	98	99	101	103	104	106	106	54	54	55	56	57	58	58
	99th	105	106	108	110	112	113	114	61	62	63	64	65	66	66
2	50th	84	85	87	88	90	92	92	39	40	41	42	43	44	44
	90th	97	99	100	102	104	105	106	54	55	56	57	58	58	59
	95th	101	102	104	106	108	109	110	59	59	60	61	62	63	63
	99th	109	110	111	113	115	117	117	66	67	68	69	70	71	71
3	50th	86	87	89	91	93	94	95	44	44	45	46	47	48	48
	90th	100	101	103	105	107	108	109	59	59	60	61	62	63	63
	95th	104	105	107	109	110	112	113	63	63	64	65	66	67	67
	99th	111	112	114	116	118	119	120	71	71	72	73	74	75	75
4	50th	88	89	91	93	95	96	97	47	48	49	50	51	51	52
	90th	102	103	105	107	109	110	111	62	63	64	65	66	66	67
	95th	106	107	109	111	112	114	115	66	67	68	69	70	71	71
	99th	113	114	116	118	120	121	122	74	75	76	77	78	78	79
5	50th	90	91	93	95	96	98	98	50	51	52	53	54	55	55
	90th	104	105	106	108	110	111	112	65	66	67	68	69	69	70
	95th	108	109	110	112	114	115	116	69	70	71	72	73	74	74
	99th	115	116	118	120	121	123	123	77	78	79	80	81	81	82
6	50th	91	92	94	96	98	99	100	53	53	54	55	56	57	57
	90th	105	106	108	110	111	113	113	68	68	69	70	71	72	72
	95th	109	110	112	114	115	117	117	72	72	73	74	75	76	76
	99th	116	117	119	121	123	124	125	80	80	81	82	83	84	84
7	50th	92	94	95	97	99	100	101	55	55	56	57	58	59	59
	90th	106	107	109	111	113	114	115	70	70	71	72	73	74	74
	95th	110	111	113	115	117	118	119	74	74	75	76	77	78	78
	99th	117	118	120	122	124	125	126	82	82	83	84	85	86	86
8	50th	94	95	97	99	100	102	102	56	57	58	59	60	60	61
	90th	107	109	110	112	114	115	116	71	72	72	73	74	75	76
	95th	111	112	114	116	118	119	120	75	76	77	78	79	79	80
	99th	119	120	122	123	125	127	127	83	84	85	86	87	87	88
9	50th	95	96	98	100	102	103	104	57	58	59	60	61	61	62
	90th	109	110	112	114	115	117	118	72	73	74	75	76	76	77
	95th	113	114	116	118	119	121	121	76	77	78	79	80	81	81
	99th	120	121	123	125	127	128	129	84	85	86	87	88	88	89
10	50th	97	98	100	102	103	105	106	58	59	60	61	61	62	63
	90th	111	112	114	115	117	119	119	73	73	74	75	76	77	78
	95th	115	116	117	119	121	122	123	77	78	79	80	81	81	82
	99th	122	123	125	127	128	130	130	85	86	86	88	88	89	90

Table 1–3 Blood Pressure Levels for Boys by Age and Height Percentile (Continued)

Age (Year)	BP Percentile	Systolic BP (mm Hg) Percentile of Height							Diastolic BP (mm Hg) Percentile of Height						
		5th	10th	25th	50th	75th	90th	95th	5th	10th	25th	50th	75th	90th	95th
11	50th	99	100	102	104	105	107	107	59	59	60	61	62	63	63
	90th	113	114	115	117	119	120	121	74	74	75	76	77	78	78
	95th	117	118	119	121	123	124	125	78	78	79	80	81	82	82
	99th	124	125	127	129	130	132	132	86	86	87	88	89	90	90
12	50th	101	102	104	106	108	109	110	59	60	61	62	63	63	64
	90th	115	116	118	120	121	123	123	74	75	75	76	77	78	79
	95th	119	120	122	123	125	127	127	78	79	80	81	82	82	83
	99th	126	127	129	131	133	134	135	86	87	88	89	90	90	91
13	50th	104	105	106	108	110	111	112	60	60	61	62	63	64	64
	90th	117	118	120	122	124	125	126	75	75	76	77	78	79	79
	95th	121	122	124	126	128	129	130	79	79	80	81	82	83	83
	99th	128	130	131	133	135	136	137	87	87	88	89	90	91	91
14	50th	106	107	109	111	113	114	115	60	61	62	63	64	65	65
	90th	120	121	123	125	126	128	128	75	76	77	78	79	79	80
	95th	124	125	127	128	130	132	132	80	80	81	82	83	84	84
	99th	131	132	134	136	138	139	140	87	88	89	90	91	92	92
15	50th	109	110	112	113	115	117	117	61	62	63	64	65	66	66
	90th	122	124	125	127	129	130	131	76	77	78	79	80	80	81
	95th	126	127	129	131	133	134	135	81	81	82	83	84	85	85
	99th	134	135	136	138	140	142	142	88	89	90	91	92	93	93
16	50th	111	112	114	116	118	119	120	63	63	64	65	66	67	67
	90th	125	126	128	130	131	133	134	78	78	79	80	81	82	82
	95th	129	130	132	134	135	137	137	82	83	83	84	85	86	87
	99th	136	137	139	141	143	144	145	90	90	91	92	93	94	94
17	50th	114	115	116	118	120	121	122	65	66	66	67	68	69	70
	90th	127	128	130	132	134	135	136	80	80	81	82	83	84	84
	95th	131	132	134	136	138	139	140	84	85	86	87	87	88	89
	99th	139	140	141	143	145	146	147	92	93	93	94	95	96	97

BP, blood pressure.

*Note: Use the child's height percentile for the age and sex from the standard growth charts found in chapter 3. A blood pressure value at the 50th percentile for the child's age, sex, and height percentile is considered the midpoint of the normal range. A reading above the 95th percentile indicates hypertension.

*The 90th percentile is 1.28 SD, the 95th percentile is 1.645 SD, and the 99th percentile is 2.326 SD over the mean.

Source: From National Heart, Lung, and Blood Institute. (2004). Blood pressure tables for children and adolescents from the fourth report on the diagnosis, evaluation, and treatment of high blood pressure in children and adolescents. Retrieved June 30, 2008, from http:// www.nhlbi.nih.gov/guidelines/hypertension/child_tbl.htm. Used with permission.

Table 1–4 Blood Pressure Levels for Girls by Age and Height Percentile*

Age (Year)	BP Percentile	Systolic BP (mm Hg) Percentile of Height							Diastolic BP (mm Hg) Percentile of Height						
		5th	10th	25th	50th	75th	90th	95th	5th	10th	25th	50th	75th	90th	95th
1	50th	83	84	85	86	88	89	90	38	39	39	40	41	41	42
	90th	97	97	98	100	101	102	103	52	53	53	54	55	55	56
	95th	100	101	102	104	105	106	107	56	57	57	58	59	59	60
	99th	108	108	109	111	112	113	114	64	64	65	65	66	67	67
2	50th	85	85	87	88	89	91	91	43	44	44	45	46	46	47
	90th	98	99	100	101	103	104	105	57	58	58	59	60	61	61
	95th	102	103	104	105	107	108	109	61	62	62	63	64	65	65
	99th	109	110	111	112	114	115	117	69	69	70	70	71	72	72
3	50th	86	87	88	89	91	92	93	47	48	48	49	50	50	51
	90th	100	100	102	103	104	106	106	61	62	62	63	64	64	65
	95th	104	104	105	107	108	109	110	65	66	66	67	68	68	69
	99th	111	111	113	114	115	116	117	73	73	74	74	75	76	76
4	50th	88	88	90	91	92	94	94	50	50	51	52	52	53	54
	90th	101	102	103	104	106	107	108	64	64	65	66	67	67	68
	95th	105	106	107	108	110	111	112	68	68	69	70	71	71	72
	99th	112	113	114	115	117	118	119	76	76	76	77	78	79	79
5	50th	89	90	91	93	94	95	96	52	53	53	54	55	55	56
	90th	103	103	105	106	107	109	109	66	67	67	68	69	69	70
	95th	107	107	108	110	111	112	113	70	71	71	72	73	73	74
	99th	114	114	116	117	118	120	120	78	78	79	79	80	81	81
6	50th	91	92	93	94	96	97	98	54	54	55	56	56	57	58
	90th	104	105	106	108	109	110	111	68	68	69	70	70	71	72
	95th	108	109	110	111	113	114	115	72	72	73	74	74	75	76
	99th	115	116	117	119	120	121	122	80	80	80	81	82	83	83
7	50th	93	93	95	96	97	99	99	55	56	56	57	58	58	59
	90th	106	107	108	109	111	112	113	69	70	70	71	72	72	73
	95th	110	111	112	113	115	116	116	73	74	74	75	76	76	77
	99th	117	118	119	120	122	123	124	81	81	82	82	83	84	84
8	50th	95	95	96	98	99	100	101	57	57	57	58	59	60	60
	90th	108	109	110	111	113	114	114	71	71	71	72	73	74	74
	95th	112	112	114	115	116	118	118	75	75	75	76	77	78	78
	99th	119	120	121	122	123	125	125	82	82	83	83	84	85	86
9	50th	96	97	98	100	101	102	103	58	58	58	59	60	61	61
	90th	110	110	112	113	114	116	116	72	72	72	73	74	75	75
	95th	114	114	115	117	118	119	120	76	76	76	77	78	79	79
	99th	121	121	123	124	125	127	127	83	83	84	84	85	86	87
10	50th	98	99	100	102	103	104	105	59	59	59	60	61	62	62
	90th	112	112	114	115	116	118	118	73	73	73	74	75	76	76
	95th	116	116	117	119	120	121	122	77	77	77	78	79	80	80
	99th	123	123	125	126	127	129	129	84	84	85	86	86	87	88

Table 1–4 Blood Pressure Levels for Girls by Age and Height Percentile (Continued)

Age (Year)	BP Percentile	Systolic BP (mm Hg) Percentile of Height							Diastolic BP (mm Hg) Percentile of Height						
		5th	10th	25th	50th	75th	90th	95th	5th	10th	25th	50th	75th	90th	95th
11	50th	100	101	102	103	105	106	107	60	60	60	61	62	63	63
	90th	114	114	116	117	118	119	120	74	74	74	75	76	77	77
	95th	118	118	119	121	122	123	124	78	78	78	79	80	81	81
	99th	125	125	126	128	129	130	131	85	85	86	87	87	88	89
12	50th	102	103	104	105	107	108	109	61	61	61	62	63	64	64
	90th	116	116	117	119	120	121	122	75	75	75	76	77	78	78
	95th	119	120	121	123	124	125	126	79	79	79	80	81	82	82
	99th	127	127	128	130	131	132	133	86	86	87	88	88	89	90
13	50th	104	105	106	107	109	110	110	62	62	62	63	64	65	65
	90th	117	118	119	121	122	123	124	76	76	76	77	78	79	79
	95th	121	122	123	124	126	127	128	80	80	80	81	82	83	83
	99th	128	129	130	132	133	134	135	87	87	88	89	89	90	91
14	50th	106	106	107	109	110	111	112	63	63	63	64	65	66	66
	90th	119	120	121	122	124	125	125	77	77	77	78	79	80	80
	95th	123	123	125	126	127	129	129	81	81	81	82	83	84	84
	99th	130	131	132	133	135	136	136	88	88	89	90	90	91	92
15	50th	107	108	109	110	111	113	113	64	64	64	65	66	67	67
	90th	120	121	122	123	125	126	127	78	78	78	79	80	81	81
	95th	124	125	126	127	129	130	131	82	82	82	83	84	85	85
	99th	131	132	133	134	136	137	138	89	89	90	91	91	92	93
16	50th	108	108	110	111	112	114	114	64	64	65	66	66	67	68
	90th	121	122	123	124	126	127	128	78	78	79	80	81	81	82
	95th	125	126	127	128	130	131	132	82	82	83	84	85	85	86
	99th	132	133	134	135	137	138	139	90	90	90	91	92	93	93
17	50th	108	109	110	111	113	114	115	64	65	65	66	67	67	68
	90th	122	122	123	125	126	127	128	78	79	79	80	81	81	82
	95th	125	126	127	129	130	131	132	82	83	83	84	85	85	86
	99th	133	133	134	136	137	138	139	90	90	91	91	92	93	93

BP, blood pressure.

*Note: Use the child's height percentile for the age and sex from the standard growth charts found in chapter 3. A blood pressure value at the 50th percentile for the child's age, sex, and height percentile is considered the midpoint of the normal range. A reading above the 95th percentile indicates hypertension.

The 90th percentile is 1.28 SD, the 95th percentile is 1.645 SD, and the 99th percentile is 2.326 SD over the mean.

Source: From National Heart, Lung, and Blood Institute. (2004). Blood pressure tables for children and adolescents from the fourth report on the diagnosis, evaluation, and treatment of high blood pressure in children and adolescents. Retrieved June 30, 2008, from http:// www.nhlbi.nih.gov/guidelines/hypertension/child_tbl.htm. Used with permission.

2 ASSESSMENT

ELEMENTS OF THE CHILD'S HISTORY

Patient identifying information: name, nickname, age, sex, ethnic origin, birth date, race, religion, contact information. Name of person providing information.

Chief complaint.

History of present illness or injury: detailed description of current health problem, including onset, type of symptoms, location, duration, severity, influencing factors, and current therapies (prescribed, over-the-counter, complementary).

Medical history: detailed description of the child's prior health status.

- Birth history: prenatal history, description of delivery, condition of baby at birth, postnatal care and concerns.
- All major past illnesses, injuries, hospitalizations, and surgeries: age at the time of each; transfusions; treatment; outcome; complication or residual problem; and the child's reaction to the event.

Current health status: typical health status, allergies, medications, immunization status, activities and exercise, sleep patterns, nutrition, safety measures used, and health maintenance care.

Family history: infectious diseases, allergies, hereditary disorders, major body system disorder, cancer, problem pregnancies, learning problems. Health status of each parent.

Review of systems: comprehensive overview of the child's health by body system (Table 2–1).

Psychosocial data: family composition, family members living in home, relationships, persons caring for child, financial resources, health insurance, description of housing and home environment, neighborhood, school or childcare arrangements, daily routines, spiritual life.

Developmental data: motor, cognitive, language, and social development; language, fine and gross motor milestones, and current skills; academic performance; interaction with other children, family members, and strangers.

Table 2–1   Review of Systems

Body Systems	Examples of Problems to Identify
General	General growth pattern, alertness, health status; easily tires, fever, sleep patterns; allergies, reaction (hives, rash, respiratory difficulty, swelling, nausea), seasonal or with each exposure
Skin and lymph	Rashes, dry skin, itching, skin color or texture changes, bruising tendency, swollen or tender lymph glands
Hair and nails	Hair loss, color or texture changes; nail growth or color abnormalities, clubbing
Head	Headaches
Eyes	Vision problems, squinting, crossed eyes, lazy eye, wears glasses; eye infections, redness, tearing, burning, rubbing, swelling eyelids
Ears	Ear infections, discharge from ears, tubes in ears; hearing loss or hearing tested; hearing aids or cochlear implants
Nose and sinuses	Nosebleeds, nasal congestion, runny nose, sinus pain or infections; difficulty breathing, snoring at night
Mouth and throat	Mouth breathing, difficulty swallowing, sore throats, strep infections; mouth odor; tooth eruption, cavities, braces; hoarseness, speech problems
Cardiac and hematologic	Heart murmur, anemia, hypertension, cyanosis, edema, chest pain
Chest and respiratory	Trouble breathing, choking episodes, cough, wheezing, cyanosis, exposure to tuberculosis, other infections
Gastrointestinal	Bowel movements, frequency, color, regularity, consistency, discomfort, constipation or diarrhea; abdominal pain, rectal bleeding, flatulence; nausea or vomiting, appetite
Urinary	Frequency, urgency, dysuria, dribbling, enuresis, strength of urinary stream; age when day and night dryness attained
Reproductive	For pubescent children
Female	Menses onset, amount, duration, frequency, discomfort, problems; vaginal discharge, breast development
Male	Puberty onset, emissions, erections, pain or discharge from penis, swelling or pain in testicles
Both	Sexual activity, use of contraception, sexually transmitted diseases
Musculoskeletal	Weakness, poor coordination, balance, tremors, abnormal gait; pain, swelling, or redness of muscles or joints, fractures
Neurologic	Seizures, fainting spells, dizziness, numbness, brain injuries; learning problems, concentration or memory problems, attention span, hyperactivity

PHYSICAL EXAMINATION TECHNIQUES

Inspection is the purposeful observation of the child's physical features and behaviors and detection of odors with your nose.

Palpation is the use of touch to identify characteristics of the skin, internal organs, and masses (texture, moistness, tenderness, temperature, position, shape, consistency, and mobility of masses and organs).

Auscultation is listening to sounds produced by the airway, lungs, stomach, heart, and blood vessels to identify their characteristics.

Percussion is striking the surface of the body, either directly or indirectly, setting up vibrations to reveal the density of underlying tissues and borders of organs.

Standard precautions are used during the physical examination.

EQUIPMENT NEEDED

Stethoscope, sphygmomanometer, otoscope, ophthalmoscope, reflex hammer, cotton balls, penlight, tongue blades, and gloves.

GENERAL APPRAISAL

Procedure[1]	Findings[2]
Observe the child's general appearance and behavior.	Well-nourished, well-developed. *Infants and young children may be fearful.*
Measure the child's weight, length or height, and head circumference, and plot on appropriate growth curves. Calculate the body mass index.	Following a consistent growth channel for all measurements. Height and weight are proportional.

[1]Italics indicates caution to take with procedure.
[2]Italics indicates abnormal findings.

ASSESSING SKIN AND HAIR CHARACTERISTICS AND INTEGRITY

Procedure[1]	Findings[2]
Inspect the skin for color and the presence of imperfections, elevations, variations, or lesions. Identify lesion characteristics (location, size, type of lesion, pattern, and discharge). Inspect the buccal mucosa and tongue when a skin color abnormality such as jaundice or cyanosis is suspected.	Even color distribution; bruises are common on the knees, shins, and lower arms from falls. See chapter 26 for skin lesion descriptions. *Suspect child abuse when bruises are on other parts of the body in various stages of healing. Pigmentation, pallor, mottling, bruises, erythema, cyanosis, or jaundice may indicate local or generalized conditions.*
Palpate skin for temperature, texture, moistness, and resilience, or turgor.	Feels cool, dry, soft, and smooth to the touch; taut, elastic, and mobile with good turgor. *Warm skin with fever or inflammation. Excessive sweating without exertion in an uncorrected congenital heart defect. Poor skin turgor with dehydration.*
Test capillary refill time.	Capillary refill is less than 2 seconds. *Prolonged times indicate poor circulation or hypovolemia.*

Inspect the scalp hair for color, distribution, and cleanliness, presence of lice, and development of pubic and axillary hair.	Hair is evenly colored, shiny. Pubic and axillary hair at expected ages. *Hair loss due to tight braids. A low neck or forehead hairline may indicate a congenital defect. Insects in scalp or eggs on hair shafts indicate head lice.*
Palpate the hair shafts for texture.	Soft or silky, with fine or thick shafts.

ASSESSING THE HEAD FOR SKULL CHARACTERISTICS AND FACIAL FEATURES

Procedure[1]	Findings[2]
Inspect the head for shape.	The skull is rounded, with a prominent occipital area. *Abnormal skull shape with premature closure of the sutures. Flat, elongated skull in low-birth-weight infants.*
Inspect the face for symmetry when child rests, smiles, talks, and cries. Draw an imaginary line down the middle of the face to compare sides.	Symmetric facial features with expressions are expected. *Facial asymmetry with paralysis of cranial nerves V and VII. Coarse facial features, wide eye spacing, or disproportionate size may indicate a congenital anomaly. Tremors, tics, and twitching of facial muscles may indicate a seizure.*

| Palpate the sutures and fontanels of the skull. | No separation of sutures, fontanel is diamond-shaped. Posterior fontanel closes by 2–3 months. |
| | *Additional bone edges may indicate a skull fracture. Bulging fontanel with increased intracranial pressure. Sunken fontanel with dehydration.* |

ASSESSING THE EYE STRUCTURES, FUNCTION, AND VISION

Procedure[1]	Findings[2]
Inspect the external eye structures (eye size and spacing, eye color). Test the function of cranial nerves II, III, IV, and VI.	Eyes are equal and appropriately sized. Sclerae are white or ivory.
	A sunken appearance with dehydration. Hypertelorism may indicate mental retardation. Blue tinge to the sclerae indicates osteogenesis imperfecta.
Inspect the eyelids for color, size, position, mobility, and condition of the eyelashes. Inspect palpebral slant. Inspect the conjunctivae.	Eyelids free of swelling or inflammation. Each lid covers part of the iris but none of the pupil. Conjunctivae are pink and glossy. No redness or excess tearing. An epicanthal fold in children of Asian descent.
	Ptosis indicates injury of cranial nerve III. Setting sun sign with hydrocephalus or retracted eyelids.

Inspect the pupils and iris for size and shape. Test pupillary response to light and accommodation.	Pupils are round, clear, and equal in size and respond to light and accommodation. *Brushfield's spots on the iris with Down syndrome.*
Inspect eye muscles for extraocular movement and corneal light reflex, and perform cover-uncover test.	Both eyes move and track together. Symmetric light reflection on corneas. No obvious movement of either eye is seen with the cover-uncover test. *Asymmetric corneal light reflex after 6 months of age with strabismus.*
Assess visual acuity with standardized charts, and assess visual fields.	Infants fixate on and track an object. *Vision acuity of 20/40 or less in either eye by 3 to 5 years, or 20/30 or less by 6 years or difference in vision of 2 lines or more between the eyes.* (American Academy of Pediatrics Committee on Practice and Ambulatory Medicine and Section of Ophthalmology, 2003).
Use an ophthalmoscope to inspect the internal eye structures.	A bilateral red reflex; pink retinas; sharply defined, round optic disc margin that is yellow to creamy pink. *A white reflex indicates a retinoblastoma.*

ASSESSING THE EAR STRUCTURES AND HEARING

Procedure[1]	Findings[2]
Inspect the position and characteristics of the pinna.	Pinna appropriately formed and positioned; auditory canals patent; no discharge. *Low-set ears may indicate a congenital renal disorder.*
Inspect the tympanic membrane with the otoscope. Assess mobility of the tympanic membrane.	Tympanic membrane is pearly gray, translucent, and mobile. Light reflex and ossicles are visible. *A bulging, red tympanic membrane without movement indicates acute otitis media.*
Screen for hearing loss with noisemakers or whispering words.	Infants turn toward the noise-maker. Children repeat the whispered words accurately.
Weber test: place a vibrating tuning fork on the child's skull at midline, and ask if the sound is heard best in one ear or both ears. Rinne test: place the vibrating tuning fork on the mastoid process and when the sound is no longer heard, move and hold the tines next to the ear. Repeat for the other ear.	Sound is heard equally in both ears with the Weber test. The child hears the air-conducted sound twice as long as the bone-conducted sound with the Rinne test.

ASSESSING THE NOSE AND SINUSES FOR AIRWAY PATENCY AND DISCHARGE

Procedure[1]	Findings[2]
Inspect the external nose for size, shape, symmetry, and midline placement on the face. Observe for nasal discharge.	The nose is midline and proportional to other facial features; symmetric nasolabial folds, no discharge. *A saddle-shaped nose with congenital defects such as cleft palate.*
Palpate the external nose for pain, break in contour, masses.	No tenderness, contour deviations, or masses.
Test for nasal patency by occluding one nostril at a time.	The child breathes through the open nostril with the mouth closed. *Nasal flaring is a sign of respiratory distress.*
Inspect the internal nose for color of the mucous membranes and the presence of any discharge, swelling, lesions, or other abnormalities. Do not touch the nasal septum with the speculum.	Mucous membranes and turbinates are dark pink and glistening; a film of clear discharge. Intact nasal septum. *Pale or bluish gray turbinates and polyps with allergies. A foul-smelling discharge in one nostril with a foreign body.*
Press up under both zygomatic arches to palpate the maxillary sinuses. Press up against the bone above both eyes to palpate the ethmoid sinuses.	No swelling or tenderness is expected. *Puffiness and swelling of the face around the sinuses and tenderness on palpation indicate sinusitis.*

ASSESSING THE MOUTH AND THROAT

Procedure[1]	Findings[2]
Inspect the lips for color, shape, symmetry, moisture, and lesions. *Do not examine the mouth if there are signs of respiratory distress, high fever, drooling, and intense apprehension as epiglottitis may be present. Inspecting the mouth may trigger an airway obstruction.*	Lips symmetric with pink color in Whites, more bluish in children of darker skin. *Pale, cyanotic, or cherry-red lips are indicators of poor tissue perfusion.*
Inspect and count the child's teeth, assess tooth eruption, and identify loose or missing teeth. Inspect the condition of the teeth.	Teeth are white; not mottled or pitted. Discolored tooth crown may indicate a carie. *Discolored tooth surface with some medications and fluorosis.*
Inspect the gums for color and adherence to the teeth.	Pink gums with a stippled or dotted appearance. *Inflammation and tenderness with infection, poor nutrition.*
Inspect mucous membranes for color and moisture. Inspect the tongue and floor of the mouth for color, moistness, size, tremors, and lesions.	Pink mucous membranes. Hyperpigmentation patches in children of darker skin. No redness, swelling, or ulcerative lesions. Tongue is pink and moist. *A protuberant tongue with various genetic conditions, such as Down syndrome. A white, adherent coating may be thrush, a* Candida *infection.*

Inspect the hard and soft palate to detect any clefts, masses, or an unusually high arch.	Palate is pink, dome-shaped arch, no cleft. Uvula hangs freely.
Palpate the palate. Test the tongue's strength by asking the child to press the tongue against a finger on the cheek.	No clefts are palpated. Good tongue strength.
Inspect the throat for color, swelling, lesions, and the condition of the tonsils. Assess the gag reflex.	Throat is pink without lesions, drainage, or swelling. Tonsils are pink without exudate, but crypts (fissures) may be seen. The uvula rises symmetrically. *Swelling or bulging in the posterior pharynx with a peritonsillar abscess.*

ASSESSING THE NECK FOR CHARACTERISTICS, RANGE OF MOTION, AND LYMPH NODES

Procedure[1]	Findings[2]
Inspect the neck for size, symmetry, swelling, and any abnormalities, such as webbing.	Neck is symmetric, no swelling. Infants have short neck with skin folds. *Webbing may indicate Turner syndrome.*
Note the head control in infants.	Infants develop head control by 2 months. *Lack of head control can result from neurologic injury.*

Palpate both sides of the neck for lymph nodes. Define the characteristics of a palpated node.	Firm, clearly defined, nontender, movable lymph nodes up to 1 cm (0.5 in.) in diameter are common. *Enlarged, firm, warm, tender lymph nodes with infection.*
Palpate the trachea by placing the thumb and forefinger on each side of the trachea near the chin and slowly slide them down the trachea. Palpate the isthmus of the thyroid, a band of glandular tissue crossing over the trachea.	The trachea is midline. Thyroid lobes are not usually palpable. *Any tracheal shift to the right or left of midline may indicate a tumor or a collapsed lung.*
Assess horizontal and vertical neck movement. Move a light or toy in all four directions when assessing infants.	Freely moves the neck and head in all four directions, no pain. *Limited horizontal motion with torticollis. Pain with neck flexion (Brudzinski sign) with meningitis.*

ASSESSING THE CHEST FOR SHAPE, MOVEMENT, RESPIRATORY EFFORT, AND LUNG FUNCTION

Procedure[1]	Findings[2]
Identify the topographic landmarks of the chest.	The intercostal spaces are the horizontal markers. The sternum and spine are the vertical landmarks.
Inspect the anterior and posterior chest for size and shape. Inspect the chest for any irregularities in shape.	The rib cage is prominent, thinner chest muscles and subcutaneous tissue. The rounded chest of infants becomes oval by 2 years.

	A rounded chest in a child may indicate a chronic obstructive lung condition. Scoliosis causes a lateral deviation of the chest.
Inspect for simultaneous chest expansion and abdominal rise. Count the respiratory rate when the child is quiet. See chapter 1 for normal respiratory rate ranges by age.	Chest movement is symmetric bilaterally, and the chest and abdomen rise simultaneously on inspiration. *Asymmetric chest rise with a collapsed lung. Retractions and a high sustained respiratory rate with respiratory distress.*
Palpate the chest motion. Palpate any depressions, bulges, or unusual chest wall shape.	Chest movement is symmetric. No tenderness, bulges, depressions, crepitus, or fractures.
Palpate the chest for tactile fremitus. Ask the child to repeat a series of words or numbers, such as Mickey Mouse or ice cream. Compare quality of vibrations side to side.	The vibration is palpated over the entire chest. *Decreased sensations when air is trapped in the lungs. Increased sensations with lung consolidation.*

Auscultate the chest for the characteristics of breath sounds, comparing side to side, and listening through the inspiratory and expiratory phase at each location. See Figure 2–1. For auscultated abnormal breath sounds, determine location, respiratory phase present, duration, intensity, and change with coughing or shifting position.

Breath sounds of equal intensity, pitch, and rhythm bilaterally. Breath sounds usually heard include the following:

- Vesicular—low-pitched, swishing, soft, short expiratory sounds.
- Bronchovesicular—medium-pitched, hollow, blowing sounds heard equally on inspiration and expiration in all age groups.
- Bronchial/tracheal—hollow, higher pitched than vesicular breath sounds.

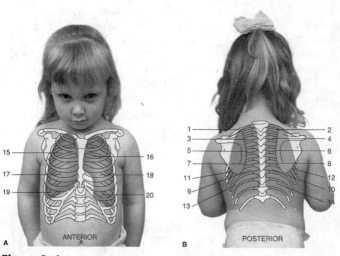

Figure 2–1 ■ Sequence for auscultating the chest.

	Absent or diminished breath sounds indicate a pneumothorax or obstruction. Abnormal breath sounds include crackles, rhonchi, and friction rubs.
Auscultate the chest while the child repeats a series of words to evaluate voice sound transmission.	Muffled, indistinct words and syllables heard throughout the chest. *Voice sounds absent with an airway obstruction. Abnormal vocal resonance characteristics include the following:* • *Whispered pectoriloquy—syllables are heard distinctly in a whisper.* • *Bronchophony—increased intensity and clarity of sounds while the words remain indistinct.* • *Egophony—transmission of the "ee" sound as a nasal "ay."*
Note the quality of the voice and other audible sounds.	*Hoarse voice or cry. Stridor is a high-pitched crowing sound heard with croup. Wheezing results from air passing through mucus or fluids in a narrowed airway.*

BREASTS

Procedure[1]	Findings[2]
Inspect the breasts. Inspect the anterior chest for supernumerary nipples (small, undeveloped nipples and areola that may be mistaken for moles).	The areola is normally round and more darkly pigmented than the surrounding skin. *Supernumerary nipples are associated with congenital renal or cardiac anomalies.*
Inspect the breasts of older children and adolescents while sitting, for stage of development.	Breast development Stage I: preadolescent, nipple is raised above the level of the breast Stage II: budding stage; areola increased in diameter, slightly elevated, usually between age 9 and 14 years Stage III: breast and areola enlarged Stage IV: areola forms a secondary elevation above that of the breast Stage V: areola is part of the general breast contour and strongly pigmented, nipple usually projects Breasts may develop at different rates and appear asymmetric. Black girls have earlier onset, followed by Mexican American girls, and then White girls (Anderson & Must, 2005). *Breast development before 6 years in Black girls and 7 years in White girls is abnormal and needs further evaluation* (Greydanus, Matytsina, & Gains, 2006).

Position the adolescent female on her back with one arm behind the neck. Palpate the breast and axilla on that side in a concentric pattern covering all quadrants and the axilla, then around the nipple. Repeat on other side.	Breast tissue feels dense, firm, and elastic. *Abnormal masses or hard nodules need further investigation but are usually not malignancies.*
Palpate the breast tissue in adolescent boys to detect any masses.	Unilateral or bilateral breast enlargement during adolescence (gynecomastia).

ASSESSING THE HEART FOR HEART SOUNDS AND FUNCTION

Procedure[1]	Findings[2]
Place the child in a reclining or semi-Fowler's position. Observe the anterior chest for movement associated with the heart's contraction.	Symmetric rib cage. The apical impulse is where the left ventricle taps the chest wall during contraction. *Bulging of the left side of the chest wall or a heave may indicate an enlarged heart.*
Palpate the precordium for pulsations, heaves, or vibrations. Use the topographic landmarks of the chest to describe their location.	Apical impulse felt as a slight tap against a fingertip. *A lift or thrill is usually abnormal. Estimate the diameter of the thrill.*

Use the bell of the stethoscope and auscultate the heart with child in both sitting and reclining positions. Note differences in heart sounds with position change. Count the apical heart rate and compare to the radial or brachial pulse. See chapter 1 for heart rate ranges by age. Assess the rhythm. If a rhythm irregularity is detected, re-assess as the child holds his or her breath.	The apical and brachial or radial pulse rates should be the same. Children often have a normal cycle of irregular rhythm associated with respiration called *sinus arrhythmia*; the rate is faster on inspiration and slower on expiration. The rhythm should become regular when the breath is held. *Other irregular rhythms are not expected.*
Auscultate heart sounds at specific listening areas on the chest wall (see Figure 2–2). S_1 is the heart sound heard simultaneously with the carotid pulsation. See Table 2–2 for best sites to auscultate S_1 and S_2. Auscultate heart sounds for quality (distinct versus muffled) and intensity (loud versus weak).	S_1 and S_2 heard in all listening areas. S_1 is produced by closure of the tricuspid and mitral valves. S_2, produced by closure of the aortic and pulmonic valves, may be heard as a single sound or a split sound. The timing of the valve closures vary with respirations, such as taking a deep breath when the S_2 split is more apparent. Heart sounds are distinct and crisp in children with a thin chest wall. *Muffling, or indistinct sounds, with a heart defect or congestive heart failure. Fixed splitting that does not vary with respiration with an atrial septal defect.*

Section I: General Information

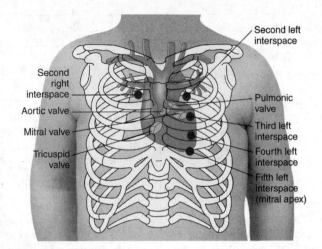

Figure 2–2 ■ Listening posts of the heart.

Table 2–2   Identification of the Sites for Auscultating the Quality and Intensity of Heart Sounds

Heart Sound	Locations Best Heard
S_1	Apex of the heart
	Tricuspid area
	Mitral area
S_2	Base of the heart
	Aortic area
	Pulmonic area
Physiologic splitting	Pulmonic area
S_3	Mitral area

| Auscultate for other unexpected heart sounds and murmurs. Note characteristics such as

• intensity,
• presence of a thrill,
• location,
• change in character with position change,
• radiation,
• timing in relation to S_1 and S_2, and
• quality. | S_3 heard in diastole, louder in the mitral area than the pulmonic area, just after S_2, is found in some children.

Murmurs, abnormal sounds produced by blood passing through a defective valve, great vessel, or other heart structure are described by grade of intensity.

Grade 1: Barely heard in a quiet room

Grade 2: Quiet, but clearly heard

Grade 3: Moderately loud, no thrill palpated

Grade 4: Loud, a thrill is usually palpated

Grade 5: Very loud, a thrill is easily palpated

Grade 6: Heard without the stethoscope in direct contact with the chest wall |
| Auscultate for a venous hum over the supraclavicular fossa above the middle of the clavicle or over the upper anterior chest with the bell of the stethoscope. | A venous hum is a continuous low-pitched hum, may be loudest during diastole or when the child stands, does not change with respiration but may be quieter when the child turns the neck. |

Assess the blood pressure; use correct cuff size for the extremity. Take two readings and average them. Compare the systolic and diastolic blood pressure reading to the values in chapter 1.	The systolic reading is the onset of Korotkoff's sounds. The diastolic reading is the fifth Korotkoff's sound or the disappearance of Korotkoff's sounds in children and adolescents. The leg blood pressure should be the same or up to 10 mm Hg higher than the arm reading.
When any concern exists about a heart condition, obtain a blood pressure reading in both an arm and a leg, and then compare the readings.	*A lower leg blood pressure reading than in the arm occurs with coarctation of the aorta.*
Palpate the pulses in both extremities to compare rate, rhythm regularity, and strength. Compare the femoral artery pulse strength with the brachial or radial pulses.	Detecting distal pulses in infants is often difficult. The femoral pulsations are stronger than or as strong as the brachial pulsations.
	A weaker femoral pulse with coarctation of the aorta.
Assess heart and tissue perfusion by observing color and capillary refill.	Mucous membranes pink. Capillary refill less than 2 seconds.
	Cyanosis with a congenital heart defect in children. Prolonged capillary refill with poor tissue perfusion or shock.

ASSESSING THE ABDOMEN FOR SHAPE, BOWEL SOUNDS, AND UNDERLYING ORGANS

Procedure[1]	Findings[2]
Inspect the abdomen's shape and contour, condition of the umbilicus and rectus muscle, and abdominal movement.	Abdomen symmetrically rounded or flat when supine; rises with inspiration and falls with expiration. An umbilical hernia or a separation of the rectus muscle up to 5 cm (2 in.) may be seen.
	A scaphoid or sunken abdomen in dehydration or with a diaphragmatic hernia in a newborn. Peristaltic waves indicate an intestinal obstruction, such as pyloric stenosis.
Auscultate the abdomen with the diaphragm of the stethoscope. Listen in each quadrant long enough to hear at least one bowel sound. Before determining that bowel sounds are absent, auscultate at least 5 minutes. Auscultate over the abdominal aorta and the renal arteries for a vascular hum or murmur.	High-pitched, tinkling, metallic bowel sounds every 10–30 seconds. No murmur.
	Absence of bowel sounds with peritonitis or a paralytic ileus. Hyperactive bowel sounds with gastroenteritis or a bowel obstruction. A murmur may indicate a narrowed artery.

While the child is supine, use indirect percussion to evaluate borders and sizes of abdominal organs and masses. Identify organ size, listening for a percussion tone change at organ borders.	Dullness over organs (liver, spleen, and a full bladder); tympany over the stomach or the intestines when an obstruction is present; resonance over other areas. The upper liver edge is near the fifth intercostal space at the right midclavicular line.
To palpate the abdomen, position the child supine with knees flexed to relax the abdominal muscles. Use the edge of your fingers plus fingerpads to palpate the entire abdomen. Watch the child's face for signs of pain.	
Use *light palpation* to evaluate the tenseness of the abdomen, the liver, any tenderness or masses, and any defects in the abdominal wall. Use a superficial, gentle touch that slightly depresses the abdomen. Palpate any bulging along the abdominal wall. Measure the diameter of the umbilical ring if open.	Abdomen is soft, no tenderness. An open umbilical muscle ring normally becomes smaller and closes by 4 years of age.

Place the fingers in the right midclavicular line at the level of the umbilicus. Gently move the side of the index finger toward the costal margin during expiration to palpate the liver. As the liver edge descends with inspiration, a flat, narrow ridge may be felt. Measure the distance of the liver edge below the right costal margin.	The lower liver edge is 2–3 cm (about 1 in.) below the right costal margin in infants and toddlers, near the costal margin in older children. *An enlarged liver, more than 3 cm (1.25 in.) below the right costal margin, with congestive heart failure or hepatic disease.*
Deep palpation is used to detect masses, define their shape and consistency, and identify tenderness in the abdomen. Press the fingers of one hand (two hands for older children) more deeply into the abdomen. Ask the child to take regular deep breaths when each area of the abdomen is palpated. Palpate for the spleen at the left costal margin in the midclavicular line. Palpate for the kidneys deep in the abdomen along each side of the spinal column. *If any abnormal mass is palpated, discontinue palpation to prevent the potential release of cancer cells.*	The spleen tip may be felt when the child takes a deep breath. The kidneys are difficult to palpate in all children, except newborns. Feces feel like a tubular mass in the lower left or right quadrant. A distended bladder feels like a firm, central, dome-shaped mass above the symphysis pubis. *The spleen is enlarged when it is easily palpated below the left costal margin. If a kidney is palpated, an abnormal mass may be present. Any fixed mass that moves laterally, pulsates, or is located along the vertebral column may be a neoplasm.*

ASSESSING THE INGUINAL AREA

Procedure[1]	Findings[2]
Inspect the inguinal area for any change in contour, comparing sides.	*A small bulging over the femoral canal in girls may be a femoral hernia. A bulging in the inguinal area in boys may be an inguinal hernia.*
Palpate the inguinal area for lymph nodes and other masses.	Lymph nodes, less than 1 cm (0.5 in.) in diameter, often present. *Tenderness, heat, or inflammation in lymph nodes with a local infection.*

ASSESSING THE GENITAL AND PERINEAL AREAS FOR EXTERNAL STRUCTURAL ABNORMALITIES

Procedure[1]	Findings[2]
Females Position young children on the parent's lap with legs spread apart. Older children can be positioned on the examining table with their knees flexed and the legs spread apart like a frog. Gloves, lubricant, and a penlight are needed for the examination. Inspect the mons pubis for the presence of pubic hair and its characteristics. See Figure 2–3A to calculate a sexual maturity rating.	Pubic hair development Stage I: preadolescent, no growth of pubic hair Stage II: initial, scarcely pigmented straight hair, especially along medial border of the labia Stage III: sparse, dark, visibly pigmented curly pubic hair on labia Stage IV: hair coarse and curly, abundant but less than adults

Inspect the external genitalia for color, size, and symmetry of the mons pubis, labia, urethra, and vaginal opening. Look for any inflammation, swelling, masses, lacerations, or discharge.

Separate the labia minora to view the vestibule and inspect for lesions or discharge. ·

An internal vaginal examination is performed by an experienced examiner when abnormal findings are noted.

Stage V: lateral spreading in triangle shape to medial surface of thighs

Stage VI: further extension laterally and upward

Pubic hair before age 8 years may indicate premature pubertal development.

In preadolescents labia minora are thin and pale, hymen is a thin membrane with a crescent-shaped opening just inside the vaginal opening, no vaginal discharge.

After puberty

Dark pink and moist labia minora; vaginal opening is approximately 1 cm (0.5 in.) when the hymen is intact; clear discharge without a foul odor; menses begin about 2 years after breast budding at sexual maturity rating 4; urethral or vaginal openings have no lesions or signs of inflammation.

In young infants, the labia minora may be fused and cover the vestibule. A foul-smelling discharge may be a foreign body or vaginal infection. Sexual abuse signs include bruising or swelling of the vulva, foul-smelling vaginal discharge, enlarged vaginal opening, and rash or lesions on perineum.

Palpate the vaginal opening with a finger of your free hand.	*If the Bartholin's and Skene's glands are palpated in preadolescents, an infection such as gonorrhea may be present.*

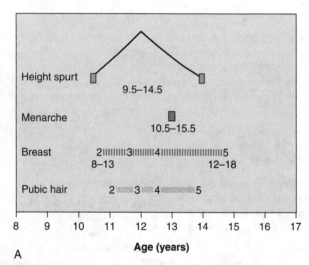

A

Figure 2–3 ■ The sexual maturity rating (SMR) is an average of the breast and pubic hair Tanner stages in females and of the genital and pubic hair Tanner stages in boys. The rating is a number between 2 and 5, as stage I is prepubertal. Determine the stage of breast and pubic hair development for females or the stage of genital and pubic hair development in males with the numbers (Tanner stages 2, 3, 4, 5) corresponding to the stages listed on the sexual maturity rating figures. The sexual maturity rating figures can then provide information about where the child is in regard to other pubertal changes such as the height spurt and menarche. **A:** Females. **B:** Males.
Source: A. Redrawn from "Variations in Pattern of Pubertal Changes in Girls," by W. A. Marshall & J. M. Tanner, 1969, *Archives of Disease in Childhood, 44,* 291; B. redrawn from "Variations in Pattern of Pubertal Changes in Boys," by W. A. Marshall & J. M. Tanner, 1970, *Archives of Diseases in Childhood, 45,* 13, with permission. *(continued)*

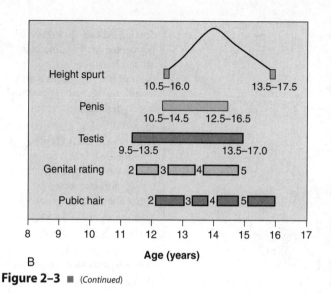

B

Figure 2–3 ■ *(Continued)*

Males	Pubic hair and external genital development
Seat boys with legs crossed in front of them to push the testicles into the scrotum.	Stage I: Preadolescent, hair present is same as that on abdomen; testes, scrotum, and penis are the same size and shape as young child
Inspect the pubertal development of the penis, scrotum, testicles, and pubic hair. Pubic hair and external genital development occur at different ages, so stage each separately from information at the right. See Figure 2–3B to assess the sexual maturity rating.	Stage II: Slightly pigmented, longer, straight pubic hair usually at base of penis, sometimes on scrotum; enlargement of scrotum and testes

	Stage III: Dark, definitely pigmented, curly pubic hair around base of penis; enlargement of penis, especially in length, further enlargement of testes, descent of scrotum
	Stage IV: Public hair adult in type, but spread no further than inguinal fold; continued enlargement of penis, sculpturing of glans, increased pigmentation of scrotum
	Stage V: Pubic hair spreads to medial surface of thighs; scrotum ample, penis reaching nearly to bottom of scrotum
	Penile enlargement occurs about 1 year after testicular enlargement. Ejaculation at sexual maturity rating 3, semen between sexual maturity ratings of 3 and 4
	Pubic hair before age 9 years or onset of testicular enlargement after age 14 years needs evaluation.

Inspect the penis for size, foreskin, hygiene, and position of the urethral meatus. Inspect the urinary stream. Use gentle traction to evaluate the degree of foreskin retraction and the meatal location and size.	The newborn penis length is 2–3 cm (1 in.). The penis is straight. Foreskin adhesions in infants and young boys, with opening adequate for a good urinary stream, is normal, even if the meatus cannot be seen. Easy foreskin retraction by age 5 years.
Avoid forcible retraction of the foreskin in the uncircumcised young boy to prevent tearing of adhesions.	The glans penis is clean and smooth with a slit-shaped urethral meatus near the tip. No discharge. Strong stream, no dribbling.
	Erythema and edema of the glans (balanitis). A round, pinpoint urethral meatus with meatal stenosis. Hypospadias or epispadias.
Inspect the scrotum for size, symmetry, presence of the testicles, and any abnormalities. To distinguish between a hydrocele and an incarcerated hernia, place a bright penlight under the scrotum and look for a red glow or transillumination.	The scrotum is loose and pendulous, with rugae, or wrinkles. A hydrocele transilluminates; a hernia does not.
	Scrotum is undeveloped with undescended testicles. Scrotal enlargement with inguinal hernia, hydrocele, torsion of the spermatic cord, or testicular inflammation.

Palpate the shaft of the penis for nodules and masses.	No nodules or masses present. The testicles are smooth and equal in size, approximately 1.0–1.5 cm (0.5 in.) in diameter until puberty, when they increase in size. The testicle is descendable if it can be moved from the inguinal canal into the scrotum. The spermatic cord is solid and smooth without tenderness.
Place your index finger and thumb over the inguinal canals on each side of the penis to keep the testicles from retracting. Gently palpate each testicle to identify the shape and size. If a testicle is not in the scrotum, palpate the inguinal canal for a soft mass. If found in the inguinal canal, try to move the testicle to the scrotum to palpate the size and shape.	
When scrotal bulging or swelling is present, palpate the scrotum to identify the characteristics of the mass and attempt to reduce it. Determine if it is unilateral or bilateral.	*An undescended testicle cannot be palpated in the inguinal canal or scrotum. A hard, enlarged, painless testicle may indicate a tumor. A scrotal mass that can be reduced may be an inguinal hernia; hydroceles and incarcerated hernias do not reduce.*
Palpate the length of the spermatic cord between the thumb and forefinger from the testicle to the inguinal canal.	
Anus and rectum	
Inspect the anus for sphincter control, inflammation, fissures, or lesions when the child is in supine or prone position.	The external sphincter is usually closed.
Lightly touch the anal opening to stimulate an anal contraction or "wink."	*Inflammation and scratch marks around the anus may indicate pinworms.*
	Absence of an anal contraction may indicate a lower spinal cord lesion.
A rectal examination is performed by an experienced examiner.	

ASSESSING THE MUSCULOSKELETAL SYSTEM FOR BONE AND JOINT STRUCTURE, MOVEMENT, AND MUSCLE STRENGTH

Procedure[1]	Findings[2]
Inspect and compare the arms and legs for alignment, contour, skin folds, length, and deformities. Count the fingers and toes. Inspect the nails and creases on the palmar surface of each hand.	Extremities of equal length, circumference, and numbers of skin folds bilaterally. Straight arm alignment with a minimal angle at the elbows. All fingers and toes present; nails are convex and pink. Multiple palmar creases. *Polydactyly or syndactyly. A single crease crossing the palm of the hand with Down syndrome. Clubbing of the nails with chronic respiratory and cardiac conditions.*
Inspect the feet for in-toeing when the infant stands and walks. Inspect the feet for alignment and the presence of an arch when the child is standing. If the toddler has bowlegs, measure the distance between the knees with ankles together when standing. To evaluate knock-knees, measure the distance between the ankles at the level of the medial malleoli with knees together when standing.	Children up to 3 years of age appear to have flat feet due to a fat pad over the arch. Older children have a longitudinal foot arch. The infant's toes turn in due to tibial torsion. By 4 years, long bone alignment is straight. Toddlers have a sequence of bowlegs (genu varum) and knock-knees (genu valgum) before the legs assume a straight alignment. No more than 3.5 cm (1.5 in.) between the knees and no more than 2 in. (5 cm) between the ankles is normal.

Inspect and compare the joints bilaterally for size, discoloration, and ease of voluntary movement.	Joints same color as surrounding skin; no swelling; flexion and extension without pain. *Extra skin folds and a larger circumference may indicate a shorter extremity. Redness, swelling, and pain with movement may indicate injury or infection.*
Palpate the bones and muscles in each extremity for muscle tone, masses, or tenderness. Palpate each joint and surrounding muscles to detect any swelling, masses, heat, or tenderness.	Muscles feel firm. No bony masses. *Doughy muscles with poor muscle tone. Rigid muscles (hypertonia) with an active seizure or cerebral palsy. A mass over a long bone with a recent fracture or a bone tumor. Tenderness, heat, swelling, and redness around a joint with injury or inflammation.*
Inspect the posture of a standing child from a front, side, and back view. Observe the height of the shoulders and hips. Ask the child to bend forward slowly at the waist, with arms extended toward the floor. Palpate each vertebra for a change in alignment.	Shoulders and hips are level; head is erect without a tilt, shoulder contour is symmetric. Thoracic convex and lumbar concave spinal curves after 6 years. No lateral curve. The lumbar concave curve flattens with forward flexion. *A lateral curve to the spine or a one-sided rib hump indicates scoliosis.*

Assess range of motion of all major joints during typical play activities (reaching for objects, climbing, and walking). Perform passive range of motion when a joint has limited active range of motion. Take care to avoid causing extra pain.	Children spontaneously move joints through the full range of motion with play activities. No pain. *Limited active and passive range of motion indicates pain, malformation, injury, inflammation of a joint, or a muscle abnormality. Increased passive range of motion with muscle weakness.*
Assess the hips of young infants for dislocation or subluxation. Assess skin fold symmetry on the upper legs. Assess knee height with feet flat on exam table. Perform the Ortolani-Barlow maneuver. With the infant supine, flex the hips and knees at a 90-degree angle. Place a hand over each knee with the thumb over the inner thigh, and the first two fingers over the upper margin of the femur. Move the infant's knees together until they touch, and then put downward pressure on one femur at a time to see if the hips dislocate. Then, slowly abduct the hips toward the exam table, one knee at a time, keeping pressure on the hip joints with the fingers in a lever-type motion.	Equal number of skin folds on each leg, knee height is even. The hips do not easily slip out of joint. The hips equally abduct, knees nearly touching the table. The iliac crests stay level when the child stands on each leg. *Signs of hip dislocation include uneven skin folds or knee heights, hip slips easily out of the joint, a palpated clunk, or hip resistance to abduction.*
Ask the child to stand on one leg and then the other.	*If the iliac crest opposite the weight-bearing leg appears lower, the hip that is bearing weight may be dislocated.*

Assess muscle strength. Observe the child in activities such as climbing, throwing a ball, clapping hands, or moving around on the bed.	The child's ability to play indicates good muscle tone and strength. Good muscle strength bilaterally.
Assess the strength of specific extremity muscles. Ask the child to squeeze your fingers tightly with each hand, push against and pull your hands, lower legs and feet, and resist extension of a flexed elbow or knee. Compare muscle strength bilaterally. When generalized muscle weakness is suspected, ask the child to stand up from the supine position.	*Unilateral muscle weakness may indicate a nerve injury.* *Bilateral muscle weakness from hypoxemia or a congenital disorder such as Down syndrome. Asymmetric weakness with cerebral palsy. Children who push their body upright from a supine position using the arms and hands have generalized muscle weakness, a sign of muscular dystrophy.*

ASSESSING THE NERVOUS SYSTEM FOR COGNITIVE FUNCTION, BALANCE, COORDINATION, CRANIAL NERVE FUNCTION, SENSATION, AND REFLEXES

Procedure[1]	Findings[2]
Observe level of consciousness and activity, including facial expressions, gestures, and interaction. Match the neurologic examination to the child's developmental stage.	Alert, curious, easily aroused from sleep. Infants and toddlers seek the security of the parent. Older children are often anxious and watch all of the examiner's actions. Toddlers follow simple directions; by 3 years, speech can be understood.

Listen to speech articulation and words used. Compare the child's performance with standards of social development and speech articulation for the child's age.	*Decreased consciousness with brain injury, seizure, infection, or brain tumor. Lack of interest may indicate a serious illness. Unusually short attention span and high activity level with attention deficit hyperactivity disorder. Delay in language and social skill development with mental retardation or hearing loss.*
Evaluate recent memory beginning at age 4 years by asking the child to remember a special name or object. Have the child recall the name or object 5–10 minutes later. Ask the child to repeat his or her address or birth date to assess remote memory.	By 5 or 6 years of age, children are able to recall this information without difficulty.
Observe the young child at play, standing on one foot, and hopping to assess coordination and balance. Use the Romberg test to assess balance in children older than age 3 years. Have the child stand with eyes closed, and stand close to catch the child if needed.	Preschool-age children extend the arms to maintain balance; older children stand with arms at their sides. Children do not stumble or fall. *Leaning to one side or falling with the Romberg test indicates poor balance, cerebellar dysfunction, or inner ear disturbance.*

Tests of coordination assess the smoothness and accuracy of movement. Assess fine motor skills in young children. After 6 years of age use the finger-to-nose, finger-to-finger, heel-to-shin, and alternating motion maneuvers.	*Jerky movements or inaccurate pointing (past pointing) indicates poor coordination.*
Inspect the child when walking from both a front and a rear view.	Level iliac crests during walking. *A limp with injury or joint disease. Staggering or falling with cerebellar ataxia. Scissoring with cerebral palsy or other spastic conditions.*
Assess cranial nerves. See Table 2–3 for procedures and expected findings.	*Abnormalities of cranial nerves with compression of an individual nerve, brain injury, or infections.*
Assess sensory function bilaterally and compare responses to stimulation. An infant's sensory function is not routinely assessed. Stroke the skin on the lower leg or arm with a cotton ball or a finger while the child's eyes are closed to test superficial tactile sensation. When the child's eyes are closed, touch the child on each arm and leg, alternating the sharp and dull ends of the tongue blade.	Equal bilateral responses. Children older than age 2 years can point to the location touched. Children older than age 4 years can distinguish between a sharp and dull sensation each time. Withdrawal responses to painful procedures indicate normal sensory function in infants. *Loss of sensation with a brain or spinal cord lesion. Inability to identify superficial touch and pain sensation indicates sensory loss.*

Table 2–3 Cranial Nerve Assessment in Infants and Children

Cranial Nerve[a]	Assessment Procedure and Normal Findings[b]
I Olfactory	Infant: Not tested.
	Child: Not routinely tested. Give familiar odors to child to smell, one naris at a time. *Identifies odors such as orange, peanut butter, and chocolate.*
II Optic	Infant: Shine a bright light in eyes. A quick blink reflex and dorsal head flexion indicate light perception.
	Child: Test vision and visual fields if cooperative. *Visual acuity appropriate for age.*
III Oculomotor ⎫	Infant: Shine a penlight at the eyes and move it side to side. *Focuses on and tracks the light to each side.*
IV Trochlear ⎬	Child: Move an object through the six cardinal points of gaze. *Tracks objects through all fields of gaze.*
VI Abducens ⎭	All ages: Inspect eyelids for drooping. Inspect pupillary response to light. *Eyelids do not droop and pupils are equal sized and briskly respond to light.*
V Trigeminal	Infant: Stimulate the rooting and sucking reflex. *Turns head toward stimulation at side of mouth and sucking has good strength and pattern.*
	Child: Observe the child chewing a cracker. Touch forehead and cheeks with cotton ball when eyes are closed. *Bilateral jaw strength is good. Child pushes cotton ball away.*
VII Facial	All ages: Observe facial expressions when crying, smiling, frowning, and so forth. *Facial features stay symmetric bilaterally.*
VIII Acoustic	Infant: Produce a loud sound near the head. *Blinks in response to sound, moves head toward sound, or freezes position.*
	Child: Use a noisemaker near each ear or whisper words to be repeated. *Turns head toward sound and repeats words correctly.*
IX Glossopharyngeal ⎫	Infant: Observe swallowing during feeding. *Good swallowing pattern.*
X Vagus ⎬	All ages: Elicit gag reflex. *Gags with stimulation.*
XI Spinal accessory	Infant: Not tested.
	Child: Ask child to raise the shoulders and turn the head side to side against resistance. *Good strength in neck and shoulders.*
XII Hypoglossal	Infant: Observe feeding. *Sucking and swallowing are coordinated.*
	Child: Tell the child to stick out the tongue. Listen to speech. *Tongue is midline with no tremors. Words are clearly articulated.*

[a]Bracketed nerves are tested together.
[b]Italics indicate normal findings.

Primitive infant reflexes	Movements are equal bilaterally.
Moro reflex: Startle the infant with a sudden noise or change in position.	The arms extend and the fingers form a C as they spread. The arms slowly move together as in a hug. The legs may make a similar movement. Present at birth and disappears by 6 months of age.
Palmar grasp: Place a finger across the infant's palm and avoid touching the thumb.	A strong grip of the finger occurs. Present at birth and disappears by 3 months of age.
Plantar grasp: Place finger across the foot at the base of the toes.	The toes curl as if to grip the finger. Present at birth and disappears at about 8 months of age.
Placing reflex: Hold the infant erect and touch the top of one foot with the edge of a table or chair.	The infant lifts the foot as if to step up on the surface. Present within days of birth and disappears at various times.
Stepping reflex: Hold the infant erect and touch the bottom of the foot on the surface of a table or chair.	The feet lift in an alternating pattern as if to walk. Present at birth and disappears between 4 and 8 weeks of age.
Tonic neck reflex: When the supine infant is relaxed, turn the head to one side. Repeat by turning the head to the opposite side.	The arm and leg on the face side extend and the opposite arm and leg flex (fencing position). Appears at 2 months and disappears by age 6 months.
	An asymmetric response may indicate a serious neurologic problem.
Superficial reflexes	
The plantar reflex tests spine levels L4 through S2. Stroke the bottom of the foot from the heel, along the lateral side of the foot and curve over the ball of the foot. Watch the toes for plantar flexion or for fanning and dorsiflexion of the big toe (Babinski response).	The Babinski response in children younger than 2 years. Plantar flexion of the toes in older children.
	A Babinski response in children older than 2 years indicates neurologic disease.

Stroke the inner thigh of each leg to stimulate the cremasteric reflex.	The testicle and scrotum rise on the stroked side with intact T12, L1, and L2 function.
Deep tendon reflexes Tap a tendon near specific joints with a reflex hammer (index finger for infants), and compare responses bilaterally. Inspect for movement in the associated joint and palpate the strength of the muscle contraction.	Bilaterally symmetric and active grade 2+ responses indicate intact spinal segments. *An absent response (grade 0) indicates decreased muscle tone and strength. Hyperactive responses (grade 4+) are associated with muscle spasticity.*
Biceps: Flex the child's arm at the elbow, and place your thumb over the biceps tendon in the antecubital fossa. Tap the thumb.	Elbow flexion with biceps muscle contraction indicates intact C5 and C6 segments.
Triceps: Flex the child's arm at the elbow and tap the triceps tendon above the elbow.	Elbow extension with triceps muscle contraction indicates intact C6, C7, and C8.
Brachioradialis: Lay the child's arm with the thumb upright over your arm. Tap the brachioradialis tendon 2.5 cm (1 in.) above the wrist.	Forearm pronation (palm facing downward) and elbow flexion indicate intact C5 and C6.
Patellar: Flex the child's knees, and tap the patellar tendon below the knee.	Knee extension with quadriceps muscle contraction indicates intact L2, L3, and L4.
Achilles: While the child's legs are flexed, support the foot and tap the Achilles tendon.	Plantar flexion with gastrocnemius muscle contraction indicates intact S1 and S2.

3 Physical Growth Charts

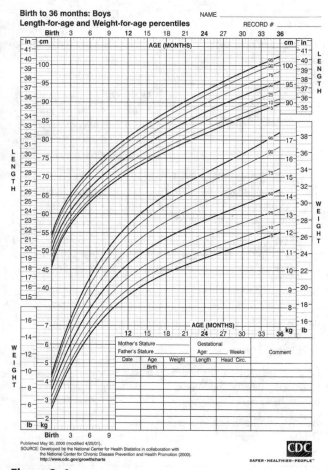

Birth to 36 months: Boys
Length-for-age and Weight-for-age percentiles

NAME _____

RECORD # _____

Published May 30, 2000 (modified 4/20/01).
SOURCE: Developed by the National Center for Health Statistics in collaboration with the National Center for Chronic Disease Prevention and Health Promotion (2000).
http://www.cdc.gov/growthcharts

SAFER · HEALTHIER · PEOPLE™

Figure 3–1 ■ Physical growth percentiles for length and weight—boys: birth to 36 months.
Source: From CDC, 2001, http://www.cdc.gov/growthcharts.

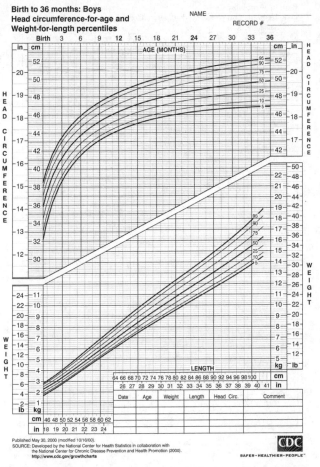

Birth to 36 months: Boys
Head circumference-for-age and
Weight-for-length percentiles

NAME _____
RECORD # _____

Figure 3–2 ■ Physical growth percentiles for head circumference, weight for length—boys: birth to 36 months.
Source: From CDC, 2001, http://www.cdc.gov/growthcharts.

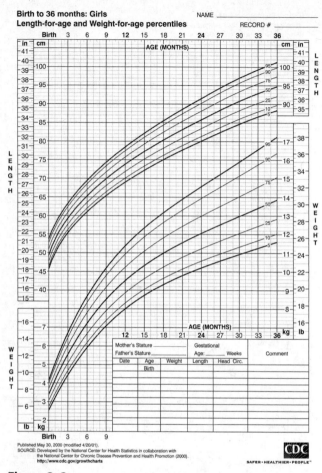

Figure 3–3 ■ Physical growth percentiles for length and weight—girls: birth to 36 months.

Source: From CDC, 2001, http://www.cdc.gov/growthcharts.

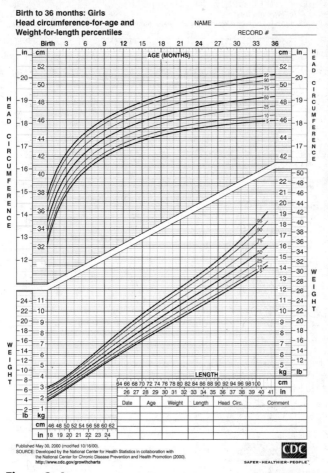

Birth to 36 months: Girls
Head circumference-for-age and
Weight-for-length percentiles

NAME _____

RECORD # _____

Published May 30, 2000 (modified 10/16/00).
SOURCE: Developed by the National Center for Health Statistics in collaboration with
the National Center for Chronic Disease Prevention and Health Promotion (2000).
http://www.cdc.gov/growthcharts

Figure 3–4 ■ Physical growth percentiles for head circumference, weight for length—girls: birth to 36 months.
Source: From CDC, 2001, http://www.cdc.gov/growthcharts.

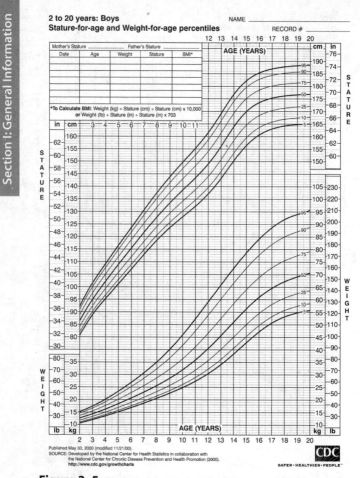

Figure 3–5 ■ Physical growth percentiles for stature and weight according to age—boys: 2 to 20 years.
Source: From CDC, 2001, http://www.cdc.gov/growthcharts.

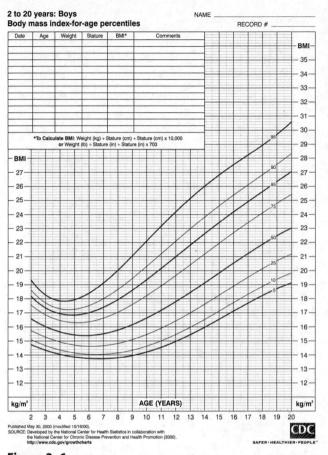

2 to 20 years: Boys
Body mass index-for-age percentiles

NAME _____

RECORD # _____

Date	Age	Weight	Stature	BMI*	Comments

*To Calculate BMI: Weight (kg) ÷ Stature (cm) ÷ Stature (cm) x 10,000
or Weight (lb) ÷ Stature (in) ÷ Stature (in) x 703

AGE (YEARS)

Published May 30, 2000 (modified 10/16/00).
SOURCE: Developed by the National Center for Health Statistics in collaboration with
the National Center for Chronic Disease Prevention and Health Promotion (2000).
http://www.cdc.gov/growthcharts

SAFER · HEALTHIER · PEOPLE™

Figure 3–6 ■ Physical growth percentiles for body mass index (BMI) according to age—boys: 2 to 20 years.
Source: From CDC, 2001, http://www.cdc.gov/growthcharts.

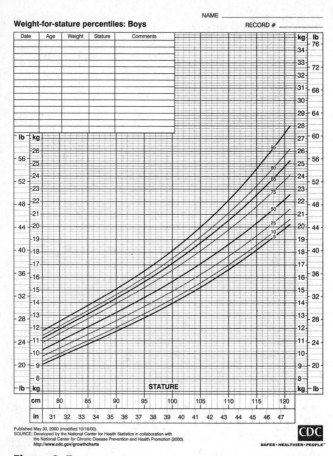

Figure 3–7 ■ Physical growth percentiles for weight for stature—boys: 2 to 20 years.
Source: From CDC, 2001, http://www.cdc.gov/growthcharts.

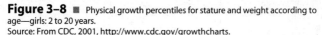
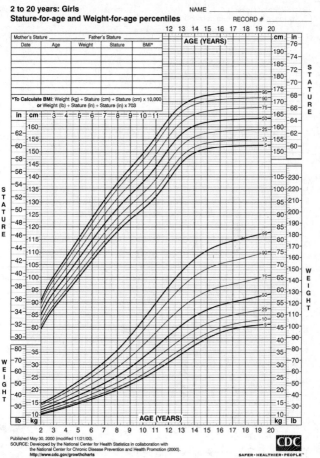

2 to 20 years: Girls
Stature-for-age and Weight-for-age percentiles

NAME _____
RECORD # _____

Figure 3–8 ■ Physical growth percentiles for stature and weight according to age—girls: 2 to 20 years.
Source: From CDC, 2001, http://www.cdc.gov/growthcharts.

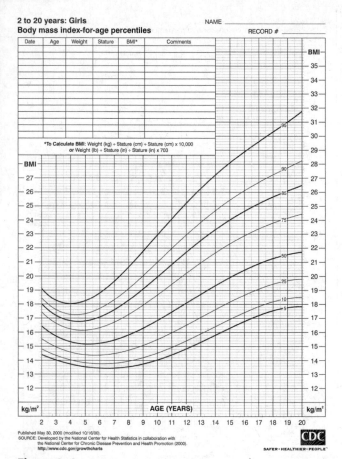

Figure 3–9 ■ Physical growth percentiles for body mass index (BMI) according to age—girls: 2 to 20 years.
Source: From CDC, 2001, http://www.cdc.gov/growthcharts.

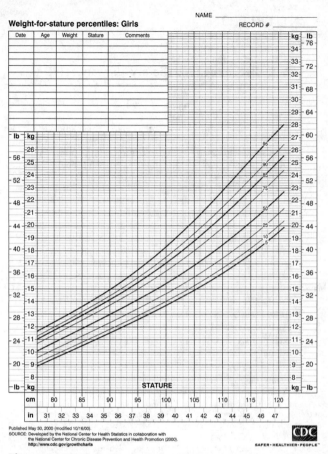

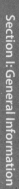

Figure 3–10 ■ Physical growth percentiles for weight for stature—girls: 2 to 20 years.
Source: From CDC, 2001, http://www.cdc.gov/growthcharts.

4 NUTRITION

Table 4–1 Recommended Dietary Allowances (RDAs)

	Age	Vitamin A (mcg/day)	Vitamin D (mcg/day)[†]	Vitamin E (mcg/day α-Tocopherol)	Vitamin K (mcg/day)	Vitamin C (mg/day)	Thiamin (mg/day)	Riboflavin (mg/day)	Niacin (mg/day)	Vitamin B_6 (mg/day)
Infants	0–6 months	400*	5*	4*	2.0*	40*	0.2*	0.3*	~0.2*	0.1*
	7–12 months	500*	5*	5*	2.5*	50*	0.3*	0.4*	~0.4*	0.3*
Children	1–3 years	300	5*	6	30*	15	0.5	0.5	6	0.5
	4–8 years	400	5*	7	55*	25	0.6	0.6	8	0.6
Males	9–13 years	600	5*	11	60*	45	0.9	0.9	12	1.0
	14–18 years	900	5*	15	75*	75	1.2	1.3	16	1.3
Females	9–13 years	600	5*	11	60*	45	0.9	0.9	12	1.0
	14–18 years	700	5*	15	75*	65	1.0	1.0	14	1.2

*Values are adequate intakes rather than RDAs. All other values on chart are RDAs.
Source: All data from *Dietary Reference Intakes: The Essential Guide to Nutrient Requirements*, by J. J. Otten, J. P. Hellwig, & L. D. Meyers (Eds.), 2006, Washington, DC: National Academies Press.

[†]In 2008, the American Academy of Pediatrics doubled the recommended intake for Vitamin D for all infants, children and adolescents, due to common deficiencies. Their recommendation is for 400 international units/day (10 mcg/day) as minimum intake for all infants, children and adolescents. [Wagner, C. L., Greer, F. R. and the Section on Breastfeeding and Committee on Nutrition (2008). Prevention of rickets and Vitamin D deficiency in infants, children and adolescents. *Pediatrics* 122(5), 1142–1152.]

Table 4–1 Recommended Dietary Allowances (RDAs)

Folate (mg/ day)	Vita-min B_{12} (mg/ day)	Cal-cium (mg/ day)	Phos phorus (mg/ day)	Magne-sium (mg/ day)	Iron (mg/ day)	Zinc (mg/ day)	Iodine (mcg/ day)	Sele-nium (mcg/ day)
65*	0.4*	210*	100*	30*	0.27*	2.0*	110*	15*
80*	0.5*	270*	275*	75*	11	3	130*	20*
150	0.9	500*	460	80	7	3	90	20
200	1.2	800*	500	130	10	5	90	30
300	1.8	1,300*	1,250	240	8	8	120	40
400	2.4	1,300*	1,250	240	11	11	150	55
300	1.8	1,300*	1,250	410	8	8	120	40
400	2.4	1,300*	1,250	360	15	9	150	55

Potassium (g/d)	Sodium (g/d)
0.4*	0.12*
0.7*	0.37*
3*	1*
3.8*	1.2*
4.5*	1.5*
4.5*	1.5*
4*	1.5*
4.7*	1.5*

Table 4-2 RDA for Protein, Carbohydrate, Fat

RDA

	Age	Protein	Carbohydrate	Polyunsaturated Fatty Acids n-6	Polyunsaturated Fatty Acids n-3	Total Fat	Fiber
Infants	0–6 months	9.1 g/day or 1.52 g/kg/day*	60 g/day	4.4 g/day	0.5 g/day	31 g/day	NE
	7–12 months	1.5 g/kg/day	95 g/day	4.6 g/day	0.5 g/day	30 g/day	NE
Children	1–3 years	13 g/day or 1.1 g/kg/day	130 g/day	7 g/day (linoleic)	0.7 g/day (α-linolenic)	NE	19 g/day
	4–8 years	0.95 g/kg/day or 19 g/day	130 g/day	10 g/day (linoleic)	0.9 g/day (α-linolenic)	NE	25 g/day
Males	9–13 years	0.95 g/kg/day or 34 g/day	130 g/day	12 g/day (linoleic)	1.2 g/day (α-linolenic)	NE	31 g/day
	14–18 years	0.85 g/kg/day or 52 g/day	130 g/day	16 g/day (linoleic)	1.6 g/day (α-linolenic)	NE	38 g/day
Females	9–13 years	0.95 g/kg/day or 34 g/day	130 g/day	10 g/day (linoleic)	1.0 g/day (α-linolenic)	NE	26 g/day
	14–18 years	0.85 g/kg/day or 46 g/day	130 g/day	11 g/day (linoleic)	1.1 g/day (α-linolenic)	NE	26 g/day

NE, not established.

*Values are adequate intakes rather than RDAs. All other values on charts are RDAs.

Note: All data from *Dietary Reference Intakes: The Essential Guide to Nutrient Requirements*, by J. J. Otten, J. P. Hellwig, & L. D. Meyers (Eds.), 2006, Washington, DC: National Academies Press.

CLINICAL MANIFESTATIONS OF DIETARY DEFICIENCIES/EXCESSES

Nutrient	Deficiency Manifestation	Excess Manifestation
Vitamin A	Night blindness Skin dryness and scaling	Headache Drowsiness Hepatomegaly Vomiting and diarrhea
Vitamin C	Abnormal hair (coiled shape) Skin abnormalities (dermatitis and lesions) Purpura Bleeding gums Joint tenderness Sudden heart failure	Usually none, excess is excreted in urine
Vitamin D	Rib abnormalities Bowed legs	Drowsiness
B vitamins	Weakness Decreased deep tendon reflexes Dermatitis	Usually none, excess is excreted in urine
Protein	Hepatomegaly Edema Scant, depigmented hair	Kidney failure
Carbohydrate	Emaciation Decreased energy Retarded growth and development	Overweight
Iron	Lethargy Slowed growth and developmental progression Pallor	Vomiting, diarrhea, abdominal pain Pallor Cyanosis Drowsiness Shock

FOOD GUIDE PYRAMID

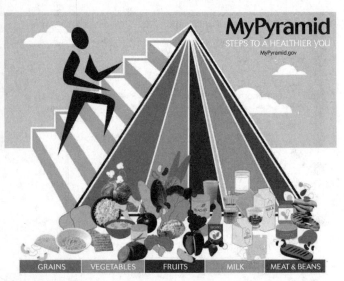

Figure 4–1 ▧ The food guide pyramid of the United States is used to provide information about amounts of foods recommended for daily intake.
Source: From U.S. Department of Agriculture and U.S. Department of Health and Human Services, 2005, http://www.mypyramid.gov/downloads/miniposter.pdf, accessed October 26, 2005. (*continued*)

GRAINS Make half your grains whole	VEGETABLES Vary your veggies	FRUITS Focus on fruits	MILK Get your calcium-rich foods	MEAT & BEANS Go lean with protein
Eat at least 3 oz. of whole-grain cereals, breads, crackers, rice, or pasta every day	Eat more dark-green veggies like broccoli, spinach, and other dark leafy greens	Eat a variety of fruit Choose fresh, frozen, canned, or dried fruit	Go low-fat or fat-free when you choose milk, yogurt, and other milk products	Choose low-fat or lean meats and poultry Bake it, broil it, or grill it
1 oz. is about 1 slice of bread, about 1 cup of breakfast cereal, or ½ cup of cooked rice, cereal, or pasta	Eat more orange vegetables like carrots and sweet potatoes Eat more dry beans and peas like pinto beans, kidney beans, and lentils	Go easy on fruit juices	If you don't or can't consume milk, choose lactose-free products or other calcium sources such as fortified foods and beverages	Vary your protein routine – choose more fish, beans, peas, nuts, and seeds

For a 2,000-calorie diet, you need the amounts below from each food group. To find the amounts that are right for you, go to MyPyramid.gov.

Eat 6 oz. every day	Eat 2½ cups every day	Eat 2 cups every day	Get 3 cups every day; for kids aged 2 to 8, it's 2	Eat 5½ oz. every day

Find your balance between food and physical activity

- Be sure to stay within your daily calorie needs.
- Be physically active for at least 30 minutes most days of the week.
- About 60 minutes a day of physical activity may be needed to prevent weight gain.
- For sustaining weight loss, at least 60 to 90 minutes a day of physical activity may be required.
- Children and teenagers should be physically active for 60 minutes every day, or most days.

Know the limits on fats, sugars, and salt (sodium)

- Make most of your fat sources from fish, nuts, and vegetable oils.
- Limit solid fats like butter, margarine, shortening, and lard, as well as foods that contain these.
- Check the Nutrition Facts label to keep saturated fats, trans fats, and sodium low.
- Choose food and beverages low in added sugars. Added sugars contribute calories with few, if any, nutrients.

MyPyramid.gov
STEPS TO A HEALTHIER YOU

USDA

U.S. Department of Agriculture
Center for Nutrition Policy and Promotion
April 2005
CNPP-15

USDA is an equal opportunity provider and employer.

Figure 4–1 ■ (Continued)

5 AVERAGE LABORATORY VALUES

Laboratory value ranges listed are approximate. Laboratories have slightly different levels of normal depending on assays performed. Always consult your local laboratory reference guide for normal values.

NORMAL VALUE RANGES: BLOOD[1]*

Albumin (S)[1]	1 mo–1 year: 2.1–4.7 g/dL
	1–18 years: 3.5–5.6 g/dL

Alkaline phosphatase (S)[1]	Age	Males	Females
	1–30 days	75–316	48–406
	1–3 yr	104–345	108–317
	4–6 yr	93–309	96–297
	7–9 yr	86–315	69–325
	10–12 yr	42–362	51–332
	13–15 yr	74–390	50–162
	16–18 yr	52–171	47–119

Blood Gases

Base excess (B)[1]	Infant: –7 to –1 mmol/L
	Child: –4 to +2 mmol/L
	Thereafter: –3 to +3 mmol/L
Bicarbonate, actual (P)[2] calculated from pH and $Paco_2$	Newborns: 17.2–23.6 mmol/L
	Children: 18–25 mmol/L
Carbon dioxide, partial pressure ($Paco_2$) (B)[1]	Newborn: 27–40 mmHg (3.6–5.3 kPa)
	Infant: 27–41 mmHg (3.6–5.5 kPa)
	Children: 32–48 mmHg (4.3–6.4 kPa)
Oxygen, partial pressure (Pao_2) (B)[1]	83–108 mmHg (11.0–14.4 kPa)

---

[1]***B,** whole blood; **P,** plasma; **S,** serum.

Oxygen saturation (B)[1]	Newborns: 85–90% Thereafter: 95–99%
pH (B)[1]	0–6 months 7.18–7.50 6–12 months 7.27–7.49

Cholesterol (S)[3]

Total cholesterol	Borderline: 170–199 mg/dL	Elevated: 200 mg/dL or higher
High-density lipoprotein	Less than 35 mg/dL	
Low-density lipoprotein	Borderline: 110–129 mg/dL	Elevated 130 mg/dL or higher
Triglycerides	Less than 150 mg/dL	

Coagulation Values

Bleeding time (Simplate)[2]	2–9 min
Fibrinogen[2]	200–500 mg/dL (5.9–14.7 micromol/L)
Partial thromboplastin time (PTT)[2]	42–54 seconds
Prothrombin time (PT)[2]	11–15 seconds
Thrombin time[2]	12–16 seconds

Electrolytes

Calcium (P, S)[1]	Newborn: 7.3–11.4 mg/dL (1.83–2.85 mmol/L) Infant and Child: 8.7–10.7 mg/dL (2.17–2.66 mmol/L)
Chloride (S, P)[1]	96–109 mmol/L

Glucose (S, P)[2]	Newborn: 30–100 mg/dL Child and Adult (fasting): 60–105 mg/dL
Magnesium (P, S)[1]	Newborn: 1.7–2.4 mg/dL (0.7–1.03 mmol/L) Infant and Child: 1.6–2.5 mg/dL (0.65–1.02 mmol/L)
Phosphorus, inorganic (S, P)[1]	Newborn: 2.7–7.2 mg/dL (0.81–2.1 mmol/L) Infant and Child: 2.5–6.5 mg/dL (0.81–2.1 mmol/L)
Osmolality (S)[1]	Newborn: 275–300 mOsm/kg Over 1 year: 280–300 mOsm/kg
Potassium (S, P)[1]	Newborn: 3.2–5.7 mmol/L Infant and Child: 3.3–4.7 mmol/L
Sodium (P, S)[1]	Newborn: 131–144 mmol/L Infant and Child: 132–141 mmol/L
Urea nitrogen (S, P)[1]	1–3 years: 4–17 mg/dL (1.1–4.6 mmol/L) 4–13 years: 6–17 mg/dL (1.6–4.6 mmol/L) 14–19 years: 7–21 mg/dL (1.9–5.7 mmol/L)

Hematology Mean Values for Children (B)

Red blood cell (RBC)[2]	$3.8–4.9 \times 10^{12}$/L
Hemoglobin (Hb)[2]	11.5–14.5 g/dL
Hematocrit (HCT)[2]	35–43%
Mean corpuscular volume[1]	72.3–90 micrometer^3
Mean corpuscular hemoglobin[1]	24.2–31 picograms
Mean corpuscular hemoglobin concentration[1]	32.7–35%

White blood cell (WBC)[2]	7.8–12.2×10^9/L

Differential[1]
   Neutrophils
   Eosinophils
   Basophils
   Lymphocyte
   Atypical lymphocytes
   Monocytes
	
	 1.2–11.1×10^9/L
	 0–0.9×10^9/L
	 0–1%
	 0.9–4.4×10^9/L
	 2–4%
	 0.3–2×10^9/L

Platelets[2]	150–400×10^9/L
Reticulocyte count (B)[1]	36.4–88.2×10^9/L
Sedimentation rate (micro) (B)[2]	1–8 mm/hr

Hemoglobin A1c (B)[1]	Normal: 4–7% Stable diabetic patients: 8–10% Young or unstable diabetic patients: 8–18%

Hematology Electrophoresis (B)[2]

Fetal hemoglobin[2]	At birth: 50%–85% of total hemoglobin At 1 year: Less than 15% of total hemoglobin Up to 2 years: Up to 5% of total hemoglobin Thereafter: Less than 2% of total hemoglobin
A_1 hemoglobin A_2 hemoglobin	96–98.5% of total hemoglobin 1.5–4% of total hemoglobin

Iron-Related Values

Ferritin (S)[1]	1–3 years: 12–501 ng/mL
	4–10 years: 25–280 ng/mL
	11–14 years: 15–112 ng/mL
	15–18 years: 10–158 ng/mL
Iron (S, P)[1]	5–11 am: 20–105 mcg/dL (3.6–18.8 micromol/L)
	5–11 pm: 20–145 mcg/dL (3.6–26 micromol/L)
Iron-binding capacity (S, P)[2]	275–458 mcg/dL (45–72 micromol/L)

| Lead (B)[1] | Less than 5.6 mcg/dL |

Thyroid Hormones

	Age	Males	Females
Thyroid-stimulating hormone (TSH) (P,S)[1] Values in milliInternational Units/mL	1–30 days 1 mo–5 yr 6–18 yr	0.64–12.75 0.67–5.97 0.52–5.08	0.8–10.83 0.59–6.78 0.51–4.91
Thyroxine (T4) (S, P)[1] Values in mcg/dL	1–30 days 1–12 mo 1–10 yr 11–18 yr	3.4–14.5 5.6–16.4 5.7–11.6 4.9–10.5	3.5–13.5 5–13.5 5.6–12.9 5.3–10.2
Thyroxine-binding globulin (TBG) (P)[1] Values in mg/L	1–12 mo 1–3 yr 4–12 yr 13–18 yr	16.2–32.9 16.4–32 16.5–29.8 13.4–25.6	17.7–32 19.3–33.8 15–30.8 13.7–28.7
Thyroxine, "free" (Free T4)(S)[1]	0–3 days: 3 days–18 yr	2–5 ng/mL 0.9–2.2 ng/mL	
Triiodothyronine (T3) (S)[1]	0–3 days 4 days–11 yr 12–18 yr	60–300 ng/dL 90–260 ng/dL 11–210 ng/dL	

NORMAL VALUE RANGES: URINE
Addis Count[2]

Red cells (12-hr specimen)	Less than 1 million
White cells (12-hr specimen)	Less than 2 million
Casts (12-hr specimen)	Less than 10,000
Protein (12-hr specimen)	Less than 55 mg

Catecholamines (Norepinephrine, Epinephrine)[1]
Values in mcg/24 hours (nmol/24 hours)

Age	Catecholamines	Norepinephrine	Epinephrine
Under 1 year	20	5.4–15.9 (32–94)	0.1–4.3 (0.5–23.5)
1–5 years	40	8.1–30.8 (48–181)	0.8–9.1 (4.4–49.7)
6–15 years	80	19–71.1 (112–421)	1.3–10.5 (7.1–57.3)
Over 15 years	100	34.4–87 (203–514)	3.5–13.2 (19.2–72.1)

Chloride[2]	Infants: 1.7–8.5 mmol/24 hr. Children: 17–34 mmol/24 hr. Adults: 140–240 mmol/24 hr.
Creatine[2]	18–58 mg/L (1.37–4.42 mmol/L)
Creatinine[1]	3–8 years: 0.11–0.68 g/24 hr 9–12 years: 0.17–1.41 g/24 hr 13–17 years: 0.29–1.87 g/24 hr Adults: 0.63–2.50 g/24 hr
Osmolality[2]	Infants: 50–600 mosm/L Older children: 50–1400 mosm/L

Phosphorus, tubular reabsorption[2]	78–97%
Potassium[2]	26–123 mmol/L
Sodium[2]	Infant: 0.3–3.5 mmol/24 hr
	Child and Adult: 5.6–17 mmol/24 hr
Specific gravity	1.010–1.030

NORMAL VALUE RANGES: SWEAT

Sodium	Normal: less than 40 mmol/L
	Patients with cystic fibrosis: greater than 60 mmol/L
Chloride	Normal: less than 40 mmol/L
	Patients with cystic fibrosis: greater than 60 mmol/L

NORMAL VALUE RANGES: CEREBROSPINAL FLUID

Protein[1]	Under 1 month: 15–153 mg/dL
	Under 3 months: 15–93 mg/dL
	Over 3 months: 15–50 mg/dL
Glucose[1]	All ages: 60–80% of blood glucose
	All ages: 41–84 mg/dL (2.28–4.66 mmol/L)

Source Modified from:
[1]*Pediatric Reference Ranges* (5th ed.), by S. J. Soldin, C. Brugnara, & E. C. Wong, 2005, Washington, DC: AACC Press.
[2]*Current Pediatric Diagnosis and Treatment* (17th ed.), by W. W. Hay, M. J. Levin, J. M. Sondheimer, R. R. Deterding, and Associate Authors, 2005, New York: Lange Medical Books/McGraw-Hill.
[3]"American Heart Association Guidelines for Primary Prevention of Atherosclerotic Cardiovascular Disease Beginning in Childhood," by R. W. Kavey, S. R. Daniels, R. M. Lauer, D. L. Atkins, L. L. Hayman, & K. Taubert, 2003, *Journal of Pediatrics, 142*(4), 368–372.

6 GROWTH, DEVELOPMENT, HEALTH PROMOTION, AND HEALTH MAINTENANCE

GROWTH AND DEVELOPMENT

General Concepts

Growth refers to an increase in physical size; growth represents quantitative changes such as height, weight, blood pressure, and number of words in the child's vocabulary.

Development refers to an increase in capability or function; developmental skills unfold in a complex manner as a relationship between the child's innate, unfolding capabilities with the stimuli and support provided in the environment.

Growth and development, or quantitative and qualitative changes in body organ functioning, ability to communicate, and performance of motor skills, unfold over time and are key components in the process of planning pediatric health care.

Each child displays a unique maturational pattern during the process of development; although the exact age at which skills emerge differs, the sequence, or order, of skill performance is uniform among children.

Development that proceeds from the head downward through the body and toward the feet is called *cephalocaudal* development.

Development that proceeds from the center of the body outward to the extremities is called *proximodistal* development.

Major theoretical frameworks used to understand and analyze the development of children include the following:

- Psychoanalytic theory of Sigmund Freud
- Psychosocial theory of Erik Erikson
- Cognitive theory of Jean Piaget
- Moral development theory of Lawrence Kohlberg
- Social learning theory of Albert Bandura
- Ecologic theory of Urie Bronfenbrenner
- Temperament theory of Stella Chase and Alexander Thomas
- Resilience theory

See Table 6–1 for a description of nursing applications related to the theories of Freud, Erikson, and Piaget.

Table 6–1   Nursing Applications of Theories of Freud, Erikson, and Piaget

Age Group	Developmental Stages	Nursing Applications
Infant (birth to 1 year)	Oral stage (Freud): The baby obtains pleasure and comfort through the mouth.	When a baby is to have nothing by mouth, offer a pacifier if not contraindicated. After painful procedures, offer a baby a bottle or pacifier, or have the mother breastfeed.
	Trust versus mistrust stage (Erikson): The baby establishes a sense of trust when basic needs are met.	Hold the hospitalized baby often. Offer comfort after painful procedures. Meet the baby's needs for food and hygiene.
		Encourage parents to room in.
		Manage pain effectively with use of pain medications and other measures.
	Sensorimotor stage (Piaget): The baby learns from movement and sensory input.	Use crib mobiles, manipulative toys, wall murals, and bright colors to provide interesting stimuli and comfort.
		Use toys to distract the baby during procedures and assessments.
Toddler (1–3 years)	Anal stage (Freud): The child derives gratification from control over bodily excretions.	Ask about toilet training and the child's rituals and words for elimination during admission history.
		Continue child's normal patterns of elimination in the hospital.
		Do not begin toilet training during illness or hospitalization.
		Accept regression in toileting during illness or hospitalization.
		Have potty chairs available in hospital and childcare centers.
	Autonomy versus shame and doubt stage (Erikson): The child is increasingly independent in many spheres of life.	Allow self-feeding opportunities.
		Encourage child to remove and put on own clothes, brush teeth, or assist with hygiene.
		If restraint for a procedure is necessary, proceed quickly, providing explanations and comfort.

Table 6–1 Nursing Applications of Theories of Freud, Erikson, and Piaget (Continued)

Age Group	Developmental Stages	Nursing Applications
Toddler (continued)	Sensorimotor stage (end); preoperational stage (beginning) (Piaget): The child shows increasing curiosity and explorative behavior. Language skills improve.	Ensure safe surroundings to allow opportunities to manipulate objects. Name objects and give simple explanations.
Preschooler (3–6 years)	Phallic stage (Freud): The child initially identifies with the parent of the opposite sex but by the end of this stage has identified with the same-sex parent.	Be alert for children who appear more comfortable with male or female nurses, and attempt to accommodate them. Encourage parental involvement in care. Plan for playtime and offer a variety of materials from which to choose.
	Initiative versus guilt stage (Erikson): The child likes to initiate play activities.	Offer medical equipment for play to lessen anxiety about strange objects. Assess children's concerns as expressed through their drawings. Accept the child's choices and expressions of feelings.
	Preoperational stage (Piaget): The child is increasingly verbal but has some limitations in thought processes. Causality is often confused, so the child may feel responsible for causing an illness.	Offer explanations about all procedures and treatments. Clearly explain that the child is not responsible for causing the illness.
School age (6–12 years)	Latency stage (Freud): The child places importance on privacy and understanding the body.	Provide gowns, covers, and underwear. Knock on door before entering. Explain treatments and procedures.
	Industry versus inferiority stage (Erikson): The child gains a sense of self-worth from involvement in activities.	Encourage the child to continue school work while hospitalized. Encourage child to bring favorite pastimes to the hospital. Help child adjust to limitations on favorite activities.

Table 6–1   Nursing Applications of Theories of Freud, Erikson, and Piaget (Continued)

Age Group	Developmental Stages	Nursing Applications
School age (continued)	Concrete operational stage (Piaget): The child is capable of mature thought when allowed to manipulate and see objects.	Give clear instructions about details of treatment. Show the child equipment that will be used in treatment.
Adolescent (12–18 years)	Genital stage (Freud): The adolescent's focus is on genital function and relationships.	Ensure access to gynecologic care for adolescent girls. Provide information on sexuality. Ensure privacy during health care. Have brochures and videos available for teaching about sexuality.
	Identity versus role confusion stage (Erikson): The adolescent's search for self-identity leads to independence from parents and reliance on peers.	Provide a separate recreation room for teens who are hospitalized. Take health history and perform examinations without parents present. Introduce adolescent to other teens with same health problem.
	Formal operational stage (Piaget): The adolescent is capable of mature, abstract thought.	Give clear and complete information about health care and treatments. Offer both written and verbal instructions. Continue to provide education about the disease to the adolescent with a chronic illness, as mature thought now leads to greater understanding.

HEALTH PROMOTION AND HEALTH MAINTENANCE

Health is a state of complete physical, mental, and social well-being and not merely the absence of disease and infirmity (World Health Organization, 1996).

Health promotion refers to activities that increase well-being and enhance wellness or health (Pender, Murdaugh, & Parsons, 2006). These activities lead to actualization of positive health potential for all individuals, even those with chronic or acute conditions.

Health maintenance (or health protection) refers to activities that preserve an individual's present state of health and that prevent disease or injury occurrence (Figure 6–1).

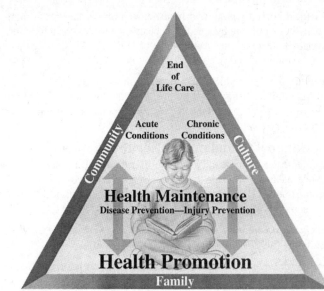

Figure 6–1 ■ The Bindler-Ball Continuum of Pediatric Healthcare for Children and Their Families. The outer bars represent the family, cultural, and community influences on the care that the child receives, either through the services sought by the family or the services provided in the community. Cultural influences include the family's decision to seek health care and follow recommendations, as well as the healthcare provider's cultural competence in caring for a child and family.

The inner categories represent the different types of health care needed by children. All children need health promotion and health maintenance services, represented by the base of the triangle. Notice the arrows representing the upward and downward movement between the levels of care as the child's condition changes.

Children may be healthy with episodic acute illnesses and injuries. Some children develop a chronic condition for which specialized health care is needed. A child's chronic condition may be well controlled, but acute episodes (e.g., with asthma) or other illnesses and injuries may occur, and the child also needs health promotion and health maintenance services to continue. Some children develop a life-threatening illness and ultimately need end-of-life care. A healthy child can also experience a catastrophic injury that causes death, and the family needs supportive end-of-life care.

Anticipatory guidance includes teaching for families to promote provision of an environment for children to assist in meeting developmental milestones.

Health supervision is the provision of services that focus on disease and injury prevention (health maintenance), growth and developmental surveillance, and health promotion at key intervals during the child's life.

A medical home or **pediatric healthcare home** is the site of comprehensive health care by a pediatric healthcare professional to ensure optimal health (National Association of Pediatric Nurse Associates and Practitioners, 2002).

Screening is a procedure used to detect the possible presence of a health condition before symptoms are apparent. It is usually conducted on large groups of individuals at risk for a condition and represents the secondary level of prevention.

U.S. National Guidelines for Health Promotion

Bright Futures, American Academy of Pediatrics (original editions by Maternal and Child Health Bureau, Health Resources and Services Administration, Department of Health and Human Services [http://www.aap.org])

The Guide to Clinical Preventive Services, U.S. Preventive Services Task Force (http://sss.ahrq.gov/clinic/uspstfix.htm)

Put Prevention Into Practice, Office of Disease Prevention and Health Promotion, Public Health Service, Department of Health and Human Services (http://www.ahcpr.gov/clinic/ppipix.htm)

Guidelines for Adolescent Preventive Services, American Medical Association (http://www.ama-assn.org)

Newborn Health Promotion and Health Maintenance
Timing of Visits

During the hospital stay, the nurse provides ongoing physical assessment of the mother and newborn, while providing education and anticipatory guidance to prepare the mother to care for herself and her newborn after hospital discharge.

If the newborn is discharged from the hospital less than 48 hours after birth, an experienced healthcare professional who is competent in newborn assessment should examine the newborn in the clinic or home setting within 48 hours of discharge (AAP, 2004).

For newborns discharged between 48 and 72 hours of age, the first follow-up visit should occur by 3 to 5 days of age.

General Observations

Welcome the family warmly.

Observe the family members that attend the visit and the interactions between them and with the new baby.

Apply information from observations to guide further questions and planned interventions.

Growth and Developmental Surveillance

For the healthy newborn, basic activities integrate surveillance of growth and development (Table 6–2), provide opportunities to work with the family, and promote the health of the newborn. These activities include:

- First bath (to remove blood and amniotic fluid from the newborn's skin and prevent transmission of microorganisms to others)
- Umbilical cord care
- Vitamin K injection (to prevent vitamin K–deficiency bleeding)
- Eye prophylaxis (administration of ophthalmic antibiotic ointment to prevent gonococcal ophthalmia neonatorum) within 1 hour of birth
- Physical assessment
- Feeding assessment
- Metabolic screen
- Hepatitis B vaccination
- Hearing screen
- Maternal syphilis screen reviewed
- Other screening test results reviewed as indicated by maternal–newborn risk factors and state regulations, including screening for human immunodeficiency virus infection (Kaye, 2006)

Table 6–2   Newborn Growth and Developmental Milestones Observed in Health Promotion and Health Maintenance Visits

Growth	Weight: baby may lose up to one-tenth of birth weight in the first week of life; birth weight should be reattained by day 10; weight gain is approximately two-thirds of an ounce per day thereafter.
	Length increases by 1–1.5 in.
	Head circumference increases by approximately 1 in.
Vision	Focuses 8–12 in. away
	Eyes wander and may cross.
	Prefers black and white or high-contrast patterns.
	Prefers the human face to all other patterns.
Hearing	Recognizes some sounds.
	May turn toward familiar sounds and voices.
	Responds to sounds with increased movement, quieting, or calming (Data from Shelov, 2004).

Source: Data from Shelov, S. P. (Ed.). (2004).

- Assessment of parental ability to adequately care for the newborn and to recognize and report signs of illness
- Administer any needed medications/immunizations.

Perform physical assessment (see chapter 2), including metabolic screening. (See chapter 22 for further information about metabolic screening.)

Perform gestational age examination (see chapter 2).

Observe for expected developmental performance (see Table 6–2).

Teach parents about expected growth and developmental milestones and ways to encourage the newborn's development.

Nutrition

Measure weight, length, head circumference, and chest circumference, and compare them to expected norms.

Assess type and amount of all feedings.

Ask about wet diapers (six to eight daily usually indicate adequate hydration).

Encourage breastfeeding as the most beneficial form of infant feeding (AAP, 2005a) to include decreased incidence of:

- Ear infections (otitis media)
- Allergies
- Diarrhea
- Vomiting
- Respiratory tract infection
- Meningitis and other infections

Teach proper mixing of formula, if used, and proper storage of breast milk.

Physical Activity

Newborn reflexes are strong and should be symmetric.

Hands are kept in tight fists and extremities flexed.

As the first month of life progresses, the baby straightens and lengthens.

Methods to encourage normal physical activity should be provided for parents:

- Position baby on stomach for supervised play periods (Graham, Kreutzman, Earl, et al., 2005). Be sure to place the baby on back when tired and starting to fall asleep.

- Allow the baby free movement of arms and hands. If the baby is swaddled, allow the hands to be outside the blanket and positioned in midline.
- Encourage appropriate toys, such as a mobile with contrasting colors and patterns; a plastic mirror; music boxes and exposure to soft music on the radio; a tape recorder or CD player; and soft toys with colors, patterns, and gentle sounds.
- Encourage switching positions when bottle feeding. Breastfeeding babies automatically feed from both sides. Parents who bottle feed may need to be reminded to promote this skill in their newborn.
- Beginning at birth, prevent flat spots on the newborn's head from supine positioning by nightly alternating the head position from left to right during sleep and occasionally changing the orientation of the newborn in relation to the activity at the doorway of the room.

Oral Health

Perform oral assessment (see chapter 2).

Instruct parents to avoid propping bottles and prolonged feedings.

Breast milk, formula, and water should be the only liquids provided.

Ask about plans for dental care and provide resources for use in the future if needed.

Mental Health

Establishing a sense of attachment is critical for the newborn's developing mental health.

Assess signs of attachment between baby and parents:
- Parent looks at the newborn frequently
- Parent has specific questions and observations about the individual characteristics of the newborn
- Parent touches, massages, or gently rubs the newborn
- Parent attempts to soothe the newborn when the newborn is upset
- Newborn looks content
- Newborn signals needs
- Newborn feeds well
- Newborn responds to parent's attempts to soothe

Provide suggestions for parents of activities that will enhance the newborn's mental health:
- Encourage your newborn to look at your face while feeding; imitate the baby's soft sounds and accommodate the baby's movements.

- Respond quickly to your baby's feeding cues, and avoid rigid feeding schedules; feeding times are unpredictable, especially in the first few months.
- Identify ways to soothe the crying newborn; babies cry for reasons other than hunger.
- Learn infant massage; for healthy infants, massage reportedly facilitates bonding, helps induce sleep in the baby, and makes parents feel relaxed while massaging their baby.
- Allow the baby to suck on fingers, hands, or a pacifier.
- Make eye contact with the baby, hold and rock the baby frequently, and read and sing to the baby. If you cannot think of what to say to the baby, talk about your day, or talk about what is happening—for example, "Are you hungry now?" "Is that milk nice and warm?" "Do you hear that dog barking outside?" "You are very alert. I like it when you look at me that way."
- Be consistent and predictable in the way you respond to the newborn's needs.

(Adapted from Hagan, Shaw, & Duncan, 2008; Shelov, 2004)

Teach parents about the sleep and wake cycles of the baby so that they can engage the newborn during alert periods.

Newborn mental health relates directly to the parent's state.

Evaluate parents, and especially mothers, for adaptation, signs of depression, and stress.

Relationships

Family adaptation begins in the prenatal period and extends into the newborn period.

Perform assessment of risk and protective factors in family relationships (Table 6–3).

Evaluate for signs of domestic abuse, substance abuse, or child neglect or abuse.

Provide ideas for activities that promote family health and positive parent–newborn interaction:

- Share newborn care activities. Recognize that you may do things differently than your partner, such as the way you change a diaper or give a bath, but, if the baby is cared for, safe, and secure, these differences in technique do not matter.
- Compliment one another on newborn caregiving strengths, such as the mother's ability to breastfeed and the partner's ability to calm the crying baby.

Table 6–3 Risk and Protective Factors in Newborn and Family Relationships

Newborn Risk Factors	Newborn Protective Factors
Preterm birth, congenital disabilities, and chronic illness	Good health
Feeding and sleep problems	Normal eating, bowel, and sleep patterns
Fussing, crying, irritability, and difficulty consoling	Positive temperament
Diminished social interactions and responsiveness	Responds to parents' attention
Undernutrition, developmental delay	Normal growth and development

Parental Risk Factors	Parental Protective Factors
Baby unplanned and unwanted at birth; potential for neglect and/or rejection	Welcome baby at birth
Financial insecurity, homelessness, and lack of knowledge about how to care for newborn	Meet newborn's basic needs for food, shelter, clothing, and health care
Cannot promote strong nurturing environment owing to serious problems, such as abusive behavior, depression, mental illness, or substance abuse	Provide a strong nurturing environment
Severe marital problems, absent parent, or frequent change of partners	Parents have positive relationship with one another, and share care of newborn
Lack of parenting skills, lack of parenting self-esteem, inability to cope with multiple roles, and inappropriate coping strategies	Strong self-esteem, developmental maturity, and knowledge of infant development
History of maltreatment as a child (risk increases with positive history) (Data from Hagan, Shaw, & Duncan, 2008)	No history of maltreatment as a child

Source: Data from Hagan, J. G., Shaw, J. S., & Duncan, P. M. (2008).

- Attend health supervision visits together as much as possible.
- Be sensitive to when your partner is overstressed and overtired. Ask how you can help, and then follow through with suggested activities. Sometimes listening is the most helpful thing you can do.
- Rest and take time for yourself. Make decisions about what must be done (paying bills, laundry, grocery shopping) and what could wait (traveling to visit grandparents, painting the house, cleaning closets). Accept help from family and friends.

- Discuss how you will raise your baby in a loving, supportive, and respectful environment.
- Discuss how you were raised and what you would like to be different in your new family. Learn about parenting strategies, and try out what feels comfortable for you.
- Keep in contact with family and friends. Maintain community ties that are important to you, such as social, religious, and cultural or recreational organizations or programs.
- Leave the baby with a trusted friend or family member, and take time to be alone once in a while. Talk about something other than the baby.
- Supervise siblings in their contacts with the newborn. Allow siblings to "help" care for the new baby in age-appropriate ways. Praise siblings for positive attention they give to the baby, and allow siblings to express their feelings about the new baby and changes in the family.
- Support one another in seeking and using community resources to strengthen parenting skills, such as classes and parenting groups.
- Cuddle, hold, and rock the baby as much as possible. Babies cannot be spoiled by too much attention.
- Take advantage of baby's time awake to play with baby. Singing, reading, and simply talking to the baby about what is happening provide developmental stimulation.

Injury and Disease Prevention

Assess parental knowledge of injury prevention strategies.

Promote healthy and safe habits by including teaching about proper and consistent use of an infant car seat and strategies to prevent falls, burns, choking, drowning, and suffocation (see Table 6–4).

Be alert for the most common neonatal conditions that require extension of the newborn hospital stay or return to the hospital—conditions associated with bilirubin metabolism, prematurity (including respiratory distress), respiratory problems, infections, and birth defects (Owens, Thompson, Elixhauser, et al., 2003).

Integrate health maintenance activities for disease prevention into the visit:
- Metabolic screening
- Hearing screening
- Eye examination
- Immunizations (hepatitis B is needed, with an additional injection of hepatitis B immune globulin if the mother is hepatitis B surface antigen–positive)

Table 6–4   Injury Prevention Topics for Newborns

Topic	Injury Prevention Teaching Topics
Car safety seat	Choose an infant-only seat or a convertible seat suitable for an infant.
	Infant rides rear-facing until at least 1 year of age and >20 lb. The safest place for all children to ride is in the back seat. Never place a rear-facing car safety seat in the front seat with an active passenger airbag.
	Use a car safety seat every time the infant is in the car.
	Read and follow the manufacturer's instructions for the car safety seat and the vehicle owner's manual for installation information.
	Dress the infant in clothes that allow the straps to go between the legs. Never place blankets under the baby. Buckle the baby into the seat and place blankets over the baby.
	To make sure the car safety seat is installed correctly and the baby is positioned correctly, go to a car seat inspection station. A certified Child Passenger Safety (CPS) technician will assist you. Find a list of certified CPS technicians by state or zip code on the National Highway Traffic Safety Administration website at http://www.nhtsa.dot.gov/people/injury/childps/contacts. Find a car safety seat inspection station at http://www.nhtsa.dot.gov/people/injury/childps/cpsfitting or 1-866-SEAT-CHECK. (AAP, 2007)
Shaken baby syndrome	Never shake a baby. Recognize that sometimes you will not be able to console your baby. Shaking a baby, even for only a few seconds, can cause serious brain damage and death.
Crib	Use a safety approved crib. Slats should be no more than 2⅜ in. apart. Mattress should be firm and fit snugly into the crib. Keep crib rails raised.
Co-sleeping	The AAP discourages co-sleeping because of the risk of sudden infant death syndrome (with overheating as a possible factor) and the danger of suffocation. Sleep with the baby nearby but not in the parental bed. If the parent must sleep with the baby, ensure that the infant is supine, separated from any soft surfaces such as pillows, and no blankets will cover the infant's head; beware of spaces between the mattress and the wall, headboard, or footboard; and do not sleep with the baby while under the influence of drugs or alcohol. The infant should never sleep in the same bed with siblings owing to the high risk of suffocation. (AAP, 2005b)
Baby toys	Use age-appropriate baby toys. Check toys for sharp edges or loose parts. Keep older siblings' toys out of baby's reach. Do not use toys with loops or string cords.

Table 6–4 Injury Prevention Topics for Newborns (Continued)

Topic	Injury Prevention Teaching Topics
Drowning	Never leave baby alone in the bathtub. If you must turn your back on the baby or leave the room, take the baby out of the tub.
Suffocation	Keep plastic bags and wrappings away from baby (take the plastic bag off the crib mattress). Shake baby powder into your hand first then apply it so the baby does not inhale it. Do not allow a baby or sibling to play with a latex balloon. Keep small objects (e.g., safety pins, coins, and small toys) out of baby's reach. Do not attach pacifiers, medals, or other objects to the crib or to the baby's body with a string or cord. Do not put the crib near blinds, curtains, or anything with a hanging cord. Do not let baby wear clothing with strings near the neck (e.g., a sweatshirt hood that ties with a cord) or a headband that could slip down and wrap around baby's neck. Use a tight-fitting crib sheet that does not come loose when the corner is pulled.
Burns	Set the hot water heater thermostat lower than 120°F. Do not smoke or drink hot liquids while holding the baby. Do not microwave bottles of formula or breast milk due to uneven heating. Do not expose baby to direct sunlight.
Falls	Keep a hand on the baby while dressing or diaper changing on a surface other than on the floor. Never leave the baby un-supervised on any high surface, such as a bed, changing table, or sofa. Always keep one hand on the baby.
Pet safety	Keep some distance between the newborn and the pet until the pet's initial reaction to the new baby is assessed. Never leave the baby unsupervised with the family dog or cat or any animal capable of harming the newborn.
Sibling supervision	Never leave your baby alone with a young sibling. When young children hold the baby, seat the child on a large soft surface, such as the couch, and supervise closely. Watch siblings for aggressive behavior toward the newborn, such as hitting or biting. Siblings may take on a caregiving role and imitate adults; watch for "feeding" of nonfood items or choking hazards.
Fire safety	Install working smoke detectors on every floor of the house and in every sleeping area. Have a fire escape plan from your house and practice it.
Poisoning	Post the universal phone number for poison control near your telephone: 1-888-222-1222.
Gun safety	Keep any gun unloaded and locked up. Keep the ammunition locked up separately from the gun. Consider not keeping a gun in the household owing to safety hazards for family members.

Table 6–4   Injury Prevention Topics for Newborns (Continued)

Topic	Injury Prevention Teaching Topics
In case of emergency	Know when and how to call your pediatric care provider.
	Know when it is appropriate to go to the emergency department.
	Take a first aid class and learn cardiopulmonary resuscitation for children and adults. (Data from Hagan, Shaw, & Duncan, 2008; AAP, 2005b; Shelov, 2004; Child Restraints, 2006; AAP 2007; NINDS, 2007.)

Source: Data from Hagan, J. G., Shaw, J. S., & Duncan, P. M. (2008).

- Prevention of secondhand smoke exposure
- Sudden infant death syndrome risk reduction
- Formula safety
- Hand hygiene
- Minimizing the newborn's exposure to disease by avoiding infant exposure to large crowds, especially in cold and flu season; covering coughs and sneezes and using good hand hygiene; alerting baby's caregiver if newborn is exposed to varicella, pertussis, or other serious communicable disease

Infant Health Promotion and Health Maintenance
General Observations

Who is bringing the baby in for care?

What are interactions like between the adults present or adults, other siblings, and the baby?

Is the baby awake or sleeping?

If awake, is the baby's body posture and alertness appropriate for age and developmental level?

Does the infant look well nourished and cared for?

Do the parents appear adequately rested, dressed, and of expected mental status?

Instruct parents to contact a provider if the infant has:
- Temperature ≥ 100.4°F (38.0°C)
- Seizure
- Skin rash, purplish spots, petechiae; change in skin color
- Change in activity or behavior that makes the parent uncomfortable

- Unusual irritability, lethargy, prolonged or unusual cry
- Failure to eat or drink
- Vomiting
- Diarrhea
- Decreased urine
- Respiratory infection or cough that concerns the parent
- Dehydration

Growth and Developmental Surveillance

Measure length, weight, and chest and head circumference. Compare to norms (see Table 6–5).

Plot findings on growth grids and evaluate percentiles (see chapter 3).

Perform physical assessment (see chapter 2).

Ask parents about care:
- Skin, nails, bathing
- Nutritional intake
- Elimination patterns
- Sleep patterns
- Activity levels and developmental milestones
- Illnesses or health conditions

Recognize types of infant sleep:
- Drowsy—flaccid posture, eyes slowly opening and closing, random movements
- Rapid eye movement or active sleep—body activity, eye movement with eyes open or closed, irregular respirations, sucking motions (30–40% of infant sleep)
- Non–rapid eye movement or quiet sleep—minimal muscle movement, eyes quiet, regular sucking motions, little motion (60–70% of infant sleep)
  (Davis, Parker, & Montgomery, 2004)

Recognize normal sleep patterns:
- Birth–3 months—10 to 16 hours daily in five periods of 30 minutes to 4 hours; by 4–6 weeks of age, a consistent sleep pattern should emerge
- 3–6 months—14 hours daily with a longer sleep at night and two to three naps
- 6–12 months—12–14 hours daily with a longer sleep at night and one to two naps
  Source: Data from Hoban. (2004)

Table 6-5 Physical Growth and Development during Infancy

Age	Physical Growth	Fine Motor Ability	Gross Motor Ability	Sensory Ability
Birth to 1 month	Gains 5–7 oz (140–200 g)/ week Grows 1.5 cm (0.5 in.) in first month Head circumference increases 1.5 cm (0.5 in.)/month	Holds hand in fist Draws arms and legs to body when crying	Inborn reflexes such as startle and rooting are predominant activity May lift head briefly if prone Alerts to high-pitched voices Comforts with touch	Prefers to look at faces and black and white geometric designs Follows objects in line of vision
2–4 months	Gains 5–7 oz (140–200 g)/ week Grows 1.5 cm (0.5 in.)/month Head circumference increases 1.5 cm (0.5 in.)/month Posterior fontanel closes Eats 120 mL/kg/24 hr (2 oz/lb/24 hr)	Holds rattle when placed in hand Looks at and plays with own fingers Readily brings objects from hand to mouth	Moro reflex fading in strength Can turn from side to back and then return Decrease in head lag when pulled to sitting; sits with head held in midline with some bobbing When prone, holds head and supports weight on forearms	Follows objects 180 degrees Turns head to look for voices and sounds
4–6 months	Gains 5–7 oz (140–200 g)/ week Doubles birth weight 5–6 months Grows 1.5 cm (0.5 in.)/month Head circumference increases 1.5 cm (0.5 in.)/month	Grasps rattles and other objects at will; drops them to pick up another offered object Mouths objects Holds feet and pulls to mouth Holds bottle	Head held steady when sitting No head lag when pulled to sitting Turns from abdomen to back by 4 months and then back to abdomen by 6 months	Examines complex visual images Watches the course of a falling object Responds readily to sounds

Table 6–5 Physical Growth and Development during Infancy (Continued)

Age	Physical Growth	Fine Motor Ability	Gross Motor Ability	Sensory Ability
4–6 months	Teeth may begin erupting by 6 months Eats 100 mL/kg/24 hr (1.5 oz/lb/24 hr)	Grasps with whole hand (palmar grasp) Manipulates objects	When held standing supports much of own weight	Recognizes own name and responds by looking and smiling Enjoys small and complex objects at play
6–8 months	Gains 3–5 oz (85–140 g)/week Grows 1 cm (0.375 in.)/month Growth rate slower than first 6 months	Bangs objects held in hands Transfers objects from one hand to the other Beginning pincer grasp at times	Most inborn reflexes extinguished Sits alone steadily without support by 8 months Likes to bounce on legs when held in standing position	Understands words such as "no" and "cracker" May say one word in addition to "mama" and "dada" Recognizes sound without difficulty
8–10 months	Gains 3–5 oz (85–140 g)/week Grows 1 cm (0.375 in.)/month	Picks up small objects Uses pincer grasp well	Crawls or pulls whole body along floor by arms Creeps by using hands and knees to keep trunk off floor Pulls self to standing and sitting by 10 months Recovers balance when sitting	
10–12 months	Gains 3–5 oz (85–140 g)/week Grows 1 cm (0.375 in.)/month Head circumference equals chest circumference Triples birth weight by 1 year	May hold crayon or pencil and make mark on paper Places objects into containers through holes	Stands alone Walks holding onto furniture Sits down from standing	Plays peek-a-boo and patty cake

Provide teaching to promote healthy sleep patterns:

- Place the baby to sleep in a quiet and darkened room.
- Have similar bedtime routines each night.
- Provide a consistent transitional object, such as a favorite blanket, each night.
- Put the baby to bed while still awake rather than after falling asleep nursing so he or she becomes accustomed to getting to sleep without nursing.
- Do not try to awaken the baby in non–rapid eye movement (quiet) sleep.
- Establish a consistent sleep routine and time; routine may involve some cuddling and rocking time but should not be vigorous, stimulating play.
- For the baby who has trouble going to sleep, remain in the room for a few minutes but do not establish eye contact; place a hand on the abdomen or chest or gently hold flailing arms and legs.

(National Sleep Foundation, 2007)

Perform recommended screening (Table 6–6).

Recognize growth and developmental milestones (Table 6–7).

Nutrition

Evaluate amount and type of feedings (breast and/or bottle).

Evaluate intake of table and finger foods.

Combine results of length and weight measurement with nutritional intakes.

Hematocrit taken during infancy, usually at 9–12 months, to rule out iron deficiency anemia.

Perform teaching to enhance nutrition (Table 6–8):

- Support breastfeeding.
- Ensure use of breast or iron-fortified formula.
- Teach recommended introduction of foods:
  - Begin at 4–6 months.
  - Introduce one food at a time and wait 4–5 days before next food.
  - Start with rice cereal or other rice source; then vegetables and fruits; then meat, tofu, and other protein sources; and then finger foods by 7–9 months.

Table 6–6   Screening during Infant Health Promotion and Health Maintenance Visits

Age	Recommended Screening Tests
1 month	Vision (follow objects, red reflex, opacities)
	Hearing (response to sound; screening by machine if not completed in the hospital)
	Physical examination with special attention to skin problems, hip dysplasia, foot position, and range of motion; mouth, abdomen, cardiac abnormality, tearing of eyes, neurologic (including child abuse), and anthropometric measurements
	Developmental milestones
	Dietary screening and stool/urine pattern assessment
	Review immunization record
2 months	As above
4 months	As above
	Vision (add cover-uncover test for strabismus); ocular mobility for lateral gaze
6 months	As above
	Vision (add ability to follow object bilaterally, corneal light reflex)
	Physical examination with special attention to muscle tone, extremities, appearance of first teeth, tympanic membrane, and testicle descent for males
9 months	As above
	Lead levels if exposure is possible
	Anemia
	Physical examination with special attention to symmetry of movement
12 months	As above
	Tuberculosis test if exposed to the disease
	Physical examination with special attention to condition of teeth

Source: Data from Hagan, Shaw, & Duncan. (2008)

Physical Activity

Observe developmental milestones.

Ask parents about opportunities for crawling, reaching for toys, and other physical activity in daily routines.

Table 6-7 Developmental Milestones Observed in Infant Health Promotion and Health Maintenance Visits

Age	Developmental Milestones
1 month	Responds to sound by startle or increased alertness
	Follows objects and human face with eyes
	Has periods of alertness and restfulness
	Comforted by touch or feeding by parent
	Has symmetrical movements and generally has arms and legs flexed
	Lifts head momentarily when prone
2 months	Above characteristics
	Makes noises, such as cooing, in response to interaction with adult
	Smiles
	Lifts head, neck, upper chest when prone
	Has increasing head control when held in sitting position
4 months	Increasing cooing and babbling
	Smiles, laughs, makes other noises during interactions
	Supports self on hands when prone
	Rolls front to back
	Touches objects and grasps rattle placed near hand
6 months	Uses sounds in repeated speech, such as bababa, dadadada
	Interested in surroundings and toys
	When pulled to sitting has no head lag
	Sits with support
	Grasps objects easily and places in mouth
	Transfers objects from one hand to other
	Bears weight on legs when held in standing position
9 months	Understands simple words and uses more sounds in babbling
	Responds to name
	Enjoys interactive games with parent
	Moves when placed on floor by crawling, creeping, or rolling repeatedly
	Sits without support
	Stands holding on to support
	Plays with toys
	Feeds self readily with fingers and tries to use cup

Table 6–7   Developmental Milestones Observed in Infant Health Promotion and Health Maintenance Visits (Continued)

Age	Developmental Milestones
12 months	Has one or more words
	Imitates sounds readily
	Increasing interactions and interest in surroundings
	Follows directions, such as saying or waving bye
	Pulls to standing, walks a few steps holding on
	Well-developed pincer grasp
	Able to drink from cup

Table 6–8   Nutrition Teaching for Infant Health Promotion and Health Maintenance Visits

Age	Nutrition Teaching
1 month	Support breastfeeding efforts.
	Teach correct formula types and preparation if used.
	Teach burping and rate of feeding information.
	Suggest water during hot weather or if family wants to use a bottle at baby's bedtime.
	Encourage families to view feedings as social interactions; emphasize importance of holding the infant and not propping bottles.
2 months	Continue above.
	Review fluid needs of infants.
	Reinforce food safety for partially used bottles of breast milk or formula.
	Use warm water for heating bottles rather than microwave to avoid burning.
	Warn against feeding honey in the first year of life.
	Begin cleaning of infant gums daily.
	Provide information about any supplements needed (e.g., iron for premature infant, vitamin D for babies not exposed to adequate sunlight).
4 months	Continue above.
	Discuss introduction of first foods between 4 and 6 months, and surveillance for symptoms of allergy or intolerance.
	Discuss changing food patterns such as increasing amounts and decreasing numbers of daily milk feedings.

Table 6–8 Nutrition Teaching for Infant Health Promotion and Health Maintenance Visits (Continued)

Age	Nutrition Teaching
6 months	Continue above.
	Reinforce proper introduction of new foods, to include rice cereal, fruits, and vegetables.
	Discuss any unusual food reactions observed.
	Introduce cup for drinking.
	Introduce soft finger foods.
	Serve juice only in a cup and limit to no more than 6 oz. daily.
	Caution about common choking foods and items.
	Provide information about fluoride supplement if water supply is not fluoridated.
9 months	Continue above.
	If mother does not continue to breastfeed, teach family to use iron-fortified formula for the first year of life.
	Encourage self-feeding of finger foods, integrating common foods for the family.
	Introduce source of protein such as tofu, cheese, mashed beans, and slivers of meats.
12 months	Continue above.
	Support mother who wishes to continue breastfeeding beyond 1 year of age.
	Encourage cups for all feedings other than breast.

Evaluate risk and protective factors for physical activity; plan interventions that enhance protective factors and alleviate risks (Table 6–9).

Perform teaching to enhance health:

- Frequent and supervised play opportunities are needed.
- Holding the infant in various positions, helping the older infant to stand, and providing positive feedback for the infant's accomplishments are encouraged.
- Toys should be placed near child to encourage movement.
- Participation in parent–infant playgroups provides stimulation for the child, provides social interaction with other infants, and increases the parent's knowledge of the child's abilities.
- Discussion of the next fine and gross motor skills anticipated.

Table 6–9   Risk and Protective Factors Regarding Physical Activity in Infancy

Risk Factors	Protective Factors
Premature birth	Meets developmental milestones at expected ages
Delayed developmental milestones	
Limited stimulation by family or other care providers	Has contact with parents, siblings, and others for significant time each day
Lack of knowledge by family about infant's physical activity needs	A supportive environment with room to play safely; stimulating surroundings
	Physically active family
Limited community resources for families with infants	Family knowledge about infant's physical activity needs
	Community programs that promote physical activity in infants and information for families

Source: Data from Patrick, Spear, & Holt. (2001)

Oral Health

Count number of teeth.

Ask about teething patterns and discomfort.

Teach healthy oral health and hazards of bottles at bedtime.

Ask about accessibility to dental care, and provide resources as needed.

Mental and Spiritual Health

Mental health is related to early experiences, inborn characteristics such as temperament and resilience, and relationships with caregivers.

Children who feel secure and have nurturing environments usually grow as expected and perform milestones at usual times (Table 6–10).

Slow growth and delayed development are sometimes related to feeding disorder of infancy and early childhood.

Stranger anxiety is manifested by crying when exposed to new people and indicates expected attachment to parents; common in second half of the first year of life.

Also in the second half of the first year of life, infants may exhibit **separation anxiety** by inconsolable crying and other signs of distress when parents are not present.

Self-regulation is the process of dealing with feelings, learning to soothe self, and focusing on activities for increasing periods of time. Infants learn early how to comfort and calm themselves.

Table 6–10 Psychosocial Development during Infancy

Age	Play and Toys	Communication
Birth to 3 months	Prefers visual stimuli of mobiles, black-and-white patterns, mirrors	Coos Babbles Cries
	Auditory stimuli are music boxes, tape players, soft voices	
	Responds to rocking and cuddling	
	Moves legs and arms while adult sings and talks	
	Likes varying stimuli—different rooms, sounds, visual images	
3–6 months	Prefers noisemaking objects that are easily grasped—e.g., rattles	Vocalizes during play and with familiar people
	Enjoys stuffed animals and soft toys with contrasting colors	Laughs
		Cries less
		Squeals and makes pleasure sounds
		Babbles multisyllabically ("mamamamama")
6–9 months	Likes teething toys	Increases vowel and consonant sounds
	Increasingly desires social interaction with adults and other children	Links syllables together
		Uses speechlike rhythm when vocalizing with others
	Soft toys that can be manipulated and mouthed are favorites	
9–12 months	Enjoys large blocks, toys that pop apart and go back together, nesting cups and other objects	Understands "no" and other simple commands
		Says "dada" and "mama" to identify parents
	Laughs at surprise toys such as jack-in-the-box	Learns one or two other words
	Plays interactive games such as peek-a-boo	Receptive speech surpasses expressive speech
	Uses push-and-pull toys	

Observe and ask about how parents provide comfort to the crying baby. Suggestions for enhanced comforting measures include:

- Offer a breastfeeding or bottle feeding, especially if the last feeding was more than 2 hours earlier.
- If feeding was recent, hold the baby in a sitting position and rub or pat the back to help expel gastric gas.
- Change the diaper if wet or soiled.
- Place a hand on the abdomen and feel for movement. If movement or passing gas is present, hold the baby against the chest, walk slowly, and pat the back.
- Swaddle the baby securely in a blanket and hold horizontally while rocking.
- Hold the baby on your lap, secure the hands in yours, and talk softly.
- Never shake or throw the baby, no matter how long the crying. Call your healthcare provider for suggestions if you feel like nothing works, and you are very frustrated.

Relationships

Social relationships are foundational to the psychosocial health of infants.

Temperament characteristics of the infant interact with the environment and other people. Common patterns of temperament include:

- Easy (moderate activity, easy to console, regular sleep and eating patterns)
- Slow to warm up (slow adaptation to new events and people or to changes in environment and schedule)
- Difficult (high activity, difficult to console, irregular sleep and eating patterns)

Assess social skills:

- Smiling
- Cooing and other sounds, words
- Response to siblings and other children
- Sleep patterns
- Childcare arrangements, playgroups

Suggest activities to parents that foster infant relationship formation:

- Encourage parents to hold, read to, and talk to babies. Positively reinforce these behaviors when observed.
- Point out the infant's abilities to respond to faces and voices, to smile and laugh, and to reflect the mood of adults in the home.
- Review sleep patterns and make recommendations for methods to plan bedtime routines.

- Be sure that parents have resources to turn to when needing assistance with infant care or other household responsibilities.

Evaluate problems in relationships:
- **Domestic violence** is a situation in which parents or adult care providers commit violent acts toward one another. Assess for domestic violence, and refer to appropriate resources.
- **Child abuse** interferes with the formation of healthy relationships. See mental health chapter (chapter 25) for assessment and interventions related to child abuse.

Injury and Disease Prevention
Car seats for infants

Review the family's routines for transporting an infant by car at every health supervision visit. Recommendations for infants from birth to 1 year, or 2–22 lb, include:
- Use only "infant-only" or rear-facing convertible seat.
- The seat must always be placed in the back seat in the rear-facing position.
- Harness straps should be at or below shoulder level.
- Be sure to follow guidelines for every trip, no matter how short.
- Have car seat and car checked by a certified Child Passenger Safety Technician (locate an inspection station at 866-732-8243 or www.seatcheck.org).
- If car seat is changed between two or more cars, it should be checked for proper installation in each car.
  (Data from National Highway Traffic Safety Administration [NHTSA], 2007; American Academy of Pediatrics, 2007.)

Perform safety teaching (Table 6–11).

Administer needed immunizations (Table 6–12).

Toddler and Preschooler Health Promotion and Health Maintenance
General Observations
Observe for signs of independence and reliance on parents.

Look at independence from adults in ambulation.

Does the parent respond to the child's questions?

Were age-appropriate toys or activities brought to the visit to help occupy the child while waiting?

Table 6–11 Injury Prevention Topics for Infancy by Age

Age	Injury Prevention Teaching Topics
1 month	Infant car safety seat guidelines. Put baby to sleep on back. Avoid loose bedding and toys in crib. Avoid bracelets, necklaces, string toys, or cords. Avoid tobacco use in the environment. Provide adult supervision of the baby at all times by trusted individuals. Test bath water temperature and never leave baby alone in the bath. Never place baby on high objects, such as counter, table, or bed; always keep one hand on the baby during activities like diaper changes to prevent falling. Wash hands correctly and often, especially before feeding or holding infant, and after providing hygiene care. Avoid contact with persons with communicable diseases. Have smoke alarms, and avoid fire hazards.
1 month	Learn infant cardiopulmonary resuscitation and airway obstruction removal. Never shake the baby. Have plans for emergency care.
2 months	As above. Use only recommended playpens or cribs and keep sides up. Avoid moldy environments. Keep baby toys cleaned. Avoid direct sunlight for the baby. Keep sharp and small objects out of baby's environment. Keep hot water heater lower than 120°F. Review emergency plan with all care providers.
4 months	As above. Get all poisonous substances out of baby's view and reach; install locks to keep them inaccessible. Do not use latex balloons or plastic bags near the baby. Never use infant walkers.
6 months	As above. If an infant-only car seat was used, switch to rear-facing convertible safety seat (intended for babies up to 40 lb) when baby is 20–30 lb or 26 in. Empty containers of water immediately after use; be sure pools or other bodies of water are locked and not accessible to baby. Use sunscreen, hat, and long sleeves when baby is in the sun.

Table 6–11   Injury Prevention Topics for Infancy by Age (Continued)

Age	Injury Prevention Teaching Topics
	Keep heavy and sharp objects out of reach; check that all poisons are locked away, including in homes visited; keep pet food and cosmetics out of reach.
	Do not drink hot liquids or eat soup while holding the baby.
	Have poison control number by phones and programmed into cell phones.
	Be alert for dangers of hot curling irons and other appliances.
	Have electrical cords out of reach and not hanging down.
	Have home and environment checked for lead hazards.
	Lower infant crib mattress if still in upper position.
	Install gates and guards on stairs and windows.
	Never use an infant walker.
9 months	As above.
	Crawl on the floor and look for hazards at baby's eye level.
	Pad sharp corners on tables and other furniture.
	Watch for tables, chairs, and other devices the baby may use for climbing to unsafe places.
	Do not leave heavy or hot objects on table with table cloths that the infant can pull.
	Use barriers for wood stoves and other heating devices.
	Do not allow siblings or other children to have the responsibility to watch the infant.
12 months	As above.
	May change to forward-facing car safety seat if baby is at least 20 lb and 1 year; install correctly and have installation checked; place in back seat and never in front seat with a passenger airbag.
	Start teaching the child to wash hands frequently, showing how.
	Provide own personal items, such as clothing and blankets, to child care providers; wash often.
	Change batteries in home smoke alarms and check system.
	Turn handles to back of stove; use back rather than front burners; watch for hot liquids.
	Check care provider setting for safety hazards.
	Remember that responsible adults should always supervise your infant, not other children.
	Peruse home once again for hazards now that the child is more active, climbing, and walking.
	Do not allow guns in the area where the young child plays or lives; guns must be unloaded, locked securely away, with ammunition locked in a separate location.

Source: Data from Hagan, Shaw, & Duncan. (2008)

Table 6–12   Routine Immunizations Recommended during Infancy

Immunization	Age Recommended
Hepatitis B	After birth up to 2 months (#1) 1–4 months (#2) 6–18 months (#3)
Diphtheria, tetanus, acellular pertussis	2, 4, and 6 months (3 doses)
Haemophilus influenzae type b	2, 4, and 6 months (3 doses; last dose is not needed if PRP-OMP [Pedvax HIB or ComVax] are used for primary series)
Inactivated poliovirus	2, 4, and 6–18 months (3 doses)
Pneumococcal	2, 4, and 6 months (3 doses)
Influenza	Annually from 6 months of age
Rotavirus	2, 4, and 6 months (3 doses)

Is the child observant of the environment and alert?

Direct greetings or questions to the child to evaluate stranger anxiety and ability to understand simple commands or questions.

What verbal skills are observed?

Comment positively about a child's traits, and encourage parents to share thoughts about the child.

Recognize that the mental health of the parents influences the environment in which the child is growing and learning, so inquire about how the family is adjusting to the growing child, and ask about the health and development of other children.

Growth and Developmental Surveillance

Measure head circumference until approximately 2 years of age.

Measure recumbent length (until approximately 2–3 years) or standing height (once the child can stand well) and weight.

Calculate body mass index, and place all measurements on growth grids (Table 6–13, Table 6–14; see also chapter 3).

Perform physical assessment (see chapter 2). Engage child by games, and leave intrusive procedures until last. Perform needed screening tests (Table 6–15).

Table 6–13 Physical Growth and Development during Toddlerhood

Age	Physical Growth	Fine Motor Ability	Gross Motor Ability	Sensory Ability
1–2 years	Gains 8 oz (227 g) or more/month Grows 3.5–5.0 in. (9–12 cm) during this year Anterior fontanel closes	By end of second year, builds a tower of four blocks Scribbles on paper Can undress self Throws a ball	Runs Walks up and down stairs Likes push and pull toys	Visual acuity 20/50
2–3 years	Gains 1.4–2.3 kg (3–5 lb)/year Grows 5.0–6.5 cm (2–2.5 in.)/year	Draws a circle and other rudimentary forms Learns to pour Learning to dress self	Jumps Kicks ball Throws ball overhand	

Table 6–14 Physical Growth and Development during Preschool

Physical Growth	Fine Motor Ability	Gross Motor Ability	Sensory Ability
Gains 1.5–2.5 kg (3–5 lb)/year Grows 4–6 cm (1.5–2.5 in.)/year	Uses scissors Draws circle, square, cross Draws at least a six-part person Enjoys art projects such as pasting, stringing beads, using clay Learns to tie shoes at end of preschool years Buttons Brushes teeth	Throws a ball overhand Climbs well Rides tricycle	Visual acuity continues to improve Can focus on and learn letters and numbers

Ask about daily life and care, such as sleeping and eating patterns, bowel movements, dental care, skin care, play patterns and toys, social interactions, and illnesses that have occurred.

Perform developmental surveillance (Table 6–16).

Instruct parents about developmental progression, and perform anticipatory guidance for skills to be learned by the child soon.

Table 6–15 Screening during Toddler and Preschooler Health Promotion and Health Maintenance Visits

Age	Recommended Screening Tests
15 months	Vision
	Hearing
	Anemia (if not previously done)
	Tuberculosis (if at risk)
	Teeth present and condition
	Physical examination with special attention to skin, gait, bruising, and other signs of possible abuse
	Developmental milestones
	Dietary screening
	Review immunization record
18 months	As above
2–3 years	As above
	Language development
	Lead exposure risk
	Hyperlipidemia risk
3–4 years	As above
	Blood pressure
	Behavioral abnormalities
4–5 years	As above
	Dental malocclusion problems

Source: Data from Hagan, Shaw, & Duncan. (2008)

Nutrition

Analyze growth patterns.

Perform nutritional assessment and dietary recall.

Ask about weaning and introduction of foods; all major food groups should be present in the diet.

Ask specific questions about dietary intake.

Perform nutrition teaching to enhance health. Topics may include dietary needs of young children, limitation of fast-food intake, food preparation and safety, avoidance of foods that can cause choking, and importance of family meals. See Table 6–17.

Table 6–16   Developmental Milestones Observed during Health Promotion and Health Maintenance Visits of Toddlers and Preschoolers

Age	Developmental Milestones
12 months	Walking alone or with help
	Enjoys social games and interactions
	Speaks one to three words and understands simple commands
	Drinks from cup and feeds self
15 months	Walks by self, crawls or walks up stairs
	Stacks two blocks
	Points to one or more body parts
	Increasingly interactive
	Explores environment
18 months	Walks with ease
	Pushes or pulls toy
	Stacks three or more blocks
	Uses spoon to eat, spilling often
	Follows directions and uses 15–20 words
2–3 years	Goes up and down steps
	Kicks ball
	Scribbles and draws lines on paper
	Imitates words and actions of adults
3–4 years	Jumps
	Rides tricycle
	Draws precise lines on paper; attempts to imitate circle, line, and cross
	Always feeds self
	Dresses self, although sometimes clothes are backward
	Has friends and plays with others
4–5 years	Recites rhymes and songs
	States name
	Draws a rudimentary person
	Builds tower of blocks and bridges with blocks
	Throws ball overhand

Table 6–17 Nutrition Teaching for Toddler and Preschooler Health Promotion and Health Maintenance Visits

Age	Nutrition Teaching
1 year	Support mother who continues to breastfeed.
	Wean child from bottle by substituting cup.
	If beginning to use cow's milk, use whole milk.
	Limit juice to 4–6 oz. daily; offer water several times daily.
	Encourage safety measures—use high chair with strap, secure child and use caution in grocery carts, and do not allow foods to be eaten in car.
	Provide information on choking and airway obstruction removal training.
	Provide food and water safety guidelines.
	Be sure all major food groups have been introduced.
	Limit high-fat and high-sugar foods.
	Review amounts of food commonly consumed and frequency of feedings.
	Review use of fluoride if water supply is not fluoridated.
2 years	Ask if the mother is still breastfeeding and support in the decision to continue or to wean the child.
	Encourage total removal of bottle if still in use.
	Ensure that all foods common to family have been offered.
	Offer child-sized eating utensils.
	Child can change to low-fat or skim milk if family desires.
	Limit milk to two to three servings daily.
	Teach parents methods for dealing with temper tantrums over food—make food available at meal and snack times only, do not force intake, and offer a variety of foods.
	Teach that child may have days of very low intake due to slowing growth rate.
3 years	Most children are weaned from breastfeeding and are drinking 1% or 2% milk.
	Teach normal intake and decreasing number of snacks.
	Engage child in food preparation and pouring liquids from small pitcher.
	Recognize that **food jags** (periods when only one or two foods are eaten) are common.
	Recognize importance of the social nature of eating; expect child to sit for a short period at meals with family.
	Meals and snacks should not be eaten while watching television.
4 years	Encourage involving child in snack selection and preparation.
	Start to teach food groups and importance of nutrition for the body.
	Alter intake as appropriate depending on weight and body mass index.
	Dairy products consumed should all be low or reduced fat.

Physical Activity

Evaluate type and amount of physical activity.

Assess motor development and coordination.

Suggestions for the family may include setting guidelines to limit television and other screen activities to a maximum of 2 hours daily to facilitate adequate physical activity time; children should not have a television and computer in their bedrooms. See Table 6–18 for risk and protective factors regarding physical activity.

Table 6–18   Risk and Protective Factors Regarding Physical Activity in Toddlerhood and Preschool

Risk Factors	Protective Factors
Developmental delay Slow development of social skills	Expected developmental progression
Limited stimulation by family or other care providers Limited social time with other children Long work hours by parents	Easily engaged socially with others Daily contact with other young children
Reluctance to try new physical activity Limited access to balls, slides, balance beams, tricycles, and other materials that foster physical activity Adequate safety gear for activities is not available	Eagerness to try new physical activity Access to balls, slides, balance beams, tricycles, and other materials that foster physical activity Adequate safety gear that properly fits child is available
Parents who have little physical activity on a daily basis Lack of knowledge by family about child physical activity needs	Family members engage in daily physical activity Family members spend time daily in physical activity with child 2 hours daily Family understands motor developmental milestones and importance of physical activity in childhood
Television or other screen activities are engaged in for more than 2 hours daily	Television and other screen activities are limited to no more than 2 hours daily
Limited community resources for childcare and physical activity Unsafe neighborhood and lack of lawns, parks, and other facilities	Neighborhood contains access to childcare which integrates physical activity Neighborhood is safe, and contains lawns, parks, and other facilities

Oral Health

Evaluate teeth for condition and number. By approximately 2 years of age, the toddler has a full set of 20 teeth. The first primary tooth is lost at approximately 6 years of age.

Inquire about dental visits. By 1 year of age, the child should have made a first visit to the dentist with continuing visits every 6 months.

Observe for caries or poor dental health. **Early childhood caries** is defined as one or more decayed, missing, or filled tooth surfaces in a child younger than 5 years of age (National Maternal and Child Oral Health Resource Center, 2004). Refer the child with early childhood caries for dental care. Assist the family without dental insurance to locate dental programs for young children.

What is the source of your drinking water? Do you know if it is fluoridated? If not, does your child take fluoride? How much? How often?

Describe how your child's teeth get brushed and how often? Do you use toothpaste? What type? How much? Is it hard for you to afford toothbrushes?

How much juice or sweetened drinks does your child have each day? Is a bottle or cup used for drinking? How many sweet foods, such as candy, gum, cookies, cake, and doughnuts, are eaten daily?

Teach the child and family dental care techniques, and provide access to toothpaste, a toothbrush, and referrals for care as needed.

Provide teaching as needed about fluoride, healthy food intake, and weaning from bottle.

Mental and Spiritual Health

Do parents communicate readily with the child?

Are interactions generally warm, caring, and loving, or are there constant criticisms of behavior? (See Table 6–19, Table 6–20.)

Does the parent seem willing to point out the child's accomplishments, or have trouble making any positive statements about the child?

Does the child appear at ease with the parent? Is the child at ease in the healthcare setting? (Toddlers often still have some stranger anxiety and may show discomfort, while preschoolers are more often eager and excited to meet you.)

The child's sense of self and mental status are related to new accomplishments. Inquire about toilet training, tooth brushing, choosing

Table 6–19   Psychosocial Development during Toddlerhood (Age 1–3 Years)

Play and Toys	Communication
Refines fine motor skills by use of cloth books, large pencil and paper, wooden puzzles	Increasingly enjoys talking
	Exponential growth of vocabulary, especially when spoken and read to
Facilitates imitative behavior by playing kitchen, grocery shopping, toy telephone	Needs to release stress by use of pounding board toy, frequent gross motor activities, and occasional temper tantrums
Learns gross motor activities by riding Big Wheel tricycle, playing with soft ball and bat, molding water and sand, tossing ball or bean bag	Likes contact with other children and learns interpersonal skills
Cognitive skills develop by educational television shows, music, stories, and books	

Table 6–20   Psychosocial Development during Preschool (Age 3–6 Years)

Play and Toys	Communication
Associative play is facilitated by simple games, puzzles, nursery rhymes, songs	All parts of speech are developed and used, occasionally incorrectly
	Communicates with a widening array of people
Dramatic play is fostered by dolls and doll clothes, play houses and hospitals, dress-up clothes, puppets	Play with other children is a favorite activity
Stress is relieved by pens, paper, glue, scissors	Health professionals can: • Verbalize and explain procedures to children
Cognitive growth is fostered by educational television shows, music, stories, and books	• Use drawings and stories to explain care • Use accurate names for bodily functions • Allow the child to talk, ask questions, and make choices

clothes and getting dressed, using crayons, or other developmental tasks.

Ask about how the parent deals with the child who is having a temper tantrum or showing other undesirable behaviors. Reinforce positive ways of helping the child set limits for self and make suggestions when parents need assistance.

Ask about sleep patterns. Most toddlers have established regular sleeping patterns with occasional night awakenings. They sleep approximately

10–12 hours at night with one or two daytime naps. The preschooler sleeps approximately 9 to 11 hours and may have one or no naps each day (Murray, Zentner, & Yakimo, 2009).

Relationships

Families with members who handle stress well and have healthy lifestyle patterns offer security for the young child.

Ask how things are going for the family in general. Inquire about siblings and whether there are any issues of concern that might influence the toddler or preschooler.

Ask about discipline techniques and whether there has been violence in the family or neighborhood.

Identify strengths in the family:
- Family time together each day
- Parents proud of child's accomplishments and knowledgeable about developmental progression
- Childcare center personnel and family members interact regularly to plan consistent approaches for the toddler and preschooler
- Teen mother of toddler enrolled in high school continuation program with childcare component

Identify risks to health:
- Mother has been diagnosed with depression
- Uncle in home uses street drugs
- Child awakens with night terrors
- Child was recently in a serious car accident
- Teen mother is estranged from own family and has few goals and resources

Observe play patterns:
- Toddlers often engage in parallel play, or side-by-side play.
- Preschoolers begin associating with other children in play and engage in dramatic play.

Assess language and communication ability, temperament, and social interactions with others.

Suggest activities that can assist in the child's development of social skills:
- Talk with and read to the child daily.
- Ensure interactions with other children and adults.
- Consider a preschool as opportunity to socialize and learn interactional skills.

- Understand the child's temperament, and structure the environment to maximize learning within the child's characteristics.

Injury and Disease Prevention

Car seats for toddlers and preschoolers:

- Car safety needs reinforcing as the types of seats change when the child reaches 20 and then 40 lb. Be certain that children from 20 to 40 lb:
  - Use a convertible forward-facing seat that has been placed in the backseat
  - Have harness straps at or above the shoulders
- Toddlers and preschoolers over 40 lb should be placed in a belt-positioning booster seat:
  - In the backseat
  - That uses both lap and shoulder belts
  - With the lap belt low and tight across the lap/upper thigh area and shoulder belt snug across the chest and shoulder
- Recommend that parents have their car seat checked by a childcare inspector. Give them the addresses of the closest inspection stations, which you can locate by going through the National Highway Traffic Safety Administration (http://www.nhtsa.dot.gov).

Assess safety hazards, and perform safety teaching (Table 6–21).

Administer needed immunizations (Table 6–22).

Ask about occurrence of acute diseases, and reinforce with teaching as needed.

Evaluate any chronic conditions, refer to resources as needed, and adjust health promotion visit to meet the child's needs.

SCHOOL-AGE CHILD HEALTH PROMOTION AND HEALTH MAINTENANCE

General Observations

The child should walk showing symmetry and ease of movement, follow instructions about where to go and taking off shoes for weighing, and demonstrate clear language skills with parent or healthcare personnel.

Observe whether the child brought a book, toy, or some other object to the visit.

How are the parents interacting with the child? What types of speech tones are used?

Table 6–21 Disease and Injury Prevention Topics for Toddlers and Preschoolers by Age

Age	Injury Prevention Teaching Topics
15 months	Wash adult and toddler hands frequently.
	Clean toys with soap and water regularly.
	Provide child's own bedding for childcare setting, and wash weekly.
	Use forward-facing car safety seat if child is 20 lb; install correctly and have installation checked; place in back seat and never in front seat with a passenger airbag.
	Empty containers of water immediately after use; be sure pools or other bodies of water are locked and not accessible.
	Use sunscreen, hat, and long sleeves in the sun.
	Keep heavy and sharp objects out of reach; check that all poisons are locked away, including in homes visited; keep pet food and cosmetics out of reach.
	Have poison control number by phones and programmed into cell phones.
	Be alert for dangers of hot curling irons and other appliances.
	Have electrical cords out of reach and not hanging down.
	Keep water temperature from 120 to 125°F.
	Have home environment checked for lead hazards.
	Secure the child in shopping carts.
	Do not let child have access to alcoholic drinks.
	Remember that responsible adults should always supervise your child, not other children.
	Know cardiopulmonary resuscitation (CPR), airway obstruction removal, and other first aid.
18 months	As above.
	Bolt heavy objects (such as bookcases and televisions) that might be pulled down securely to the wall.
	Be cautious of the toddler near machinery in the yard, such as lawn mowers and farm equipment.
	Use a helmet on the child when taking on the back of a bicycle.
	Check batteries in home smoke alarms, CO or radon monitors, and check systems monthly; change batteries on a scheduled basis as recommended by manufacturer.
	Ask care providers about discipline methods; do not allow corporal punishment.
2–3 years	As above.
	When the child is 40 lb, switch to a belt-positioning booster seat, using vehicle lap and shoulder belt; place in rear seat.
	Teach hand washing after toileting and other activities.
	Clean potty chair thoroughly.

Table 6–21   Disease and Injury Prevention Topics for Toddlers and Preschoolers by Age (Continued)

Age	Injury Prevention Teaching Topics
	Keep guns unloaded and locked away in a different locked place than ammunition; have trigger locks installed.
	Teach how to cross streets.
	Provide a helmet for riding tricycles.
	Check playgrounds for safety hazards and ensure cushioned surfaces under equipment.
3–4 years	As above.
	Do not let child play unsupervised.
	Know CPR, airway obstruction removal, and other first aid for the child who has become a preschooler.
4–5 years	As above.
	Continue teaching safety skills to the child.
	Continue supervising when near streets and water sources.
	Teach safety around strangers (never go with a stranger; find a trusted person like parent or police).

Source: Data from Hagan, Shaw, & Duncan. (2008)

Is there mutual respect, or are parents and the child ignoring each other or having disagreements?

Does the child communicate readily and at age level?

Is the child appropriately dressed? Adequately nourished? Well rested and alert?

Ask the child to describe a typical day to obtain clues about daily life.

Growth and Developmental Surveillance

Measure height and weight, calculate body mass index, and evaluate percentiles on growth grids (Table 6–23).

Perform physical assessment (see chapter 2). Explain what you are doing and why: "I'm listening to your heart with this stethoscope and counting how many times it beats in a minute. Have you heard your heart? When have you noticed it beating hard?"

Table 6–22 Routine Immunizations Recommended during Toddlerhood and Preschool Age

Immunization	Age Recommended
Hepatitis B	6–18 months (administer No. 3 if series not completed during infancy)
Hepatitis A	Series of two doses with first at 12 months and second at least 6 months later
Diphtheria, tetanus, acellular pertussis	15–18 months (No. 4) 4–6 yrs (No. 5)
Haemophilus influenzae type b	12–15 months (No. 4 or will be No. 3 for PRP-OMP type that requires only three doses for whole series)
Inactivated poliovirus	4–6 years (No. 4)
Measles, mumps, rubella	12–15 months (No. 1)
Varicella	12–18 months (#1) 4–6 years (#2)
Pneumococcal	12–15 months (No. 4)
Influenza	Annually from 6–23 months

PRP-OMP, polyribosylribitol phosphate–outer membrane protein.
Note: Schedule may need to be adapted if child did not receive all recommended immunizations during infancy. See Centers for Disease Control and Prevention and American Academy of Pediatrics for recommended catch-up schedules (http://www.cdc.gov and http://www.aap.org).

Table 6–23 Physical Growth and Development during School Age

Physical Growth	Fine Motor Ability	Gross Motor Ability	Sensory Ability
Gains 1.4–2.2 kg (3–5 lb)/year	Enjoys craft projects	Rides two-wheeler	Can read
Grows 4–6 cm (1.5–2.5 in.)/year	Plays card and board games	Jumps rope	Able to concentrate for longer periods on activities by filtering out surrounding sound
		Roller skates or ice skates	

Concentrate on skills that influence performance in school. Vision, hearing, muscular strength, and coordination are examples of areas that impact school performance.

Inquire about injuries, illnesses, and health practices.

Perform recommended screening tests (Table 6–24).

Table 6–24 **Screening during School-Age Health Promotion and Health Maintenance Visits**

Age	Recommended Screening Tests	
5 years	Vision	Hyperlipidemia risk
	Hearing	Blood pressure
	Lead exposure risk	Urinalysis
	Anemia	Tuberculosis (if at risk)
6–8 years	Vision	Hyperlipidemia risk
	Hearing	Blood pressure
	Lead exposure risk	Tuberculosis (if at risk)
8–10 years	Vision	Blood pressure
	Hearing	Tuberculosis (if at risk)
	Hyperlipidemia risk	
10–12 years	Vision	Blood pressure
	Hearing	Tuberculosis (if at risk)
	Hyperlipidemia risk	

Source: Data from Hagan, Shaw, & Duncan. (2008)

Direct observations, history questions, and questionnaires that parents complete are methods for developmental surveillance. See Table 6–25 for expected developmental milestones during school age.

Perform teaching to enhance sleep patterns, knowledge of normal growth and development patterns, and use of community resources.

Nutrition

Recognize that children are increasingly independent in food choices. They may come home alone and prepare snacks. Vending machines are often available at schools.

Evaluate nutritional patterns because habits are being formed that will impact nutrition and health in general in the years to come. Good choices help to promote health—to maintain weight at a recommended level, provide nutrients for adequate growth and activity, and prevent onset of some chronic diseases. On the other hand, poor choices can lead to being overweight and its accompanying problems—lack of adequate calcium and resultant osteoporosis, eating disorders, or lack of energy for brain growth and optimal performance in school.

Table 6–25 Developmental Milestones Observed during Health Promotion and Health Maintenance Visits of School-Age Children

Age	Developmental Milestones
5 years	Independent in bathroom and dressing activities
	Ties shoes, buttons
	Runs well, jumps, may skip, balances on one foot for 10 seconds
	Pours fluids well, uses hands to catch ball
	Prints some letters, first name
	Draws triangle, square, three- to five-part person
	Knows full name, address, phone
6–8 years	Skilled in physical activities, such as running, skipping, jumping, hopping
	Learns to ride bicycle
	Can cut, paste, write all letters
	Reads
8–10 years	Has increasingly longer periods of concentration for both physical activity and school or other quiet activity
	Can throw objects far and with accurate aim
	Increased coordination
	Develops hobbies, such as model building, musical instrument, video production, building with wood, needle work
10–12 years	Fine and gross motor skills similar to adult in ability
	Writes well, adept at computer use
	Some clumsiness may develop as prepubertal growth spurt begins

Integrate some questions for the parent and child into the visit that provide clues about diet.

Plan nursing interventions to enhance knowledge about foods, family participation in good nutritional practices, and access to healthy foods.

Physical Activity

Observe developmental milestones and coordination.

Ask about participation in school and community sports and other types of physical activity.

Evaluate risk and protective factors for physical activity; plan interventions that enhance protective factors and alleviate risks (Table 6–26).

Table 6–26 Risk and Protective Factors Regarding Physical Activity in School-Age Children

Risk Factors	Protective Factors
Limited role modeling of daily physical activity by parents and other family members	Expected developmental skill level
	Feels self-confident in ability and physical appearance
Limited facilities in the neighborhood to encourage activity, such as parks, skate board facilities, rinks, and ball courts	Willing to try new activities
	Sets goals for learning physical skills
Inadequate financial resources to join clubs or pay for organized sports	Parents exercise daily and exercise with the child some of this time in setting the child can see
School cuts to physical education programs and recess	Parents set expectation that everyone in family will choose a physical activity and engage in it regularly
School tryouts for sports that eliminate all but the best players in certain sports	Schools provide physical education each day with a variety of offerings; student gets to choose and set goals for some activities
Reluctance to try new activity	Schools schedule recess or physical activity breaks twice daily
Worry about competence and physical appearance	Sports teams are leveled so that all students desiring to play a particular sport, such as soccer, are able to do so
Television viewing or other screen activities for >2 hours daily	Adequate safety gear that properly fits child is available
Developmental delay and special needs	Neighborhood provides access to parks, skateboard facilities, rinks, ball courts, and other facilities
	Family has adequate financial resources to pay for health club or organized sports
	Television viewing and other screen activities limited to ≤ 2 hours daily

Source: Data from Patrik, Spear, & Holt. (2001)

Perform teaching to enhance health:
- Encourage participation of parents and siblings in physical activity to serve as role models.
- Help the child to identify interests for activity, and refer to community resources as needed.
- Encourage parent participation in schools to urge for daily physical education for all children.
- Assist in planning and adapting activities for the child who has a physical disability.

Oral Health

Evaluate number and condition of primary and secondary teeth.

Evaluate oral care and access to dental professionals.

Assess intake of snacks with sugar/carbohydrates.

Reinforce teaching for dental hygiene—brushing, flossing, and care of braces.

Refer to dental professionals if needed.

Mental and Spiritual Health

Assess the child's self-concept and all of its facets by observing the child and asking questions that provide clues to the child's view of self. Ask about school activities, sports, interests, and what the family does together. Observe for prepubertal physical growth and development. Ask about exposure to screen (television, game) activities and violence in the neighborhood, family, or school. Ask the child whether bullying occurs at school.

Be observant for and ask parents about any concerns that might signal mental illness—high levels of stress, unusual reactions to events, mood swings, anxiety, depression, eating disorder.

Perform teaching as needed:

- Expected body changes
- Need for friends and meaningful activities
- Continuing need for adequate rest and sleep (8–12 hours daily)
  - Teach sleep hygiene, those behaviors that foster a regular and sufficient sleep pattern and daytime alertness (Edelman & Mandle, 2006).

Relationships

The family remains an important anchor while peers become increasingly important to self-identity (Table 6–27).

Ask about family members and peers with whom the child interacts regularly.

Ask children about how they handle disagreements.

Consider the child's temperament, and work with the family to adapt the environment to best support individual characteristics (i.e., a quiet study place for a child who has difficulty studying, several activities for the child who thrives on socializing with others).

Table 6–27   Psychosocial Development during School Age (Age 6–12 Years)

Activities	Communication
Gross motor development is fostered by ball sports, skating, dance lessons, water and snow skiing/boarding, biking	Mature use of language
	Ability to converse and discuss topics for increasing lengths of time
A sense of industry is fostered by playing a musical instrument, gathering collections, starting hobbies, playing board and video games	Spends many hours at school and with friends in sports or other activities
	Health professionals can:
	• Assess child's knowledge before teaching
Cognitive growth is facilitated by reading, crafts, word puzzles, school work	• Allow the child to select rewards following procedures
	• Teach techniques such as counting or visualization to manage difficult situations
	• Include both parent and child in healthcare decisions

Suggest activities to enhance relationships:

- Encourage regular family activities.
- Ensure parents know families of friends and where the child is spending time.
- Foster the parent's active involvement in the child's school.

Injury and Disease Prevention

Evaluate correct use of car safety system for age and size.

Ask about injuries that have occurred, and adapt teaching to address prevention.

Examine safety risks and perform safety teaching (Table 6–28).

Be sure the child uses helmet and other safety gear for sports.

Evaluate for signs of disease or problems, such as frequent illness, bruising, fatigue, pain, vision or hearing problems, headaches, lack of coordination, or changes in school or other performance.

Immunizations are generally up to date for school-age children. However, some children may have missed earlier doses due to illness or missed healthcare visits. Evaluate the immunization record to be sure it meets all recommendations. Some of the most common immunization needs at this time are:

- Hepatitis B (whole series or a missed third shot)

Table 6–28 Injury Prevention Topics for School-Age Children

Age	Injury Prevention Teaching
5–8 years	Use a booster seat, properly positioned in the back seat of the car; use lap and shoulder belts.
	Never place the child in a front car seat with a passenger airbag.
	Be sure the child knows how to swim and works on these skills regularly.
	Protect the child with sunscreen when outside.
	Check smoke alarms, and keep them in proper function.
	Have an escape plan in case of fire in the home.
	Keep poisons, electrical appliances, and fire starters locked.
	Keep firearms unloaded and locked; store ammunition in separate locked location; have trigger locks installed on guns; keep dangerous knives locked.
	Provide protective gear for bicycling and other activities, and insist that it be worn.
	Teach safety precautions for bicycling and other activities.
	Teach safety with strangers.
	Provide list of people a child can approach if feeling threatened by touch or other experience.
	Choose care providers carefully; occasionally pick up child earlier than expected; ask policies about discipline and do not leave child with someone who uses corporal punishment.
	Be sure the child knows emergency numbers, names, and plans.
	Review carefully any hazardous event that has occurred with the child, and summarize what was done correctly and how response could be improved.
	Limit screen time to 2 hours daily; do not allow violent games or viewing.
	Review behavior with strangers regularly, such as not getting in cars and not engaging in phone or Internet conversations.
8–10 years	Continue to reinforce other teaching described above, including the child in teaching fully, and enlarging responsibility to the child with increasing age.
	Car booster seat used until child sits upright against back seat with bent knees over edge of seat; insist on use of lap and shoulder belts.
	Do not place child in front seat of car with a passenger airbag.
	Do not allow child to operate power tools or machinery.

Table 6–28   Injury Prevention Topics
for School-Age Children (Continued)

Age	Injury Prevention Teaching
10–12 years	Continue to reinforce teaching described above.
	Parents and child should attend class on cardiopulmonary resuscitation and airway obstruction removal.
	Avoid high noise levels, such as when listening to music through earphones.

Source: Data from Hagan, Shaw, & Duncan. (2008)

- Hepatitis A (two doses if not previously administered)
  - Tetanus and diphtheria and acellular pertussis (Tdap) at the 11- to 12-year visit
- Polio and measles-mumps-rubella (if booster doses of each were not given before school entry)
- Varicella, if not given earlier and the child has not had the disease
- Certain vaccines for children at high risk, such as pneumococcal, influenza, meningococcal

Evaluate the general health and condition of children with chronic healthcare needs.

Intervene to perform necessary screening for disease, and teach to promote health.

Adolescent Health Promotion and Health Maintenance
General Observations

As you call the adolescent back for care, observe whether parents or friends are present, or if the teen is alone. Watch to see if a parent or friend is present and if that person comes with the teen when called. If someone comes with the teen, be alert that you may need to provide some private time by asking the other person to wait outside for a moment. Reassure the parents that you will talk with them about any of their concerns and questions. Provide them with an opportunity to ask questions and get information also.

Be alert, quiet, and sensitive in working with adolescents. Initial observations guide the interaction with the teen. Someone who appears nervous needs a confident, reassuring approach. Provide privacy for issues that may be sensitive, such as weighing the overweight teen or providing information on birth control.

Observe clothing, hygiene, nutritional status, appearance of being rested or fatigued, and social skills.

Growth and Developmental Surveillance

Measure height and weight, calculate body mass index, and evaluate percentiles on growth grids (Table 6–29).

Perform physical assessment (see chapter 2). Some particular parts of the examination to include for teens are scoliosis screening; sexual maturity rating (Tanner stages); breast examination; testicular examination; testing for sexually transmitted diseases (among those sexually active); pelvic examination and pap smear (for sexually active females); hematocrit for anemia annually in menstruating adolescents; hearing screening at 12, 15, and 18 years; blood pressure annually; lipid screening for those with family history of early heart disease or other risk factors; and tuberculosis screening for those in high-risk areas.

See Table 6–30 for a summary of health assessments.

Sexually active teens should be screened annually for:

- Chlamydia
- Gonorrhea
- Trichomoniasis
- Human papilloma virus
- Herpes simplex virus
- Bacterial vaginosis

Table 6–29 Physical Growth and Development during Adolescence

Physical Growth	Fine Motor Ability	Gross Motor Ability	Sensory Ability
Variation in age of growth spurt During growth spurt, girls gain 7–25 kg (15–55 lb) and grow 2.5–20.0 cm (2–8 in.); boys gain approximately 7.0–29.5 kg (15–65 lb) and grow 11–30 cm (4.5–12.0 in.)	Skills are well developed	New sports activities attempted and muscle development continues Some lack of coordination common during growth spurt	Fully developed

Table 6–30   Screening during Health Promotion and Health Maintenance Visits of Adolescents

Age	Recommended Mental Health/Behavioral Screening	Recommended Physical Health Screening Tests
11–14 years	Use of tobacco and alcohol	Vision
	History of abuse	Hearing
	Unsatisfactory school performance	Anemia
	History of depression or other mental health problems	Lipids
		Blood pressure
	History of violence or risk taking	Urinalysis
	History of multiple personal or family stresses	Tuberculosis (if at risk)
	Loneliness or lack of friends	Pap smear (for sexually active females)
		Breast examination
		Sexually transmitted disease risks
15–17 years	As above	As above
18–21 years	As above	As above
	Difficulty with job	Offer pelvic examination for all females even if not sexually active

Source: Data from Hagan, Shaw, & Duncan. (2008)

Source: Data from Hagan, Shaw, & Duncan. (2008)

Individuals should be screened for syphilis if requesting testing or meeting any of these criteria:

- History of sexually transmitted infections
- More than one sexual partner in past 6 months
- Intravenous drug use
- Sexual intercourse with a partner at risk
- Sex in exchange for drugs or money
- Homelessness
- Males—sex with other males
- Syphilis—residence in areas where disease is prevalent
- Human immunodeficiency virus/acquired immunodeficiency syndrome—blood or blood product transfusion before 1985.

All individuals from 13 to 64 years should be offered a voluntary HIV test at each healthcare encounter. Those at high risk of infection

Section II: Nursing Care in the Community/Hospital

(under 20 years and sexually active, over 20 years with inconsistent use of barrier protection and a new or more than one sex partner in last 3 months) should be retested annually (Branson, 2006).

Integrate questions pertinent to the adolescent years and teaching throughout the health promotion/health maintenance visit.

Nutrition

Although nutrition is important, a fast lifestyle and focus on eating with peers can provide dietary challenges; high-caloric and high-fat intake and inadequate calcium, iron, and zinc are frequent.

Perform nutritional assessments and identify teaching needs.

Plan interventions that involve teaching:
- Getting five fruits and vegetables daily
- Including whole-grain products to replace refined products whenever possible
- The importance of eating three meals each day, including breakfast and lunch
- Eating together as a family several times weekly, which enhances quality food intake
- How to plan menus and prepare foods for balanced intake
- Limiting refined sugar and high-fat intake (e.g., soft drinks and fried foods) to maintain weight at recommended level
- Including two to three servings of dairy products daily to enhance bone formation and decrease chance of osteoporosis as an adult
- Using resources for treatment of eating disorders if they are identified

Physical Activity

Physical activity decreases as youth progress through the adolescent years.

Inquire about frequency and length of moderate and vigorous exercise, including school- and community-based sports, as well as other activities.

Ask whether the school requires daily physical activity.

Identify risk and protective factors for physical activity (Table 6–31).

Teach importance of 30–60 minutes of moderate to vigorous physical activity daily for mental and physical health.

Assist the teen to identify meaningful activity that can be performed regularly.

Table 6–31 Risk and Protective Factors Regarding Physical Activity in Adolescence

Risk Factors	Protective Factors
Lives in isolated setting with little opportunity for contact with other teens	Has opportunities for participation in physical activity at home, at school, and in the community
Has a developmental disability that impairs physical movement	Likes physical activity
Does not like physical activity	Has exercised during all of childhood, often with parents
Has a pattern and history of low activity levels	Knowledgeable about benefits of activity; committed to maintaining exercise patterns
Is overweight	
Does not feel competent in most sports	
Limited financial resources to pay registration fees or buy protective gear for sports	Has many friends living close who participate in physical activity
Family members who have little physical activity	Youth and parents agree to a limit of 2 hours daily of screen time
Parents who are not active in school sports and committees	Availability of financial and other resources for sports gear and protective equipment
Parents who do not like physical activity and have had low levels while their teen was growing up	Parents participate in regular physical activity and encourage the adolescent to do so also
Parents who have little time or facilities for exercise or always exercise at a club out of view of their family	Neighborhood and community provide physical activity options
Lack of youth and parent knowledge about physical activity needs and benefits	Public policies maintain parks, green spaces, biking trails, and playgrounds
Lack of neighborhood programs for physical activity promotion	Programs are available for adolescents with developmental disabilities or other healthcare needs
Presence of neighborhood hazards and unsafe areas	

Source: Data from Hagan, Shaw, & Duncan. (2008)

Oral Health

Ask about oral hygiene practices.

Examine number and condition of teeth.

Reinforce need for daily brushing and flossing and dental appointments every 6 months.

Fluoride supplements may be discontinued by approximately 14 years.

Refer for dental care if resources are needed.

Mental and Spiritual Health

Self-concept, self-esteem, and self-regulation remain key to mental health formation (Table 6–32).

Ask about meaningful activities and about disappointments and how they were handled.

Evaluate body image and sexuality.

Ask about discipline and interactions with parents.

Encourage parents to:

- Gradually increase the teen's independence. If there is success with growing responsibility, the teen may be ready for more. If the teen misuses independence (perhaps by staying out too late, having a party at home without parents present, lying about location on an evening out), there should be clear limits and loss of privilege.
- Be willing to talk with and hear the teen's story. On the other hand, do not be talked out of consequences for the teen's bad decisions.
- Recognize that driving a car, staying out late, and other activities are not a given. They are privileges for responsibility displayed.
- Comment on a teen's behavior rather than making belittling comments about them as a person.
- Realize that the teen is establishing independence and that the relationship will change. Be consistent and loving as your adolescent tries out and learns about limits and the self.

Evaluate for signs of depression, substance abuse, or other mental health problems. See Table 6–33 for common signs. Refer teen for treatment when needed.

Table 6–32 Psychosocial Development during Adolescence (Age 12–18 Years)

Activities	Communication
Sports—ball games, gymnastics, water and snow skiing/boarding, swimming, school sports	Increasing communication and time with peer group—movies, dances, driving, eating out, attending sports events
School activities—drama, yearbook, class office, club participation	
Quiet activities—reading, school work, television, computer, video games, music	Applying abstract thought and analysis in conversations at home and school

Table 6–33 Signs of Depression and Substance Abuse in Adolescents

Depression	Substance Abuse
Changes in behavior, school performance, sleep, and appetite	Changes in behavior, school performance, sleep, and appetite
Physical complaints	Accidents and other unexplained events
Loss of interest in usual activities	Lack of responsibility
Difficulty in motivating self and setting goals	Labile mood and attitude
	Hopelessness
Change in friends	Depression
Feelings of worthlessness	Feelings of ambivalence
Consideration of death or suicide	A variety of physical changes depending on the substance

Source: Data from Jellinek, Patel, & Froehle. (2007)

Many teens do not get the recommended hours of sleep. Make the following recommendations:

- Try to keep to similar hours for sleeping so your body is accustomed to them.
- Avoid caffeine in the late afternoon and evening.
- Do homework early, and relax a bit before going to bed.
- Plan 1 day each weekend to simply relax and have few demands on your time.

Ask about meaning in life, and refer to spiritual resources as needed.

Relationships

Parents are sources of guidance and reassurance, while increasingly close ties emerge with friends.

Assess type and quality of relationships with friends.

Ask about family relationships.

Be alert for signs of domestic abuse.

Some helpful tips for adolescents include:

- Most teens get frustrated with their parents at times; list some things you like and some you don't like about your family.
- Be sure to focus complaints on specific issues, such as wanting a later curfew, rather than telling your parents they don't know anything.

- Most parents, like kids, want to know what they do right; tell your parents occasionally things that are going well or that you appreciate.
- Talk to your parents; if you don't feel you can, find another adult you respect, such as an older sibling, a teacher, counselor, or clergy.

Injury and Disease Prevention

Injury is the greatest health hazard for adolescents, so injury prevention must be integrated into every health contact with youth.

The major hazard is automobile crashes. Inquire about seat belt use and driving practices.

Motorcycles, four-wheelers, boats, jet skis, farm machinery, and tools are other sources of injury. Ask about the youth's exposure, and teach about avoiding alcohol and drug use, use of safety gear, and precautions to be employed.

Review the teen's activities and injury hazards, such as falls, burns, accidental shooting, extreme sports, and date violence.

Teach about hazards and protective measures.

Teens are generally healthy and may be seen only rarely in healthcare settings. Some common problems include:
- Acne and skin infections
- Body piercing and tattooing
- Sports overuse injuries
- Constipation and diarrhea
- Dental problems

Other observations may signal more serious health concerns and need to be referred for further evaluation. Some examples include:
- Scoliosis
- Anemia
- Excessive tiredness
- Bruising
- Sexually transmitted diseases
- Eating disorder
- Abuse or severe bullying

Perform teaching about disease prevention measures, such as weight control, avoidance of smoking, and use of sunscreen (Table 6–34).

Table 6–34   Injury Prevention Topics for Adolescents

Topic	Teaching
Driving	Always wear seat and shoulder belt.
	Do not drink and drive or ride with others who do.
	Do not talk on a cell phone as you drive.
	Do not drive when you are tired.
	Drive with parents or other adults for several months in winter driving conditions if you live where there is snow, ice, or heavy rains.
	Keep your car in good repair.
Sun	Wear sunscreen.
	Limit time outside, especially early in summer.
Machinery	Learn how to use power tools correctly.
	Always have someone near when you use tools or machinery.
Emergency care	Learn first aid, cardiopulmonary resuscitation, and airway obstruction removal.
Water safety	Learn to swim well.
	If you supervise younger children near water, never leave them alone, even for a minute.
Fires	Do not play with fire.
	Follow guidelines to avoid igniting gasoline.
	Test smoke alarms in your house every 6 months, and change batteries annually.
Firearms	Know and follow rules to keep firearms locked with ammunition locked in a separate place.
	Never take out a gun to show a friend unless your parent is also present.
	Take firearm safety classes if you hunt or target shoot.
Hearing	Avoid loud music, especially for long periods and through ear phones.
Sports	Wear protective gear recommended for your sport.
Abuse	Report any abuse to an adult you trust.
	Date with other couples whenever possible, and report date rape.
	Do not drink or take drugs.

Source: Data from Hagan, Shaw, & Duncan. (2008)

Many adolescents have not had immunizations since approximately school-entry time, so their record should be carefully reviewed. Some questions to ask to determine immunizations needed by adolescents include:

- When was the last tetanus-diphtheria (TD) booster? It is recommended every 10 years if no wounds have required an update in the interim. So, if the child received it at age 5 years, a booster is needed at 15 years. A Tdap (tetanus-diphtheria and acellular pertussis) booster is given at the preferred age of 11 to 12 years. If a dose of TD was given during adolescence, wait for at least 5 years, and administer one dose of Tdap.
- Was a second measles-mumps-rubella administered? A second dose may not have been routine when teens were younger, so they may need it now.
- Has hepatitis A been administered?
- Has the youth had hepatitis B vaccine? This is important for all youth, and some may not have received it as infants.
- Did the youth have a clear history of varicella disease? If not, the vaccine is needed.
- Human papilloma virus vaccine (3-dose series) is recommended for females from 11 to 12 years, or for those 13 to 26 years not previously immunized.
- Annual influenza vaccine is recommended.

7 IMMUNIZATION SCHEDULES

RECOMMENDED IMMUNIZATION SCHEDULES FOR CHILDREN AND ADOLESCENTS

In Figures 7–1, 7–2, and 7–3, vaccines are listed under the routinely recommended ages. Bars indicate range of acceptable ages for vaccination.

Recommended Immunization Schedule for Persons Aged 0 Through 6 Years—United States • 2009

For those who fall behind or start late, see the catch-up schedule

Vaccine ▼ Age ►	Birth	1 month	2 months	4 months	6 months	12 months	15 months	18 months	19–23 months	2–3 years	4–6 years
Hepatitis B[1]	HepB	HepB				HepB					
Rotavirus[2]			RV	RV	RV						
Diphtheria, Tetanus, Pertussis[3]			DTaP	DTaP	DTaP		DTaP				DTaP
Haemophilus influenzae type b[4]			Hib	Hib	Hib	Hib					
Pneumococcal[5]			PCV	PCV	PCV	PCV				PPSV	
Inactivated Poliovirus			IPV	IPV		IPV					IPV
Influenza[6]						Influenza (Yearly)					
Measles, Mumps, Rubella[7]						MMR		see footnote 7			MMR
Varicella[8]						Varicella		see footnote 8			Varicella
Hepatitis A[9]						HepA (2 doses)				HepA Series	
Meningococcal[10]											MCV

Range of recommended ages

Certain high-risk groups

This schedule indicates the recommended ages for routine administration of currently licensed vaccines, as of December 1, 2008, for children aged 0 through 6 years. Any dose not administered at the recommended age should be administered at a subsequent visit, when indicated and feasible. Licensed combination vaccines may be used whenever any component of the combination is indicated and other components are not contraindicated and if approved by the Food and Drug Administration for that dose of the series. Providers should consult the relevant Advisory Committee on Immunization Practices statement for detailed recommendations, including high-risk conditions: http://www.cdc.gov/vaccines/pubs/acip-list.htm. Clinically significant adverse events that follow immunization should be reported to the Vaccine Adverse Event Reporting System (VAERS). Guidance about how to obtain and complete a VAERS form is available at http://www.vaers.hhs.gov or by telephone, 800-822-7967.

Figure 7–1 ■ Recommended immunization schedule for children 0 to 6 years, United States, 2009.
Source: Centers for Disease Control and Prevention. (2009)

Footnotes

Recommended Immunization Schedule for Persons Aged 0 Through 6 Years—United States • 2009

1. Hepatitis B vaccine (HepB). *(Minimum age: birth)*
At birth:
- Administer monovalent HepB to all newborns before hospital discharge.
- If mother is hepatitis B surface antigen (HBsAg)-positive, administer HepB and 0.5 mL of hepatitis B immune globulin (HBIG) within 12 hours of birth.
- If mother's HBsAg status is unknown, administer HepB within 12 hours of birth. Determine mother's HBsAg status as soon as possible and, if HBsAg-positive, administer HBIG (no later than age 1 week).

After the birth dose:
- The HepB series should be completed with either monovalent HepB or a combination vaccine containing HepB. The second dose should be administered at age 1 or 2 months. The final dose should be administered no earlier than age 24 weeks.
- Infants born to HBsAg-positive mothers should be tested for HBsAg and antibody to HBsAg (anti-HBs) after completion of at least 3 doses of the HepB series, at age 9 through 18 months (generally at the next well-child visit).

4-month dose:
- Administration of 4 doses of HepB to infants is permissible when combination vaccines containing HepB are administered after the birth dose.

2. Rotavirus vaccine (RV). *(Minimum age: 6 weeks)*
- Administer the first dose at age 6 through 14 weeks (maximum age: 14 weeks 6 days). Vaccination should not be initiated for infants aged 15 weeks or older (i.e., 15 weeks 0 days or older).
- Administer the final dose in the series by age 8 months 0 days.
- If Rotarix® is administered at ages 2 and 4 months, a dose at 6 months is not indicated.

3. Diphtheria and tetanus toxoids and acellular pertussis vaccine (DTaP). *(Minimum age: 6 weeks)*
- The fourth dose may be administered as early as age 12 months, provided at least 6 months have elapsed since the third dose.
- Administer the final dose in the series at age 4 through 6 years.

4. *Haemophilus influenzae* type b conjugate vaccine (Hib). *(Minimum age: 6 weeks)*
- If PRP-OMP (PedvaxHIB® or Comvax® [HepB-Hib]) is administered at ages 2 and 4 months, a dose at age 6 months is not indicated.
- TriHiBit® (DTaP/Hib) should not be used for doses at ages 2, 4, or 6 months but can be used as the final dose in children aged 12 months or older.

5. Pneumococcal vaccine. *(Minimum age: 6 weeks for pneumococcal conjugate vaccine [PCV]; 2 years for pneumococcal polysaccharide vaccine [PPSV])*
- PCV is recommended for all children aged younger than 5 years. Administer 1 dose of PCV to all healthy children aged 24 through 59 months who are not completely vaccinated for their age.

Section II: Nursing Care in the Community/Hospital

Footnotes

Recommended Immunization Schedule for Persons Aged 0 Through 6 Years—United States • 2009

- Administer PPSV to children aged 2 years or older with certain underlying medical conditions (see *MMWR* 2000;49[No. RR-9]), including a cochlear implant.

6. **Influenza vaccine.** *(Minimum age: 6 months for trivalent inactivated influenza vaccine [TIV]; 2 years for live, attenuated influenza vaccine [LAIV])*
   - Administer annually to children aged 6 months through 18 years.
   - For healthy nonpregnant persons (i.e., those who do not have underlying medical conditions that predispose them to influenza complications) aged 2 through 49 years, either LAIV or TIV may be used.
   - Children receiving TIV should receive 0.25 mL if aged 6 through 35 months or 0.5 mL if aged 3 years or older.
   - Administer 2 doses (separated by at least 4 weeks) to children aged younger than 9 years who are receiving influenza vaccine for the first time or who were vaccinated for the first time during the previous influenza season but only received 1 dose.

7. **Measles, mumps, and rubella vaccine (MMR).** *(Minimum age: 12 months)*
   - Administer the second dose at age 4 through 6 years. However, the second dose may be administered before age 4, provided at least 28 days have elapsed since the first dose.

8. **Varicella vaccine.** *(Minimum age: 12 months)*
   - Administer the second dose at age 4 through 6 years. However, the second dose may be administered before age 4, provided at least 3 months have elapsed since the first dose.
   - For children aged 12 months through 12 years the minimum interval between doses is 3 months. However, if the second dose was administered at least 28 days after the first dose, it can be accepted as valid.

9. **Hepatitis A vaccine (HepA).** *(Minimum age: 12 months)*
   - Administer to all children aged 1 year (i.e., aged 12 through 23 months). Administer 2 doses at least 6 months apart.
   - Children not fully vaccinated by age 2 years can be vaccinated at subsequent visits.
   - HepA also is recommended for children older than 1 year who live in areas where vaccination programs target older children or who are at increased risk of infection. See *MMWR* 2006;55(No. RR-7).

10. **Meningococcal vaccine.** *(Minimum age: 2 years for meningococcal conjugate vaccine [MCV] and for meningococcal polysaccharide vaccine [MPSV])*
    - Administer MCV to children aged 2 through 10 years with terminal complement component deficiency, anatomic or functional asplenia, and certain other high-risk groups. See *MMWR* 2005;54(No. RR-7).
    - Persons who received MPSV 3 or more years previously and who remain at increased risk for meningococcal disease should be revaccinated with MCV.

The Recommended Immunization Schedules for Persons Aged 0 Through 18 Years are approved by the Advisory Committee on Immunization Practices (www.cdc.gov/vaccines/recs/acip), the American Academy of Pediatrics (http://www.aap.org), and the American Academy of Family Physicians (http://www.aafp.org).
DEPARTMENT OF HEALTH AND HUMAN SERVICES • CENTERS FOR DISEASE CONTROL AND PREVENTION

Recommended Immunization Schedule for Persons Aged 7 Through 18 Years—United States • 2009

For those who fall behind or start late, see the schedule below and the catch-up schedule

Vaccine ▼ Age►	7–10 years	11–12 years	13–18 years	
Tetanus, Diphtheria, Pertussis[1]	see footnote 1	Tdap	Tdap	
Human Papillomavirus[2]	see footnote 2	HPV (3 doses)	HPV Series	Range of recommended ages
Meningococcal[3]	MCV	MCV	MCV	
Influenza[4]		Influenza (Yearly)		
Pneumococcal[5]		PPSV		
Hepatitis A[6]		HepA Series		Catch-up immunization
Hepatitis B[7]		HepB Series		
Inactivated Poliovirus[8]		IPV Series		
Measles, Mumps, Rubella[9]		MMR Series		Certain high-risk groups
Varicella[10]		Varicella Series		

This schedule indicates the recommended ages for routine administration of currently licensed vaccines, as of December 1, 2008, for children aged 7 through 18 years. Any dose not administered at the recommended age should be administered at a subsequent visit, when indicated and feasible. Licensed combination vaccines may be used whenever any component of the combination is indicated and other components are not contraindicated and if approved by the Food and Drug Administration for that dose of the series. Providers should consult the relevant Advisory Committee on Immunization Practices statement for detailed recommendations, including high-risk conditions: http://www.cdc.gov/vaccines/pubs/acip-list.htm. Clinically significant adverse events that follow immunization should be reported to the Vaccine Adverse Event Reporting System (VAERS). Guidance about how to obtain and complete a VAERS form is available at http://www.vaers.hhs.gov or by telephone, 800-822-7967.

Figure 7-2 ■ Recommended immunization schedule for individuals 7 to 18 years, United States, 2009.
Source: Centers for Disease Control and Prevention. (2009)

Footnotes

Recommended Immunization Schedule for Persons Aged 7 Through 18 Years—United States • 2009

1. **Tetanus and diphtheria toxoids and acellular pertussis vaccine (Tdap).** *(Minimum age: 10 years for BOOSTRIX® and 11 years for ADACEL®)*
   - Administer at age 11 or 12 years for those who have completed the recommended childhood DTP/DTaP vaccination series and have not received a tetanus and diphtheria toxoid (Td) booster dose.
   - Persons aged 13 through 18 years who have not received Tdap should receive a dose.
   - A 5-year interval from the last Td dose is encouraged when Tdap is used as a booster dose; however, a shorter interval may be used if pertussis immunity is needed.

2. **Human papillomavirus vaccine (HPV).** *(Minimum age: 9 years)*
   - Administer the first dose to females at age 11 or 12 years.
   - Administer the second dose 2 months after the first dose and the third dose 6 months after the first dose (at least 24 weeks after the first dose).
   - Administer the series to females at age 13 through 18 years if not previously vaccinated.

3. **Meningococcal conjugate vaccine (MCV).**
   - Administer at age 11 or 12 years, or at age 13 through 18 years if not previously vaccinated.
   - Administer to previously unvaccinated college freshmen living in a dormitory.
   - MCV is recommended for children aged 2 through 10 years with terminal complement component deficiency, anatomic or functional asplenia, and certain other groups at high risk. See *MMWR* 2005;54(No. RR-7).
   - Persons who received MPSV 5 or more years previously and remain at increased risk for meningococcal disease should be revaccinated with MCV.

4. **Influenza vaccine.**
   - Administer annually to children aged 6 months through 18 years.
   - For healthy nonpregnant persons (i.e., those who do not have underlying medical conditions that predispose them to influenza complications) aged 2 through 49 years, either LAIV or TIV may be used.
   - Administer 2 doses (separated by at least 4 weeks) to children aged younger than 9 years who are receiving influenza vaccine for the first time or who were vaccinated for the first time during the previous influenza season but only received 1 dose.

Footnotes

Recommended Immunization Schedule for Persons Aged 7 Through 18 Years—United States • 2009

5. Pneumococcal polysaccharide vaccine (PPSV).
- Administer to children with certain underlying medical conditions (see *MMWR* 1997;46[No. RR-8]), including a cochlear implant. A single revaccination should be administered to children with functional or anatomic asplenia or other immunocompromising condition after 5 years.

6. Hepatitis A vaccine (HepA).
- Administer 2 doses at least 6 months apart.
- HepA is recommended for children older than 1 year who live in areas where vaccination programs target older children or who are at increased risk of infection. See *MMWR* 2006;55(No. RR-7).

7. Hepatitis B vaccine (HepB).
- Administer the 3-dose series to those not previously vaccinated.
- A 2-dose series (separated by at least 4 months) of adult formulation Recombivax HB® is licensed for children aged 11 through 15 years.

8. Inactivated poliovirus vaccine (IPV).
- For children who received an all-IPV or all-oral poliovirus (OPV) series, a fourth dose is not necessary if the third dose was administered at age 4 years or older.
- If both OPV and IPV were administered as part of a series, a total of 4 doses should be administered, regardless of the child's current age.

9. Measles, mumps, and rubella vaccine (MMR).
- If not previously vaccinated, administer 2 doses or the second dose for those who have received only 1 dose, with at least 28 days between doses.

10. Varicella vaccine.
- For persons aged 7 through 18 years without evidence of immunity (see *MMWR* 2007;56[No. RR-4]), administer 2 doses if not previously vaccinated or the second dose if they have received only 1 dose.
- For persons aged 7 through 12 years, the minimum interval between doses is 3 months. However, if the second dose was administered at least 28 days after the first dose, it can be accepted as valid.
- For persons aged 13 years and older, the minimum interval between doses is 28 days.

The Recommended Immunization Schedules for Persons Aged 8 Through 18 Years are approved by the Advisory Committee on Immunization Practices (www.cdc.gov/vaccines/recs/acip), the American Academy of Pediatrics (http://www.aap.org), and the American Academy of Family Physicians (http://www.aafp.org).

DEPARTMENT OF HEALTH AND HUMAN SERVICES • CENTERS FOR DISEASE CONTROL AND PREVENTION

Section II: Nursing Care in the Community/Hospital

Catch-up Immunization Schedule for Persons Aged 4 Months Through 18 Years Who Start Late or Who Are More Than 1 Month Behind—United States • 2009

The table below provides catch-up schedules and minimum intervals between doses for children whose vaccinations have been delayed. A vaccine series does not need to be restarted, regardless of the time that has elapsed between doses. Use the section appropriate for the child's age.

Vaccine	Minimum Age for Dose 1	CATCH-UP SCHEDULE FOR PERSONS AGED 4 MONTHS THROUGH 6 YEARS			
		Minimum Interval Between Doses			
		Dose 1 to Dose 2	Dose 2 to Dose 3	Dose 3 to Dose 4	Dose 4 to Dose 5
Hepatitis B[1]	Birth	4 weeks	8 weeks (and at least 16 weeks after first dose)		
Rotavirus[2]	6 wks	4 weeks	4 weeks[2]		
Diphtheria, Tetanus, Pertussis[3]	6 wks	4 weeks	4 weeks	6 months	6 months[3]
Haemophilus influenzae type b[4]	6 wks	4 weeks if first dose administered at younger than age 12 months 8 weeks (as final dose) if first dose administered at age 12-14 months No further doses needed if first dose administered at age 15 months or older	4 weeks[4] if current age is younger than 12 months 8 weeks (as final dose)[4] if current age is 12 months or older and second dose administered at younger than age 15 months No further doses needed if previous dose administered at age 15 months or older	8 weeks (as final dose) This dose only necessary for children aged 12 months through 59 months who received 3 doses before age 12 months	
Pneumococcal[5]	6 wks	4 weeks if first dose administered at younger than age 12 months 8 weeks (as final dose for healthy children) if first dose administered at age 12 months or older or current age 24 through 59 months No further doses needed for healthy children if first dose administered at age 24 months or older	4 weeks if current age is younger than 12 months 8 weeks (as final dose for healthy children) if current age is 12 months or older No further doses needed for healthy children if previous dose administered at age 24 months or older	8 weeks (as final dose) This dose only necessary for children aged 12 months through 59 months who received 3 doses before age 12 months or for high-risk children who received 3 doses at any age	
Inactivated Poliovirus[6]	6 wks	4 weeks	4 weeks	4 weeks[6]	
Measles, Mumps, Rubella[7]	12 mos	4 weeks			
Varicella[8]	12 mos	3 months			
Hepatitis A[9]	12 mos	6 months			

		CATCH-UP SCHEDULE FOR PERSONS AGED 7 THROUGH 18 YEARS		
		4 weeks	4 weeks if first dose administered at younger than age 12 months 6 months if first dose administered at age 12 months or older	6 months if first dose administered at younger than age 12 months[11]
Tetanus, Diphtheria/ Tetanus, Diphtheria, Pertussis[10]	7 yrs[10]			
Human Papillomavirus[11]	9 yrs	Routine dosing intervals are recommended[11]		
Hepatitis A[9]	12 mos	6 months		
Hepatitis B[1]	Birth	4 weeks	8 weeks (and at least 16 weeks after first dose)	
Inactivated Poliovirus[6]	6 wks	4 weeks	4 weeks	4 weeks[6]
Measles, Mumps, Rubella[7]	12 mos	4 weeks		
Varicella[8]	12 mos	3 months if the person is younger than age 13 years 4 weeks if the person is aged 13 years or older		

Figure 7-3 ■ Catch-up immunization schedule for individuals 4 months to 18 years who start late or who are more than 1 month behind.
Source: Centers for Disease Control and Prevention. (2009)

Footnotes

Catch-up Immunization Schedule for Persons Aged 4 Months Through 18 Years Who Start Late or Who Are More Than 1 Month Behind— United States • 2009

1. **Hepatitis B vaccine (HepB).**
   - Administer the 3-dose series to those not previously vaccinated.
   - A 2-dose series (separated by at least 4 months) of adult formulation Recombivax HB® is licensed for children aged 11 through 15 years.

2. **Rotavirus vaccine (RV).**
   - The maximum age for the first dose is 14 weeks 6 days. Vaccination should not be initiated for infants aged 15 weeks or older (i.e., 15 weeks 0 days or older).
   - Administer the final dose in the series by age 8 months 0 days.
   - If Rotarix® was administered for the first and second doses, a third dose is not indicated.

3. **Diphtheria and tetanus toxoids and acellular pertussis vaccine (DTaP).**
   - The fifth dose is not necessary if the fourth dose was administered at age 4 years or older.

4. ***Haemophilus influenzae* type b conjugate vaccine (Hib).**
   - Hib vaccine is not generally recommended for persons aged 5 years or older. No efficacy data are available on which to base a recommendation concerning use of Hib vaccine for older children and adults. However, studies suggest good immunogenicity in persons who have sickle cell disease, leukemia, or HIV infection, or who have had a splenectomy; administering 1 dose of Hib vaccine to these persons is not contraindicated.
   - If the first 2 doses were PRP-OMP (PedvaxHIB® or Comvax®), and administered at age 11 months or younger, the third (and final) dose should be administered at age 12 through 15 months and at least 8 weeks after the second dose.
   - If the first dose was administered at age 7 through 11 months, administer 2 doses separated by 4 weeks and a final dose at age 12 through 15 months.

5. **Pneumococcal vaccine.**
   - Administer 1 dose of pneumococcal conjugate vaccine (PCV) to all healthy children aged 24 through 59 months who have not received at least 1 dose of PCV on or after age 12 months.
   - For children aged 24 through 59 months with underlying medical conditions, administer 1 dose of PCV if 3 doses were received previously or administer 2 doses of PCV at least 8 weeks apart if fewer than 3 doses were received previously.
   - Administer pneumococcal polysaccharide vaccine (PPSV) to children aged 2 years or older with certain underlying medical conditions (see *MMWR* 2000;49[No. RR-9]), including a cochlear implant, at least 8 weeks after the last dose of PCV.

Footnotes

Catch-up Immunization Schedule for Persons Aged 4 Months Through 18 Years Who Start Late or Who Are More Than 1 Month Behind— United States • 2009

6. Inactivated poliovirus vaccine (IPV).
- For children who received an all-IPV or all-oral poliovirus (OPV) series, a fourth dose is not necessary if the third dose was administered at age 4 years or older.
- If both OPV and IPV were administered as part of a series, a total of 4 doses should be administered, regardless of the child's current age.

7. Measles, mumps, and rubella vaccine (MMR).
- Administer the second dose at age 4 through 6 years. However, the second dose may be administered before age 4, provided at least 28 days have elapsed since the first dose.
- If not previously vaccinated, administer 2 doses with at least 28 days between doses.

8. Varicella vaccine.
- Administer the second dose at age 4 through 6 years. However, the second dose may be administered before age 4, provided at least 3 months have elapsed since the first dose.
- For persons aged 12 months through 12 years, the minimum interval between doses is 3 months. However, if the second dose was administered at least 28 days after the first dose, it can be accepted as valid.
- For persons aged 13 years and older, the minimum interval between doses is 28 days.

9. Hepatitis A vaccine (HepA).
- HepA is recommended for children older than 1 year who live in areas where vaccination programs target older children or who are at increased risk of infection. See *MMWR* 2006;55(No. RR-7).

10. Tetanus and diphtheria toxoids vaccine (Td) and tetanus and diphtheria toxoids and acellular pertussis vaccine (Tdap).
- Doses of DTaP are counted as part of the Td/Tdap series
- Tdap should be substituted for a single dose of Td in the catch-up series or as a booster for children aged 10 through 18 years; use Td for other doses.

11. Human papillomavirus vaccine (HPV).
- Administer the series to females at age 13 through 18 years if not previously vaccinated.
- Use recommended routine dosing intervals for series catch-up (i.e., the second and third doses should be administered at 2 and 6 months after the first dose). However, the minimum interval between the first and second doses is 4 weeks. The minimum interval between the second and third doses is 12 weeks, and the third dose should be given at least 24 weeks after the first dose.

Information about reporting reactions after immunization is available online at http://www.vaers.hhs.gov or by telephone, 800-822-7967. Suspected cases of vaccine-preventable diseases should be reported to the state or local health department. Additional information, including precautions and contraindications for immunization, is available from the National Center for Immunization and Respiratory Diseases at http://www.cdc.gov/vaccines or telephone, 800-CDC-INFO (800-232-4636).

DEPARTMENT OF HEALTH AND HUMAN SERVICES • CENTERS FOR DISEASE CONTROL AND PREVENTION

Section II: Nursing Care in the Community/Hospital

SUGGESTED INTERVALS BETWEEN IMMUNE GLOBULIN ADMINISTRATION AND MEASLES (ANY MEASLES VACCINE) OR VARICELLA IMMUNIZATIONS

Indication for Immunoglobulin	Dose (Including mg IgG per kg Body Weight)	Interval, Month*
Tetanus (as TIG)	250 Units (10 mg IgG/kg), IM	3
Hepatitis A prophylaxis (as IG)		
Contact prophylaxis	0.02 mL/kg (3.3 mg IgG/kg), IM	3
International travel	0.06 mL/kg (10 mg IgG/kg), IM	3
Hepatitis B prophylaxis (as HBIG)	0.06 mL/kg (10 mg IgG/kg), IM	3
Rabies prophylaxis (as RIG)	20 International Units/kg (22 mg IgG/kg), IM	4
Varicella prophylaxis (as VariZIG)	125 Units/10 kg (maximum 625 Units) (20–40 mg IgG/kg), IM	5
Measles prophylaxis (as IG)		
Standard	0.25 mL/kg (40 mg IgG/kg), IM	5
Immunocompromised host	0.5 mL/kg (80 mg IgG/kg), IM	6
RSV immune globulin (monoclonal antibody), Synagis	15 mg/kg (monoclonal) IM	None
Cytomegalovirus Immune Globulin	150 mg/kg maximum IV	6
RSV-IGIV	750 mg/kg IV	9

Blood transfusion		
Washed RBCs	10 mL/kg (Negligible IgG) IV	0
RBCs, adenine-saline added	10 mL/kg (10 mg IgG/kg) IV	3
Packed RBCs	10 mL/kg (20–60 mg IgG/kg) IV	5
Whole blood	10 mL/kg (80–100 mg IgG/kg) IV	6
Plasma or platelet products	10 mL/kg (160 mg IgG/kg) IV	7
Replacement (or therapy) of immune deficiencies (as IGIV)*	300–400 IV	8
ITP (as IGIV)	400 mg/kg IV	8
ITP	1 g/kg IV	10
Kawasaki syndrome	2 g/kg IV	11

Note: HBIG, hepatitis B immunoglobulin; IG, immunoglobulin; IgG, immunoglobulin G; IGIV, immunoglobulin intravenous; ITP, immune thrombocytopenic purpura; MMR, measles-mumps-rubella; RBCs, red blood cells; RIG, rabies immunoglobulin; RSV, respiratory syncytial virus; TIG, tetanus immunoglobulin; VariZIG, varicella-zoster immunoglobulin.

*Measles and varicella vaccination is recommended for children with asymptomatic or mildly symptomatic human immunodeficiency virus (HIV) infection but is contraindicated for persons with severe immunosuppression from HIV or any other immunosuppressive disorder.

Source: From *Guide to Contraindictions and Vaccinations Guide,* Centers for Disease Control and Prevention, 2004, retrieved July 3, 2008, from http://www.cdc.gov/vaccines/recs/vac-admin/contraindications.htm.

VACCINE ADVERSE EVENT REPORTING SYSTEM

The Vaccine Adverse Event Reporting System (VAERS) tracks serious vaccine reactions, and compensation for a family may be provided when a link between an immunization and a serious adverse effect is found. The adverse events reportable for specific vaccines are listed below. To report an adverse event, go to https://secure.vaers.org/VaersDataEntryintro.htm. The report can be submitted by Internet, mail, or fax.

NATIONAL VACCINE INJURY COMPENSATION PROGRAM—VACCINE INJURY TABLE, FEBRUARY 1, 2007

Vaccine	Adverse Event Covered	Time Period for First Symptom or Manifestation of Onset—for Compensation
Tetanus toxoid-containing vaccines (e.g., DTaP, Tdap, DTP-Hib, DT, Td, or TT)	Anaphylaxis or anaphylactic shock Bacterial neuritis Any acute complication or sequela (including death) of above events	0–4 hours 2–28 days Not applicable
Pertussis antigen-containing vaccines (e.g., DTaP, Tdap, DTP, P, DTP-Hib)	Anaphylaxis or anaphylactic shock Encephalopathy (or encephalitis) Any acute complication or sequela (including death) of above events	0–4 hours 0–72 hours Not applicable

Measles, mumps, rubella virus-containing vaccines in any combination (e.g., MMR, MR, M, R)	Anaphylaxis or anaphylactic shock	0–4 hours
	Encephalopathy (or encephalitis)	5–15 days
	Any acute complication or sequela (including death) of above events	Not applicable
Rubella virus-containing vaccines (e.g., MMR, MR, R)	Chronic arthritis	7–42 days
	Any acute complication or sequela (including death) of above events	Not applicable
Measles virus-containing vaccines (e.g., MMR, MR, M)	Thrombocyto-penia purpura	7–30 days
	Vaccine strain measles viral infection in an immunodeficient recipient	0–6 months
	Any acute complication or sequela (including death) of above events	Not applicable
Polio inactivated virus-containing vaccines (e.g., IPV)	Anaphylaxis or anaphylactic shock	0–4 hours
	Any acute complication or sequela (including death) of above events	No limit

(Continued)

Vaccine	Adverse Event Covered	Time Period for First Symptom or Manifestation of Onset—for Compensation
Hepatitis B antigen-containing vaccines	Anaphylaxis or anaphylactic shock Any acute complication or sequela (including death) of above events	0–4 hours No limit
Haemophilus influenzae type B polysaccharide conjugate vaccines	No condition specified for compensation	Not applicable
Varicella vaccine	No condition specified for compensation	Not applicable
Rotavirus vaccine	No condition specified for compensation	Not applicable
Vaccines containing live, oral, rhesus-based rotavirus	Intussusception Any acute condition or sequela (including death) of above event	0–30 days Not applicable

Pneumococcal con-jugate vaccine	No condition specified for compensation	Not applicable
Any new vaccine recommended by the Centers for Disease Control and Prevention for routine administration to children after publication by Secretary, HHS of notice of coverage.[a]		

[a]As of December 1, 2004, hepatitis A vaccines were added to the Vaccine Injury Table under this category. As of July 1, 2005, *trivalent* influenza vaccines were added to the Table under this category. As of February 1, 2007, meningococcal (conjugate and polysaccharide) and human papillomavirus (HPV) vaccines have been added to the Table under this category. For aids to interpret the defined conditions, go to the following website: http://www.hrsa.gov/osp/vaccinecompensation.

Source: From *National Childhood Vaccine Injury Act Vaccine Injury Table,* Health Resources and Services Administration Office of Special Programs, 2007, accessed July 3, 2008, from http://www.hrsa.gov/vaccinecompensation/table.htm.

8 PEDIATRIC FLUID AND DOSAGE CALCULATIONS

I. Principles of Pediatric Fluid Calculation
   A. Solutions
      1. Intravenous (IV) flow rates are most frequently calculated in microdrops in pediatrics. For all companies, 60 microdrops = 1 mL of solution. For macrodrops, generally 10 or 15 drops = 1 mL of solution. Check the manufacturer information for macrodrops in 1 mL of fluid for the company your unit uses.

      Flow rate is calculated using the following formula:

      $$\text{Drops/minute} = \frac{\text{Total volume ordered} \times \text{drops/minute}}{\text{Total infusion time (minutes)}}$$

      For example, if 250 mL of fluid were to be administered by microdrop over 3 hours, the drops per minute would be calculated as follows:

      $$\text{Drops/minute} = \frac{250 \times 60}{180}$$

      $$= \frac{15,000}{180}$$

      $$= 83.3$$

      The IV flow rate in this example would be adjusted to administer 83 drops/minute.

      2. When microdrip tubing is used, because 60 drops = 1 mL and there are 60 minutes in an hour, the formula to use is drops/minute = mL/hour. For example, if a child needed 250 mL to be delivered in 6 hours, the problem would be calculated as follows:

      $$\frac{250 \text{ mL}}{6 \text{ hours}} = 41.67 \text{ mL/hour}$$

      Therefore, the rate is set at 42 drops/minute.

      3. IV pumps are generally used in pediatrics. Regulation of dosage is easier and safer with use of these pumps. Pumps usually calculate the required flow rate in milliliters per

hour. So, if 500 mL of IV fluid needed to be delivered in 8 hours:

$$\frac{500 \text{ mL}}{8 \text{ hours}} = 62.5 \text{ mL/hour}$$

Therefore, the pump would be set at 62 or 63.

Refer to chapter 13 in this handbook for information about maintenance and replacement calculation of fluids for children, and guidelines for oral rehydration therapy. See *Clinical Skills Manual for Pediatric Nursing* for details about medication administration.

II. Principles of Pediatric Dosage Calculation
   A. A certain number of milligrams of a drug is specified for each kilogram of body weight. This is commonly written as *mg/kg*. Dosages can be prescribed for a **dose** or for a **day.** For example, a pain medication may be written as x mg/kg/dose as needed every 6 hours. When looking up a medication in a drug book, the maximum amount is usually listed as x mg/kg/day; in this case all of the day's doses need to be added together to check if the daily dose is within recommended levels. For intravenous medications, the medication is commonly diluted. Check for the recommendations for dilution, such as "Dilute x mg of medication in y mL of fluid and infuse over z minutes."
   B. A certain number of milligrams of a drug is specified for each square meter of body surface area. This is commonly written as *mg/m²*.
   C. Rules for calculation of pediatric dosages using adult doses and considering the age or weight of the child have sometimes been used in the past. These are not considered safe or accurate and should not be used.

III. Guidelines for Medication Administration
   A. Before giving any medication to a child, ask yourself these questions:
      • How will the drug be absorbed, metabolized, and excreted?
      • How will the child's illness and developmental physiology influence the absorption, metabolism, and excretion of the drug?
      • Is the child unusually small or large for age (body mass index under 5th percentile or over 95th percentile? The medication dose may need to be altered from usual levels by the prescriber.

- Is the child taking other drugs that will interact or compete with this drug for use and excretion?
- What dose should be given?
- What are the child's pulse, temperature, respiratory rate, blood pressure, skin color and condition, fluid status, and behavior? (Document in the medical record.)

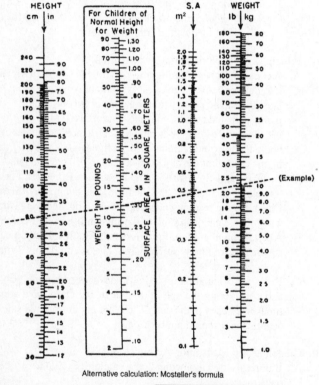

Alternative calculation: Mosteller's formula

$$\text{Surface area (m}^2) = \sqrt{\frac{\text{Height (cm)} \times \text{Weight (kg)}}{3600}}$$

Figure 8-1 ■ The body surface area is indicated at the intersection of a straight line connecting the height and weight column with the surface area column; if the patient is roughly average size, it is determined by the weight alone (enclosed area).
Nomogram is modified from data of E. Boyd by C.D. West. See also G. L. Briars & B. J. Bailey, Surface area estimation: Pocket calculator v nomogram. Arc Dis Child 1994; 70, 246–7.
Source: Reprinted by permission from Kliegman, R.M., Behrman, R.E., Jenson, H.B., & Stanton, B.F. (2007). *Nelson Textbook of Pediatrics* 18th ed. Philadelphia: Saunders Elsevier.

B. After giving any medication to a child, ask these questions:
- What time, route, amount, and site (for injections) were used for medication administration? (Document in the medical record.)
- What amount of fluid was used for dilution of an intravenous medication, and over what time period was it administered? (Document in the medical record.)
- What pertinent physical findings, such as changes in condition, lack of expected results, side effects, or unusual effects of the drug, are observed? (Document in the medical record.)
- Are there recommendations to obtain blood levels of the drug for establishing the therapeutic dose?
- How can results of this therapy be shared with other health professionals?

C. Confirm correct drug and dose with every medication given, and properly document procedure.
  1. Always check dosage prescribed against safe dosage ranges. Nurses are liable legally for any drug they administer. Use the Six Patient Rights of Medication Administration (see number 3).
  2. Identify each child carefully to avoid giving a medication to the wrong child. In the hospital, check identification bands, and, in the office or outpatient setting, have the parent and/or child provide verbal identification. Verify allergy history.
  3. Use the Six Patient Rights of Medication Administration. Nurses should follow these six "Rights" when administering medications to help prevent errors:
     a. The Right Drug
     b. By the Right Route
     c. In the Right Dose
     d. To the Right Patient
     e. At the Right Time
     f. With the Right Documentation
  4. Document immediately after administration, including the drug, dose, time, route, and site, as well as the name and title of the person who administered the medication. Check the child's response to the medication, and document the response as needed.
  5. In patient-specific documentation, including clinical documentation, order forms, progress notes, and consultation and operative reports, certain abbreviations should not be

used because of the potential problem of misinterpretation. For example, avoid U, IU QD, QOD, and use instead *unit, international unit, daily*, and *every other day*. Always use a zero before a decimal point, but never use a zero after a decimal point in a medication dosage. Additional recommendations about abbreviations to avoid can be found on the Joint Commission on Accreditation of Healthcare Organization's website (http://www.jcaho.org) and on the ISMP Medication Safety Alert website (http://www.ismp.org).

6. The American Academy of Pediatrics has adopted a policy statement titled *Prevention of Medication Errors in the Pediatric Inpatient Setting*. The statement lists recommendations regarding hospital-wide system actions and guidelines, prescriber actions and guidelines, prescriber education and communication, pharmacy action and guidelines, nursing actions and guidelines, nursing education and communication, patients, and families. The nursing actions and guidelines follow:

- Check medication calculations with another professional member of the healthcare team.
- Confirm patient identity before administration of each dose.
- Be familiar with medication ordering and dispensing systems.
- Verify drug orders before medication administration.
- Unusually large or small volumes or dosage units for a single patient dose should be verified.
- When a patient, parent, or caregiver questions whether a drug should be administered, listen attentively, answer questions, and double-check the medication order.
- Remain familiar with the operation of medication administration devices and the potential for error with such devices, particularly patient-controlled analgesia or infusion pumps.

Source: Data from "Prevention of Medication Errors in the Pediatric Inpatient Setting," Committee on Drugs and Committee on Hospital Care, 2003, 2007 (Policy Reaffirmed May 1, 2007), *Pediatrics, 112*, 431–436.

9 PAIN ASSESSMENT TOOLS

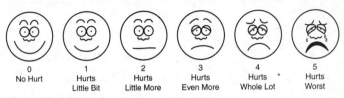

0	1	2	3	4	5
No Hurt	Hurts Little Bit	Hurts Little More	Hurts Even More	Hurts Whole Lot	Hurts Worst

Figure 9–1 ■ Wong-Baker Faces Pain Rating Scale.
Source: From Hockenberry MJ, Wilson D: Wong's essentials of pediatric nursing, ed. 8, St. Louis, 2009, Mosby. Used with permission. Copyright Mosby.
From "Pain in Children: Comparison of Assessment Scales," by D. L. Wong & C. M. Baker, 1988, *Pediatric Nursing, 14*, 9–16.

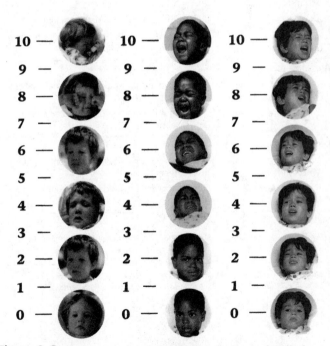

Figure 9–2 ■ Source: From Caucasian version of the Oucher, developed and copyrighted by Judith E. Beyer, RN, PhD, 1983; African-American version of the Oucher, developed and copyrighted by Mary J. Denyes, RN, PhD, and Antonio M. Villarruel, RN, PhD, 1990; and Hispanic version of the Oucher, developed and copyrighted by Antonio M. Villarruel, RN, PhD, 1990, with permission.

Table 9–1   Neonatal Infant Pain Scale

Characteristic	Scoring Criteria
Facial Expression	
0 = Relaxed muscles	Restful face with neutral expression
1 = Grimace	Tight facial muscles; furrowed brow, chin, and jaw (At low gestational ages, infants may have no facial expression)
Cry	
0 = No cry	Quiet, not crying
1 = Whimper	Mild moaning, intermittent cry
2 = Vigorous cry	Loud screaming, rising, shrill, and continuous (Silent cry may be scored if infant is intubated, as indicated by obvious facial movements)
Breathing Patterns	
0 = Relaxed	Relaxed, usual breathing pattern maintained
1 = Change in breathing	Change in drawing breath: irregular, faster than usual, gagging, or holding breath
Arm Movements	
0 = Relaxed/restrained (with soft restraints)	Relaxed, no muscle rigidity, occasional random movements of arms
1 = Flexed/extended	Tense, straight arms; rigid; or rapid extension and flexion
Leg Movements	
0 = Relaxed/restrained (with soft restraints)	Relaxed, no muscle rigidity, occasional random movements of legs
1 = Flexed/extended	Tense, straight legs; rigid; or rapid extension and flexion
State of Arousal	
0 = Sleeping/awake	Quiet, peaceful sleeping; or alert and settled
1 = Fussy	Alert and restless or thrashing; fussy

Source: From "The Development of a Tool to Assess Neonatal Pain," by J. Lawrence, D. Alcock, D. P. McGrath, et al., 1993, *Neonatal Network, 12*(6), 61, with permission.

Table 9–2 FLACC Behavioral Pain Assessment Scale

Categories	Scoring		
	0	1	2
Face	No particular expression or smile	Occasional grimace or frown; withdrawn, disinterested	Frequent to constant frown, clenched jaw, quivering chin
Legs	Normal position or relaxed	Uneasy, restless, tense	Kicking or legs drawn up
Activity	Lying quietly, normal position, moves easily	Squirming, shifting back and forth, tense	Arched, rigid, or jerking
Cry	No cry (awake or asleep)	Moans or whimpers, occasional complaint	Crying steadily, screams or sobs; frequent complaints
Consolability	Content, relaxed	Reassured by occasional touching, hugging, or being talked to; distractible	Difficult to console or comfort

How to Use the FLACC

In patients who are awake: observe for 1–5 minutes or longer. Observe legs and body uncovered. Reposition patient or observe activity. Assess body for tenseness and tone. Initiate consoling interventions if needed.

In patients who are asleep: observe for 5 minutes or longer. Observe body and legs uncovered. If possible, reposition the patient. Touch the body, and assess for tenseness and tone.

Face

- Score 0: a relaxed face, makes eye contact, or shows interest in surroundings.
- Score 1: a worried facial expression with eyebrows lowered, eyes partially closed, cheeks raised, and mouth pursed.
- Score 2: deep furrows in the forehead, closed eyes, an open mouth, and deep lines around nose and lips.

Legs

- Score 0: muscle tone and motion in the limbs are normal.
- Score 1: increased tone, rigidity, or tension and intermittent flexion or extension of the limbs.
- Score 2: hypertonicity, the legs are pulled tight, exaggerated flexion or extension of the limbs, and tremors.

Table 9–2   FLACC Behavioral Pain Assessment Scale (Continued)

Activity

- Score 0: moves easily and freely and shows normal activity or restrictions.
- Score 1: shifts positions; appears hesitant to move; demonstrates guarding, a tense torso, or pressure on a body part.
- Score 2: in a fixed position, rocking; or demonstrates side-to-side head movement or rubbing of a body part.

Cry

- Score 0: no cry or moan, awake or asleep.
- Score 1: occasional moans, cries, whimpers, or sighs.
- Score 2: frequent or continuous moans, cries, or grunts.

Consolability

- Score 0: calm and does not require consoling.
- Score 1: responds to comfort by touching or talking in 30 seconds to 1 minute.
- Score 2: requires constant comforting or is inconsolable.

Interpreting the Behavioral Score

Each category is scored on the 0–2 scale, which results in a total score of 0–10.

0 = Relaxed and comfortable	**4–6** = Moderate pain
1–3 = Mild discomfort	**7–10** = Severe discomfort or pain or both

FLACC is the acronym for five categories assessed: face, legs, activity, cry, and consolability. Source: From "The FLACC: A Behavioral Scale for Scoring Postoperative Pain in Young Children," by S. I. Merkel, T. Voepel-Lewis, J. R. Shayevitz, & S. Malviya, 1997, *Pediatric Nursing, 23*(3), 293–297, used with permission. The FLACC scale was developed by Sandra Merkel, MS, RN, Terri Voepel-Lewis, MS, RN, and Shobha Malviya, MD, at C. S. Mott Children's Hospital, University of Michigan Health System, Ann Arbor, MI.

10 POISON CONTROL INFORMATION

EMERGENCY MANAGEMENT FOR POISONING

1. Stabilize the child. Assess ABCs (airway, breathing, and circulation). Provide ventilatory support and supplemental oxygen.
2. Perform a rapid physical examination, start an IV infusion, draw blood for toxicology screen, and apply a cardiac monitor.
3. Obtain a history of the ingestion, including substance ingested, where child was found, by whom, position, when, how long unsupervised, history of depression or suicide, allergies, and any other medical problems.
4. Reverse or eliminate the toxic substance using the appropriate method:
   a. Antidotes and agonists
      Mucomyst (for acetaminophen poisoning)
      Digibind (for digoxin poisoning)
      Narcan (for opioid overdose)
      Romazicon (for benzodiazepine overdose)
   b. Gastric lavage
      - A gastric tube is inserted through the mouth; nasal insertion may be needed in some cases.
      - Normal saline solution is instilled and aspirated until the return is clear. This is considered a less effective method of removing ingested substances from the stomach than vomiting. It is reserved for children with central nervous system depression, diminished or absent gag reflex, or unwillingness to cooperate with other measures.
      - This method is contraindicated in children who have ingested alkaline corrosive substances, as insertion of the tube may cause esophageal perforation.
      - Used in children who have ingested acids to decrease continued damage and potential perforation of the stomach and intestines.
   c. Activated charcoal
      - Given to absorb and remove any remaining particles of toxic substances.
      - Usual dosage administration is 1 g/kg of body weight.
      - A commercial preparation of activated charcoal is administered orally or through a gastric tube.

- Available as a ready-to-drink solution in an opaque container.
- May be mixed with apple juice or soda if protocol allows to encourage consumption.
- Use a covered cup and straw when giving orally to prevent the child from seeing the black liquid and to minimize spillage.
- Administer activated charcoal only after the child has stopped vomiting, because aspiration of charcoal is damaging to lung tissue.
- Should not be administered for ingestion of caustic substances or hydrocarbons.

  d. Cathartics
- Hasten excretion of a toxic substance and minimizes absorption. The most commonly used cathartic is magnesium sulfate.

5. Perform other measures depending on the child's condition, the nature of the ingested substance, and the time since ingestion. They may include diuresis, fluid loading, cooling or warming measures, anticonvulsive measures, antiarrhythmic therapy, hemodialysis, or exchange transfusions.

6. Constantly evaluate the child's total condition to maintain airway, breathing, and circulation. Therapeutic management is adjusted as needed to treat the evolving condition.

7. Consider the family's emotional status. Provide information about the child, involve them in care when possible, and arrange for support persons and services to be available to them.

Table 10-1 Clinical Manifestations of Commonly Ingested Toxic Agents

Type	Sources	Clinical Manifestations	Clinical Therapy
Corrosives (strong acids and alkaline products that cause chemical burns of mucosal surfaces)	Batteries Household cleaners Clinitest tablets Denture cleaners Bleach Toilet bowl cleaners	Severe burning pain in mouth, throat, or stomach Swelling of mucous membranes; edema of lips, tongue, and pharynx (respiratory obstruction) Violent vomiting; hemoptysis Drooling; inability to clear secretions Signs of shock Anxiety Agitation	Do not induce vomiting! Dilute toxin with water to prevent further damage Give activated charcoal
Hydrocarbons (organic compounds that contain carbon and hydrogen; most are distillates of petroleum)	Gasoline Kerosene Furniture polish Lighter fluid Paint thinners	Gagging Choking Coughing Nausea Vomiting Alteration in sensorium (lethargy) Weakness Respiratory symptoms of pulmonary involvement, tachypnea, cyanosis, retractions, grunting	Do not induce vomiting! (Aspiration of hydrocarbons places child at high risk for pneumonia.) Use gastric lavage if severe central nervous system and respiratory impairment are present Use of activated charcoal is controversial Provide supportive care Decontaminate skin by removing clothing and cleansing skin

Table 10–1 Clinical Manifestations of Commonly Ingested Toxic Agents (Continued)

Type	Sources	Clinical Manifestations	Clinical Therapy
Acetaminophen	Many over-the-counter products	Nausea Vomiting Sweating Pallor Hepatic involvement (pain in upper right quadrant, jaundice, confusion, stupor, coagulation abnormalities)	Induce vomiting or perform gastric lavage, depending on amount ingested Administer charcoal or NAC (concentrated form of Mucomyst), which binds with the metabolite, preventing absorption and protecting the liver
Salicylate	Products containing aspirin	Nausea Disorientation Vomiting Dehydration Diaphoresis Hyperpnea Hyperpyrexia Bleeding tendencies Oliguria Tinnitus Convulsions Coma	Depends on amount ingested Induce vomiting Administer intravenous sodium bicarbonate, fluids, and vitamin K

Table 10–1 Clinical Manifestations of Commonly Ingested Toxic Agents (Continued)

Type	Sources	Clinical Manifestations	Clinical Therapy
Mercury	Broken thermometers Chemicals Paints Pesticides Fungicides	Tremors Memory loss Insomnia Weight loss Diarrhea Anorexia Gingivitis	Similar to that for lead poisoning (see text discussion)
Iron	Multiple vitamin supplements and therapeutic iron tablets	Vomiting Hematemesis Diarrhea Bloody stools Abdominal pain Metabolic acidosis Shock Seizures Coma	Induce vomiting Administer intravenous fluids and sodium bicarbonate Deferoxamine chelation therapy

Table 10–2 Clinical Manifestations of Lead Poisoning

Class I (less than 9 mcg/dL)	Generally asymptomatic although subtle neurological effects may be present with any exposure
Class IIA (10–14 mcg/dL) and IIB (15–19 mcg/dL)	Mild impairment in growth, fine motor skills, and cognition Anemia
Class III (20–44 mcg/dL)	General fatigue and motor impairment Difficulty concentrating Paresis or paralysis, tremor Headache Diffuse abdominal pain, vomiting, weight loss, constipation Anemia
Class IV (45–69 mcg/dL)	Colic (intermittent, severe abdominal cramps), anorexia, vomiting Hyperirritability Increased lethargy Lead line (blue-black) on gingival tissue
Class V (greater than 70 mcg/dL)	Encephalopathy, which may lead abruptly to seizures, changes in consciousness, coma, and death Ataxia

Note: mcg/dL = micrograms per deciliter
Source: Adapted from *Lead Toxicity Clinical Evaluation*, Agency for Toxic Substances and Disease Registry, 2006, Atlanta: Author.

11 EMERGENCY ASSESSMENT OF THE CHILD

INITIAL IMPRESSION

Make a quick initial impression of the severity or urgency of the child's condition using visual and auditory clues to make a rapid judgment. Be concerned if the following signs are noted.

Appearance

Poor eye contact, little interaction with parent or caregiver, no interest in toys or objects

Little spontaneous movement and poor muscle tone

Inconsolability

Weak, hoarse cry or muffled voice

Signs of Respiratory Distress

Nasal flaring, retractions, and head bobbing

Abnormal airway sounds, such as stridor, wheezing, grunting, snoring, or muffled or hoarse speech

Refusal to lie down or tripod positioning, sitting with the head and neck extended

Impaired Circulation

Pallor, mottled skin, cyanosis. In children of darker skin, the mucous membranes are usually pink, regardless of skin color.

NEXT STEPS

Analyze information from appearance, breathing effort, and circulation to evaluate the child's physiologic stability. The greater the number of abnormal findings present, the more serious the child's condition.

When an emergency condition exists, alter the sequence of assessment to identify the presence of a life-threatening condition.

- Airway—for example, if the airway is obstructed, no oxygen can enter the child's system.
- Breathing—for example, if there is lung damage, the child may be unable to ventilate and support gas exchange.

- Circulation—for example, hemorrhage may reduce blood volume and circulation to the brain and other vital organs.

Interrupt assessment as soon as a potential life-threatening physiologic condition is identified to provide the needed care.

Resume assessment when the physiologic condition is stabilized.

Reassess the airway, breathing, and circulation every 5 minutes.

ASSESSING THE ABCs (AIRWAY, BREATHING, AND CIRCULATION)

Airway Assessment

Is the infant or child crying or talking?

Are there any airway sounds?

Could the tongue be blocking the airway?

Does the chest rise?

Airway Management

Open the airway in cases of airway obstruction.

Perform a chin lift or a jaw thrust to lift the tongue out of the pharynx.[1]

Insert an oropharyngeal airway to maintain the airway in an unconscious child.[1]

Suction secretions and blood.

Assist with insertion of an endotracheal tube to maintain and secure the airway.[1]

Use a bag valve mask or perform rescue breathing with a mouth and nose barrier, and give two slow breaths if the chest does not rise.[1]

Reposition the child's head with the chin lift or jaw thrust if the head does not rise, and give two slow breaths again.

Initiate procedures for removing a foreign body obstruction if the chest still does not rise.[1]

Breathing Assessment

What is the effort associated with breathing?

How does the respiratory rate compare with the expected rate for age?

---

[1]This technique and others mentioned in this chapter can be found in the *Skills Manual* (Bindler & Ball, 2007).

What sounds are heard when auscultating the chest?

Are there any penetrating chest injuries? Are there any rib fractures? Are there any marks on the chest indicating injury?

Breathing Management

Provide high-concentration oxygen. Use a nonrebreather mask (a face mask with a reservoir bag) that enables delivery of 60–90% oxygen at a flow rate of 12–15 L/minute when the mask maintains a tight seal on the face.[1]

Assist ventilation with a resuscitation bag connected to oxygen when the child has minimal or no respiratory effort. Use only enough pressure and air volume to make the chest rise.[1]

Assist with insertion of a nasogastric or orogastric tube to keep the stomach deflated and to reduce the risk for vomiting.[1]

Cover any open chest wound with an occlusive dressing, taped on three sides.

Assist with chest-tube insertion when a pneumothorax is present.[1]

Circulatory Assessment

What is the circulation to the skin? What is the skin color? What is the capillary refill time?

Is there any bleeding or potential internal bleeding? How much blood has been lost?

Is the child possibly dehydrated?

What is the heart rate? What is the blood pressure? Are the peripheral pulses palpable?

Circulation Management

When bradycardia is present, provide oxygen, and assist ventilation as described under Breathing Management.

Attach a cardiorespiratory monitor. Monitor the heart rate during interventions to see whether the heart rate increases and stabilizes.[1]

Establish an intravenous (IV) line to provide emergency medications. Alternatively, small amounts of some medications can be administered down the endotracheal tube.

Initiate cardiac compressions if no pulse can be palpated or the pulse rate is less than 60 beats/minute in an infant or child with poor tissue perfusion.[1]

Assist with defibrillation of the infant or child with ventricular fibrillation or pulseless ventricular fibrillation. Place the appropriate size pads or paddles (with conducting gel) to the child's chest so that the heart is between them. A starting dose of 2 J/kg is recommended, increasing to 4 J/kg if ventricular fibrillation persists after the first shock (American Heart Association, 2005).[1]

Control bleeding with direct pressure using a gloved hand, and elevate the body part if it is safe to do so. Apply pressure to an arterial pressure point proximal to the injury to slow the flow of bleeding in cases of hemorrhage.

When hypovolemic shock is present, quickly administer 20 mL/kg of lactated Ringer's or normal saline. Reassess the heart rate, capillary refill, and responsiveness for the next 5–15 minutes to determine the child's response and the need for additional IV fluid, albumin, or blood. Give additional fluids or blood until the circulatory system is stabilized.

Disability (Neurologic) Assessment

What is the infant's or child's level of responsiveness using the AVPU (alert/verbal/painful/unresponsive) scale? What is the Glasgow Coma Scale score?

Check the pupils for size, symmetry, and reactivity to light.

Has the child had a seizure?

Is the child moving spontaneously? Is the child flaccid? Is any abnormal posturing present?

Disability Management

If the child has a brain injury, ensure oxygenation with assisted ventilation at the appropriate respiratory rate for the infant or child. Hyperventilation is not routinely recommended, but it may be used for brief periods in cases of increased intracranial pressure (Adelson, Bratton, Camey, et al., 2003). Administer a benzodiazepine medication if the child has had a seizure.

If spinal cord injury is suspected, immobilize the head in neutral position, and prevent movement of other parts of the body.

Exposure Assessment

Perform a rapid inspection of the entire body, when the child's condition is stabilized, to identify any additional injuries.

Check for the presence of pulses in extremities distal to the injury.

Stabilize in place any object impaling a part of the body.

Assess the child's pain level.

Exposure Management

Keep the child warm with heat lamps and warmed IV fluids to maintain a neutral temperature.

HISTORY

Obtain an abbreviated history of the event leading to the emergency. The acronym for this history is SAMPLE:

Signs and symptoms—onset and nature of the symptoms

Allergies—any known allergies

Medications—names and doses of prescribed and over-the-counter medications, including aerosol medications and complementary therapies

Past medical problems—any significant health conditions, hospitalizations, and immunizations

Last food or liquid—when the infant or child last ate or had liquids, including bottle or breastfeeding

Events leading to the injury or illness—progression of illness over time, activities contributing to injury

12 INFECTIOUS AND COMMUNICABLE DISEASES

CHICKENPOX (VARICELLA)

Epidemiology

Caused by varicella-zoster, human herpesvirus 3. Wild virus cases and breakthrough cases occur in vaccinated children.

Transmitted by direct viral contact with mucous membrane or conjunctiva primarily through airborne spread of secretions and direct lesion contact. Incubation period is 14 to 21 days.

Communicable 5 days before the onset of the rash until all lesions have crusted over.

Clinical Manifestations

Acute onset of mild fever, malaise, anorexia, headache, mild abdominal pain, and irritability; occur before eruption of lesions.

Itchy; begins as a macule on an erythematous base, progresses to a papule, then to a clear, fluid-filled vesicle. Eruption lasts 1 to 5 days. Lesions of all stages present. Crusts may remain for 1 to 3 weeks. A more severe rash with eczema or sunburn.

Lesions begin on the trunk, scalp, and face and spread to the rest of the body. Ulcerative lesions on mucous membranes may lead to decreased fluid intake and dehydration.

Clinical Therapy

Provide supportive medical management for healthy children.

Oral and intravenous acyclovir for immunocompromised patients, for adolescents, and for children with chronic cutaneous and pulmonary diseases, treated with chronic salicylate therapy, or oral or aerosol corticosteroids (American Academy of Pediatrics, 2006, p. 713).

Varicella-zoster immunoglobulin is given, up to 4 days after exposure, to newborns of infected mothers, premature neonates exposed postnatally, or to immunocompromised, unimmunized children up to 4 days after exposure (Marin, Güris, Chaves, et al., 2007).

Immunize children after 12 months of age. The vaccine can be given within 72 hours of exposure to prevent or reduce severity of the disease.

Complications: secondary infection, cellulitis, lymphadenitis, local abscesses, sepsis, encephalitis, pneumonia, thrombocytopenia, hepatitis, glomerulonephritis, arthritis, meningitis, and Reye syndrome. Significant illness or death for immunocompromised children. The disease is more severe when steroids have been given during the incubation period (American Academy of Pediatrics, 2006, p. 711).

Nursing Management
Assessment
Observe for complications such as drowsiness, meningeal signs, respiratory distress, and dehydration. Disorientation and restlessness may indicate viral encephalitis.

Monitor for acyclovir side effects: nausea, vomiting, diarrhea, abdominal pain, as well as allergic skin reactions or headache. Monitor renal function.

Implementation
Use airborne and contact precautions.

Isolate all children with a history of recent varicella exposure who are admitted to the hospital.

Isolate the child treated at home from children who are medically fragile or immunocompromised, immunocompromised adults, and women early in pregnancy.

Notify the school or childcare facility of the child's illness.

Give nonaspirin antipyretics to control fever.

Reduce itching with oral antihistamines, oatmeal and Aveeno baths, or Caladryl lotion. Keep the child's fingernails short and clean.

Change bed linens frequently.

ERYTHEMA INFECTIOSUM (FIFTH DISEASE)
Epidemiology
Caused by human parvovirus B19.

Transmitted by respiratory secretions and blood. Incubation period is 6 to 14 days.

Most communicable the week before symptom onset.

Clinical Manifestations
Stage 1: Flu-like illness (headache, chills, malaise, nausea, body ache) for 2 to 3 days, followed by symptom-free days.

Stage 2: A week later, a fiery-red rash appears on the cheeks and circumoral pallor. One to four days later, a lace-like symmetric, erythematous, maculopapular rash appears on the trunk and limbs, spreading proximal to distal. The palms and soles are spared.

Stage 3: The rash fades but reappears if the skin is irritated or exposed to sunlight over 1 to 3 weeks. The rash may be mildly pruritic.

Clinical Therapy

Provide supportive care.

Complications: children with hemolytic conditions may develop a transient aplastic crisis and need a blood transfusion. Immunodeficient patients may be treated with intravenous immunoglobulin therapy (American Academy of Pediatrics, 2006, p. 486).

Nursing Management

Isolate the hospitalized child with immunosuppression or aplastic crisis. Use standard and droplet precautions.

Control fever with nonaspirin antipyretics.

Use antipruritics or oatmeal or Aveeno baths if the rash is pruritic.

Encourage rest and offer frequent fluids. Provide quiet diversionary activities.

Avoid direct sunlight; use protective, light, loose clothing if sunlight exposure cannot be avoided.

The child may attend school or child care.

Explain the three stages of rash development to parents.

HAEMOPHILUS INFLUENZAE TYPE B

Epidemiology

Caused by coccobacilli *Haemophilus influenzae* bacterium, which has several serotypes and can be encapsulated or nonencapsulated.

Transmitted by direct contact or droplet inhalation. Unknown incubation period.

Communicable for 3 days from onset of symptoms.

Clinical Manifestations

Starts with a viral upper respiratory infection. The organism passes through the mucosal barrier to directly invade the bloodstream.

Several severe invasive illnesses may result: meningitis, epiglottitis, pneumonia, septic arthritis, cellulitis, and sepsis (in infants). Other illnesses include sinusitis, otitis media, bronchitis, and pericarditis.

Clinical Therapy

Treatment includes antibiotic therapy. Rifampin may be given to unprotected household contacts (not pregnant women).

Immunize infants, beginning at 2 months of age.

Complications: severe sequelae and death may occur in young infants from meningitis, epiglottitis, sinusitis, pneumonitis, and cellulitis.

Nursing Management

Use droplet precautions until 24 hours after the initiation of antibiotics.

Administer nonaspirin antipyretics to help the child feel more comfortable.

Perform nursing care measures specific to the illness caused by the organism.

Inform family members that rifampin turns urine and other body fluids orange, and it will cause stains.

LYME DISEASE

Epidemiology

Caused by *Borrelia burgdorferi*, a spirochete.

Transmitted by a tick bite. The tick must feed for 36 hours to transmit the disease. Incubation period is 1 to 55 days after the infected tick bites. A rash in 48 hours is an allergic reaction or infection, not Lyme disease.

Not contagious from person to person. Infection does not induce immunity.

Clinical Manifestations

A flat or raised red area that progresses to partial clearing in the center, with a bull's eye appearance, usually at least 5 cm in diameter. May look like a bruise in dark-skinned patients. Spontaneously resolves within 4 weeks.

Stage 1 (localized): malaise, fatigue, headache, stiff neck, mild fever, and muscle and joint aches lasting 5 to 21 days.

Stage 2 (early disseminated), 1 to 4 months after the bite: multiple erythema migrans, cranial nerve palsies, arthralgia, headache, fatigue, and meningitis.

Stage 3 (late disseminated), months later: Lyme arthritis and central nervous system changes.

Clinical Therapy

Localized disease: antibiotics for 2 to 3 weeks—amoxicillin or cefuroxime axetil for children 8 years of age or younger and doxycycline or tetracycline for children older than age 8 years.

Disseminated disease: oral or IV antibiotics (depending upon body system involved) for up to 4 weeks.

Complications: arm and leg weakness, Bell's palsy, encephalopathy, optic neuropathy, meningitis, severe headaches, and cognitive and behavioral changes; chronic arthritis; disorders of the peripheral nerves.

Nursing Management

Use standard precautions if the child is hospitalized.

Educate parents about need to take all medications and to avoid sun exposure if doxycycline is used.

Encourage the use of nonaspirin analgesics and antipyretics.

Promote rest and discourage vigorous activities, as the child may tire easily.

Educate parents and children to avoid tick-infested areas and wear protective clothing, check for ticks after every outing, remove ticks as soon as possible, and clean the area with soap and water.

Tell parents to mark the date of tick bite on the calendar and monitor the child's health for flu-like symptoms over the next 30 days. Encourage them to seek medical attention promptly if symptoms develop.

MEASLES (RUBEOLA)

Epidemiology

Caused by *Morbillivirus*, a member of the paramyxovirus group.

Passive immunity is active in the infant until age 12 to 15 months.

Transmitted by airborne, respiratory droplets and contact with infected persons. Incubation period is approximately 8 to 12 days.

Communicable 3 to 5 days before the rash until 4 days after the rash appears.

Clinical Manifestations

Prodromal phase of 3 to 5 days, with high fever, conjunctivitis, coryza, cough, anorexia, and malaise.

Koplik's spots (small, irregular, bluish-white spots on a red background) on the buccal mucosa approximately 2 days before and after the onset of the rash.

Characteristic dark red, blotchy, maculopapular rash becomes confluent; usually appears 2 to 4 days after onset of prodromal phase; begins on the face and spreads to the trunk and extremities. Symptoms gradually subside in 4 to 7 days.

Other symptoms include anorexia, malaise, fatigue, photophobia, and generalized lymphadenopathy.

Clinical Therapy

Treatment is supportive. Antibiotics for bacterial secondary infections.

Immunize children after 12 months of age. Immunoglobulin, administered up to 6 days after exposure, may help prevent the disease in susceptible persons.

Complications: diarrhea, otitis media, bronchopneumonia, bronchitis, laryngotracheobronchitis, and encephalitis. Children who are malnourished, medically fragile, and immunosuppressed have most complications.

Nursing Management

Maintain airborne precautions while contagious. Limit visitors to those immunized or immune.

Use a cool-mist vaporizer to help clear respiratory passages.

Give nonaspirin antipyretics for fever, antipruritics for itching, and antitussives may be ordered to control coughing.

Assess lungs carefully, as pneumonia is a common complication.

Offer cool liquids frequently to maintain fluid intake. Blended, pureed, and mashed foods are most easily tolerated.

Keep skin clean and dry. Bathe without soaps.

Keep lights dim, and cover windows if the child has photophobia.

Maintain bed rest. Elevate the head of the bed. Keep the room cool with good air circulation. Provide light, nonirritating blankets. Provide diversional activities.

MONONUCLEOSIS

Epidemiology

Caused by Epstein-Barr virus, a member of the herpesvirus group.

Transmitted by direct contact with infected oropharyngeal or by blood transfusion. Incubation period is 10 to 50 days.

Communicable for an indetermined period; asymptomatic carriage is common (American Academy of Pediatrics, 2006, p. 287).

Clinical Manifestations

Young children may be irritable but otherwise asymptomatic.

Malaise, headache, anorexia, abdominal pain, fatigue, and fever for 2 to 3 days, followed by lymphadenopathy and a painful sore throat. A maculopapular rash may be seen in a few cases. Hepatosplenomegaly may occur.

Self-limited syndrome lasts 2 to 3 weeks. Weakness and lethargy may continue for several months.

Clinical Therapy

Provide supportive treatment.

Corticosteroids for massive splenomegaly, myocarditis, hemolytic anemia, or tonsillar swelling leads to an impending airway obstruction.

Antibiotics (ampicillin and amoxicillin) should be avoided, as a nonallergic rash often develops (American Academy of Pediatrics, 2006, p. 288).

Complications: encephalitis, aseptic meningitis, Guillain-Barré syndrome, splenic rupture, respiratory failure, and thrombocytopenia; are rare. In immunodeficient children, fatal infections or lymphomas can develop.

Nursing Management

Use standard precautions. Maintain bed rest during acute phase.

Give nonaspirin antipyretics and analgesics for fever and sore throat. Offer warm salt water for gargling. Offer soft foods and encourage fluids.

Teens should avoid kissing until the fever has been gone for several days.

Avoid contact sports until the liver and spleen are normal, approximately 4 weeks.

Allow return to school when the fever and sore throat have resolved.

MUMPS (PAROTITIS)

Epidemiology

Caused by *Rubulavirus*, in the paramyxovirus family.

Passive immunity until age 12 to 15 months.

Transmitted by contact with respiratory secretions. The incubation period is 12 to 25 days.

Communicable 1 to 2 days before parotid swelling until 9 days after swelling subsides.

Clinical Manifestations

Malaise, low-grade fever, earache, headache, pain with chewing, decreased appetite and activity, bilateral or unilateral parotid gland swelling that peaks about the third day.

Meningeal signs (stiff neck, headache, and photophobia) in approximately 15% of patients.

Clinical Therapy

Provide supportive therapy.

Immunize children after 12 months of age.

Complications: orchitis may occur in postpubertal males; sterility is relatively rare (American Academy of Pediatrics, 2006, p. 465). Oophoritis, pancreatitis, aseptic meningoencephalitis, thrombocytopenia, cerebellar ataxia, and hearing impairment may occur.

Nursing Management

Use standard and droplet precautions. Avoid exposure to immunocompromised individuals.

Assess for headache, stiff neck, vomiting, and photophobia (meningeal irritation).

Give nonaspirin analgesics and antipyretics to control fever and pain.

Encourage fluid intake. Avoid foods and beverages that increase salivary flow (citrus, spices, and candies); they cause pain. Offer soft and blended foods; chewing and swallowing are painful.

Apply warm or cool compresses, whichever is preferred, to the parotid area.

Provide scrotal supports if testicular swelling occurs.

Keep children out of school or child care until 9 days after parotid swelling begins. Encourage diversional activities.

PERTUSSIS (WHOOPING COUGH)

Epidemiology

Caused by *Bordetella pertussis*.

Transmitted by respiratory droplets and direct contact with respiratory mucus membrane discharge. Incubation period is 7 to 21 days.

Communicable 1 week after exposure until 5 to 7 days after starting antibiotic therapy; most contagious before the paroxysmal stage.

Clinical Manifestations

Catarrhal stage: nasal congestion, a runny nose, low-grade fever, and a mild nonproductive cough lasting approximately 2 weeks.

Paroxysmal stage: spasms of paroxysmal coughing followed by inspiration, stridor, or "whooping" that may last 1 to 4 weeks. Young infants may have apnea rather than "whooping." Cough spasm may lead to flushing, cyanosis, vomiting, and profuse drainage from the nose, eyes, and mouth.

Convalescent stage: up to 6 weeks when paroxysms gradually subside.

Adolescents may have an upper respiratory infection with persistent coughing spasms lasting longer than 7 days.

Clinical Therapy

Treatment with antibiotics (erythromycin and other macrolides) and corticosteroids, if ordered.

Provide supportive care.

Immunize infants starting at 2 months of age. A vaccine is approved for preteens and adolescents.

Complications: pneumonia, atelectasis, otitis media, encephalopathy, seizures, and death. Highest rate of mortality and complications in infants younger than 1 year.

Nursing Management

Use droplet precautions until 5 to 7 days after antibiotics are started.

Closely monitor respirations and oxygen saturation. The smaller the child, the greater the risk for respiratory distress and apnea. Remain with the child during coughing spells, when hypoxic and apneic episodes are most likely. Give oxygen if ordered. Have emergency equipment available.

Provide humidification. Gentle suctioning may be necessary.

Give nonaspirin antipyretics for fever.

Encourage frequent rest periods.

Monitor for dehydration. Encourage fluids. Sucking may trigger the coughing spell. Intravenous hydration if oral intake not tolerated.

Allow the child to eat desired foods in small, frequent feedings.

Teach parents to watch for signs of respiratory failure and dehydration if the child is managed at home. Provide emotional support to parents.

ROSEOLA (EXANTHEM SUBITUM, SIXTH DISEASE)

Epidemiology
Caused by herpesvirus type 6.

Transmitted by respiratory secretions of healthy individuals. Incubation period is 9 to 10 days. Lifelong persistent infection and virus shedding in healthy individuals (American Academy of Pediatrics, 2006, p. 376).

Clinical Manifestations
Sudden, high fever up to 40.5°C (105°F) for 3 to 8 days, but the child has normal appetite and behavior.

A characteristic pale pink, discrete, maculopapular rash starts on the trunk and spreads to the face, neck, and extremities after the fever stage. The rash can last for 1 to 2 days. May have mild upper respiratory symptoms and cervical and occipital lymphadenopathy.

Clinical Therapy
Provide supportive treatment.

Complications: children may have febrile seizures during high fever stage. Encephalopathy may develop in rare cases.

Nursing Management
Use standard precautions.

Give nonaspirin antipyretics to control fever. Encourage fluids.

Observe for seizure activity during the acute febrile periods.

Reassure parents that the rash will disappear in a few days.

RUBELLA (GERMAN MEASLES)

Epidemiology

Caused by an RNA virus, a member of the family Togaviridae, genus *Rubivirus*.

Transmitted by droplet spread, direct contact with infected persons, or contact with articles soiled by nasal secretions. Incubation period is 14 to 21 days (most commonly 16 to 18 days).

Communicable from approximately 7 days before until approximately 4 days after the onset of the rash.

Clinical Manifestations

Mild disease with a characteristic pink, nonconfluent, maculopapular rash that appears on the face, progresses to the neck, trunk, and legs, and disappears in the same order.

Prodromal symptoms of low-grade fever, headache, malaise, coryza, sore throat, anorexia, and Forschheimer spots (discrete, erythematous pinpoint or larger lesions on the soft palate) are seen 1 to 5 days before the rash.

Generalized lymphadenopathy involving the postauricular, suboccipital, and posterior cervical areas is common up to 7 days before the rash.

Clinical Therapy

Provide supportive treatment.

Immunize infants beginning at age 12 months. Immunize susceptible females of childbearing age.

Complications: arthritis in adolescents, encephalitis, and congenital rubella syndrome.

Nursing Management

Maintain standard and droplet precautions. Isolate from pregnant women.

Give nonaspirin analgesics and antipyretics for any pain and fever.

Encourage fluids. Provide food and beverage choices.

Provide quiet activities.

Exclude children from child care or school until 7 days after rash onset. Notify school and childcare facility of child's illness.

STREPTOCOCCUS A

Epidemiology

Caused by various M-protein groups of group A alpha- and beta-hemolytic streptococci. Different strains are associated with pharyngeal and pyodermal infections, rheumatic fever, and acute glomerulonephritis.

Transmitted by contact with respiratory secretions for pharyngitis or skin lesions for pyoderma. Incubation period for pharyngeal infection is usually 2 to 5 days and for pyodermal infection is usually 7 to 10 days.

Communicable for weeks in untreated pharyngeal infections, or for 24 hours after antibiotics are started.

Clinical Manifestations

Pharyngeal infection: abrupt onset with a sore throat, dysphagia, malaise, high fever, chills, headache, abdominal pain, anorexia, and vomiting. A beefy red pharynx with exudate (strep throat) and tender cervical nodes. Palatal petechiae may be seen.

Scarlet fever: a characteristic erythematous, sandpaper rash appearing 12 to 48 hours after onset of symptoms, starting on the neck and spreading to the trunk and extremities. In 3 to 4 days, the rash begins to fade and the tips of the toes and fingers begin to peel. The classic strawberry tongue is seen on day 4 or 5.

Pyodermal infection: lesions (impetigo) that are honey-colored crusts at the site of open lesions.

Clinical Therapy

Diagnosis is by a rapid strep test or a culture of secretions from the pharynx and tonsils.

Pharyngeal infection: oral penicillin V or erythromycin if the child is allergic to penicillin.

Pyodermal infection: topical mupirocin ointment.

Complications: acute otitis media, sinusitis, peritonsillar or retropharyngeal abscess, cervical lymphadenitis, acute rheumatic fever, acute glomerulonephritis, toxic shock syndrome, bacteremia, and necrotizing fasciitis or myositis.

Nursing Management

Maintain droplet precautions for pharyngeal infections and contact precautions for skin lesions for 24 hours after beginning antibiotics.

Promote bed rest during the febrile stage. Give nonaspirin antipyretics to control fever. Teach parents signs of a worsening condition.

For pharyngeal infections, offer warm salt water for gargling, a soft diet, and nonacidic beverages. Encourage fluids. Provide cool, clear liquids. Swallowing may be difficult.

Explain to parents the importance of the child's taking antibiotics for the full number of days prescribed.

Encourage other family members with sore throats to have throat cultures taken.

For impetigo, teach the parents to wash the skin, remove crusts, and apply antibiotic ointment.

13 ALTERATIONS IN FLUID AND ELECTROLYTE FUNCTION

Table 13–1 Clinical Manifestations of Extracellular Fluid Volume Deficit

Etiology	Clinical Manifestations
Decreased fluid volume	Weight loss
	Sunken fontanel (infant)
Inadequate circulating blood volume to offset the force of gravity when in upright position	Postural blood pressure drop (older children)
	Dizziness
Decreased intravascular volume	Delayed capillary refill time
	Flat neck veins when supine (older children)
Inadequate circulation to the brain	Dizziness, syncope
Inadequate circulation to the kidneys	Oliguria
Cardiac reflex response to decreased intravascular volume	Thready, rapid pulse
Decreased interstitial fluid volume	Decreased skin turgor

Table 13–2 Severity of Clinical Dehydration

Clinical Assessment	Mild	Moderate	Severe
Percent of body weight lost	Up to 5% (40–50 mL/kg)	6–9% (60–90 mL/kg)	10% or more (100+ mL/kg)
Level of consciousness	Alert, restless, thirsty	Irritable or lethargic (infants and very young children); alert, thirsty, restless (older children and adolescents)	Lethargic to comatose (infants and young children); often conscious, apprehensive (older children and adolescents)
Blood pressure	Normal	Normal or low; postural hypotension (older children and adolescents)	Low to undetectable

Table 13–2   Severity of Clinical Dehydration (Continued)

Pulse	Normal	Rapid	Rapid, weak to nonpalpable
Skin turgor	Normal (immediate or within 2 second return after pinching skin)	Poor; 2–3 second return after pinching skin	Very poor; 3–4 second return after pinching skin
Mucous membranes	Moist	Dry	Parched
Urine	May appear normal	Decreased output (less than 1 mL/kg/hr); dark color; increased specific gravity	Very decreased or absent output
Thirst	Slightly increased	Moderately increased	Greatly increased unless lethargic
Fontanel	Normal	Sunken	Sunken
Extremities	Warm; normal capillary refill of less than 2 seconds	Delayed capillary refill (3–5 sec)	Cool, discolored; delayed capillary refill (greater than 5 sec)
Respirations	Normal	Normal or rapid	Changing rate and pattern
Eyes	Normal	Slightly sunken; decreased tears	Deeply sunken; absent tears

Source: Data from Aehlert, 2005; and Kliegman, Behrman, Jenson, et al., 2007.

Table 13–3 Normal Serum Values for Electrolytes in Infants and Youth*

	Newborn	Infant and Child
Sodium	131–144 mmol/L	132–141 mmol/L
Potassium	Premature 4.5–7.2 mmol/L Term 3.2–5.7 mmol/L	3.3–4.7 mmol/L
Calcium (total)	Premature1.7–2.3 mmol/L Term 2.1–2.64 mmol/L or 8.4–10.6 mg/dL	2.12–2.64 mmol/L or 8.5–10.6 mg/dL
Magnesium	0.65–1.02 mmol/L or 1.6–2.5 mg/dL	0.7–1.1 mmol/L or 1.6–2.7 mg/dL

* Laboratories may have slightly different levels of normal depending on assays performed. Always consult the normal values for your particular laboratory.
Source: Data from Soldin, 2005.

Table 13–4 Normal Blood pH and Gases

	Infants	Children	Adolescents
Arterial blood pH	7.18–7.50	7.27–7.49	7.35–7.41
Arterial blood oxygen partial pressure	60–70 mm Hg (8.0–9.3 pKa)	80–108 mm Hg (10.7–14.4 pKa)	80–100 mm Hg (10.7–13.3 pKa)
Arterial blood carbon dioxide partial pressure	27–41 mm Hg (3.6–5.5 pKa)	32–48 mm Hg (4.3–6.4 pKa)	32–48 mm Hg (4.3–6.4 pKa)
Arterial blood bicarbonate	19–24 mmol/L	18–25 mmol/L	20–29 mmol/L

Source: Data from Soldin, 2005.

Box 13-1   Oral Rehydration Therapy Guidelines

Calculate the specific amounts required for individual children based on the guidelines below and instruct parents in terminology they understand. Provide measuring devices, with proper amounts marked.

- Children with diarrhea and no dehydration should be continued on age-appropriate diets.
- For minimal dehydration, if the child weighs less than 10 kg, give 60–120 mL oral rehydration solution (ORS) for each diarrheal stool or vomiting episode; if over 10 kg in weight, give 120–240 mL ORS for each diarrheal stool or vomiting episode. Meanwhile, continue breastfeeding, or resume age-appropriate diet after initial hydration.
- Start slowly, administering 3–5 mL in a small cup or spoon every few minutes. Increase amounts gradually if no vomiting occurs.
- Recommend or provide samples of oral rehydration therapy solutions. Suggest ready-to-feed or powdered forms for choice by parents.
- For moderate dehydration, give 50–100 mL/kg oral rehydration therapy in first 3–4 hours and replace fluids lost in each stool/vomiting episode.
- For severe dehydration, the child is hospitalized and treated with intravenous fluids. When hydrated adequately or concurrently with intravenous rehydration, begin oral rehydration therapy with 50–100 mL/kg of fluid in 4 hours and stool replacement as described above.
- Recalculate fluid needs after first 4 hours and adjust as needed. If the child is not taking increased fluids and not otherwise improving by this time, contact healthcare provider.
- When rehydration is complete, resume normal diet.

Source: Data from "Managing Acute Gastroenteritis Among Children: Oral Rehydration, Maintenance, and Nutritional Therapy," 2004, *Pediatrics 114,* 507.

Box 13-2 Calculation of Fluid Needs

1. First, calculate the maintenance fluid needs of the child, according to the following guidelines:

Usual Weight	Maintenance Amount
Up to 10 kg	100 mL/kg/24 hr
11–20 kg	1,000 mL + (50 mL/kg for weight above 10 kg)/24 hr
Over 20 kg	1,500 mL + (20 mL/kg for weight above 20 kg)/24 hr

2. Next, calculate replacement fluid for that lost. To calculate the child's percentage of weight loss:
   - Subtract the child's present weight from the original weight to find the loss.
   - Divide the loss by the child's original weight.
   - Multiply the percentage of body weight loss (in %) × 10 to reach the mL/kg/24 hour requirement.
3. Finally, calculate continued losses and add to the total maintenance and replacement needs.

Note: These fluid needs are for normal children who have a problem causing dehydration. In special circumstances, such as very-low-birth-weight infants, or children with problems such as renal disease, the maintenance amounts need to be adjusted. Consult with specialists treating the child and specialized references to learn about fluid needs in these situations.

14 ALTERATIONS IN EYE, EAR, NOSE, AND THROAT FUNCTION

DISORDERS OF THE EYE

Infectious Conjunctivitis

Conjunctivitis is an inflammation of the conjunctiva, the clear membrane that lines the inside of the lid and sclera. There are several types of conjunctivitis, depending on the cause of inflammation. Bacteria, viruses, allergies, trauma, or irritants cause the conjunctiva to become swollen and red, with a clear, yellow, or white discharge.

Clinical Manifestations

Symptoms depend on the type of conjunctivitis and provide clues to diagnosis.

Bacterial conjunctivitis in an infant younger than 30 days of age is called *ophthalmia neonatorum*. These infections are usually acquired from the mother during vaginal delivery as a result of contact with infected vaginal discharge containing organisms such as *Chlamydia trachomatis* and *Neisseria gonorrhoeae*. Redness, swelling, and exudate are characteristic.

Bacterial conjunctivitis can occur in older children as well. It is characterized by edema of the eyelid, red conjunctiva, and enlarged preauricular lymph glands. There is usually mucopurulent exudate that causes matting, making the eyes difficult to open on awakening. Older children with conjunctivitis complain of itching or burning, mild photophobia, and a feeling of scratching under the lids.

Viral conjunctivitis may cause redness, swelling, and tearing of the eyes. Adenoviruses are common causes. Herpesviruses may be accompanied by herpes lesions on the face and are serious viral infections.

In allergic conjunctivitis, the child complains of intense itching. Eyes are red and swollen, with watery discharge; the conjunctivae have a "cobblestone" appearance. This condition is not infectious and is simply related to allergy.

Diagnostic Tests

Diagnosis is based on the history and symptoms.

Cultures may be taken, especially in infants or in cases suspected of being unusual bacterial illness or herpesviruses.

A Gram stain of discharge and conjunctival scraping for potential *Chlamydia* infection or herpes may be performed.

Clinical Therapy

Clinical therapy includes routine prophylaxis of all infants to prevent ophthalmia neonatorum; penicillin, tetracycline, erythromycin, or povidone-iodine ointments may be used.

Antibiotic eye medication in droplet or ointment form for bacterial infection can be used; fluoroquinolones are frequently used.

For gonococcal conjunctivitis in newborns, ceftriaxone is recommended; the disease is resistant to penicillin.

Chlamydial infections are treated with oral erythromycin or tetracycline.

Viral conjunctivitis is treated with comfort measures such as cleaning drainage away with a warm clean cloth, avoiding bright lights, and avoiding reading.

Herpes simplex virus infections of the eye are treated promptly by an ophthalmologist, neonatologist, or others trained in treating this serious disease. Topical drugs are used and often are combined with a systemic antiviral agent such as acyclovir. Neonatal herpes simplex virus is treated vigorously with parenteral acyclovir for 14 days (or longer if central nervous system involvement is found on lumbar puncture) and with topical ophthalmic medication (trifluridine, iododeoxyuridine, or vidarabine). Recurrent lesions may necessitate suppressive or prophylactic treatment with oral acyclovir (American Academy of Pediatrics, 2006).

If an allergen is diagnosed as the cause of conjunctivitis, systemic or topical antihistamines, or topical steroids and vasoconstrictors, may be prescribed (Abelson & Granet, 2006). Decongestants can be combined with systemic antihistamines for short-term therapy. More current treatment involves use of mast cell stabilizers in children over 3 years to decrease the activation of mast cells that accompanies allergic reactions.

Nursing Management

Assess eyes of infants and children for any signs of conjunctivitis.

Refer the child to an ophthalmologist or other care provider for diagnosis and treatment.

Administer eye medications as prescribed.

Isolate children infected with bacterial or viral agents from others in the hospital; they should be kept home from school for bacterial conjunctivitis until treated with antibiotics for 24 hours.

Be alert for infections in childcare and school settings so that spread to other children can be minimized.

Teach parents correct administration of medications, comfort measures, and proper hygiene to prevent spread of infection to others.

Visual Disorders
Clinical Manifestations

In hyperopia (farsightedness), light rays focus posterior to the retina, resulting in an inability to focus on nearby objects.

In myopia (nearsightedness), light rays focus anterior to the retina, resulting in an inability to focus on far objects.

In astigmatism, light rays are refracted differently depending on their place of entry to the eye because the curvature of the cornea or lens is not uniformly spherical, causing blurred images.

Strabismus is an abnormal deviation or misalignment of the eye, usually inward or outward due to a weak eye muscle; the eyes are misaligned so that binocularity of vision does not occur.

In amblyopia, or reduced vision of the eye, generally one eye has much poorer vision than the other, resulting in loss of binocularity.

A cataract is opacity of the lens that is present at birth or develops during childhood.

Glaucoma is increased intraocular pressure that changes the structure of the eye and can lead to visual impairment and blindness if untreated.

Depending on the disorder and severity, the child may have asymmetric eye movements, have asymmetric light reflex, hold the head to one side, squint, have watering eyes or headaches, and/or show developmental delays.

See Table 14–1 for further detail on clinical manifestations of visual disorders.

Diagnostic Tests

Diagnostic tests include those for visual acuity and developmental testing, as well as ophthalmologic examination.

Table 14–1   Clinical Manifestations of Visual Disorders

Etiology	Clinical Manifestations
Strabismus Can be congenital or acquired.	Eyes appear misaligned to observer.
Seen in up to 4% of all children; 30–50% of children with strabismus develop amblyopia.	May occur only when child is tired.
Most common types:	Symptoms include squinting and frowning when reading; closing one eye to see; having trouble picking up objects; dizziness and headache.
Esotropia: inward deviation of eyes ("crossed eyes").	Corneal light reflex and cover-uncover tests confirm diagnosis.
Exotropia: outward deviation of eyes ("wall eyes"). Strabismus	Child may have no other abnormalities, but certain conditions such as cerebral palsy, hydrocephalus, Down syndrome, and seizure disorder are more commonly accompanied by strabismus.
	If treatment is begun before 24 months of age, amblyopia (reduced vision in one or both eyes) may be prevented.
Amblyopia ("lazy eye") Reduced vision in one or both eyes; affects up to 4% of children.	Symptoms are the same as for strabismus.
Can result from anything that causes visual deprivation to one eye. The most common causes are untreated strabismus, with the child "tuning out" the image in deviating eye, congenital cataract, or uncorrected refractive errors causing visual differences between eyes.	Vision testing can be used to diagnose condition.
Cataracts Occur when all or part of lens of eye becomes opaque, which prevents refraction of light rays onto retina.	Can affect one or both eyes and may be congenital or acquired.
Seen in 2/10,000 newborns. Congenital cataract	Clouding of lens indicates presence of cataract; however, cataracts are not always visible to naked eye.
	Symptoms include distorted red reflex, symptoms of vision loss (see Strabismus), white pupil.
	May be present alone but sometimes associated with fetal alcohol syndrome, Turner syndrome, and Down syndrome.

Table 14–1   Clinical Manifestations of Visual Disorders (Continued)

Etiology	Clinical Manifestations
Glaucoma	
Increased intraocular pressure damages eye and impairs visual function; ciliary body of eye produces aqueous fluid that flows between iris and lens into anterior chamber; if enough fluid accumulates, blindness results; affects 1 in 100,000 newborns.	Symptoms of congenital glaucoma include tearing, blinking, corneal clouding, eyelid spasms, and progressive enlargement of eye; photophobia (extreme sensitivity to light).
May be congenital (occurring in first 3 years of life) or juvenile (occurring from 3–30 years) and affect one or both eyes.	Symptoms of juvenile glaucoma include constant bumping into objects in child's periphery (painless visual field loss); seeing halos around objects.
Congenital glaucoma	Diagnosis is made using tonometer, which measures intraocular pressure.

Source: Data from Donahue, 2007.

Clinical Therapy

Refraction errors are commonly treated by compensatory corrective lenses (glasses or contact lenses).

Clinical therapy for strabismus includes compensatory lenses, occlusion therapy, surgery, and visual therapy (eye exercises).

Amblopia is treated with compensatory lenses, occlusion therapy, visual therapy, and sometimes atropine eye drops.

Cataracts are treated by surgical lens removal with lens implant and/or corrective lenses.

Surgery is used to reduce intraocular pressure in glaucoma, followed by corrective lenses; medications to reduce pressure are sometimes effective.

Nursing Management

Assessment

Observe for

- Visual acuity.
- Symmetry of eye movement.
- Ability to follow objects in all planes.
- Symmetry of light reflex.
- Developmental progression.

Obtain a complete and thorough history.

Table 14–2   Assessment Questions for Identifying Visual Disturbances in Children

Infant	Young Child	School-Age Child
Ask the parents the following:	Ask the parents the following:	Ask the parents the following:
Does your baby follow an object from one side to the other?	Does your child follow you with his or her eyes as you come into a room?	Does your child like to look at pictures and read?
What is your baby's reaction when you are directly in front and close?	Are other objects followed with ease?	Does your child hold toys or books close or sit very close to the television?
Does the baby seem to notice an object to the right and left sides?	Do both eyes work together or does one seem to wander off?	Does your child squint or rub the eyes?
Do your baby's eyes ever appear to move asymmetrically?	At what age did your baby sit, stand, and walk?	Is he or she performing at grade level in all subjects?
What is your baby learning to do right now?	Does your child have any difficulty picking up objects?	Has your child demonstrated any learning difficulties?
	Do the child's eyes appear crossed in photos?	Does he or she use a computer, watch television, or play computer games?
		Does your child play sports and games at the same level of ability as peers?

Examine for risk factors such as prematurity and low birth weight.

See Table 14–2 for assessment of visual disorders.

Implementation
Refer all abnormalities to eye specialist.

Teach importance of prescribed treatments.

Teach correct care for compensatory lenses, postsurgical care, and medication instillation.

Encourage interactions and skills that promote development.

Retinopathy of Prematurity
Clinical Manifestations
Retinopathy of prematurity occurs when immature blood vessels in the retina constrict and become necrotic. This condition, most

common in infants of low birth weight or of short gestation who have other health problems and receive assisted ventilation, can heal completely or lead to mild myopia or retinal detachment and blindness.

Arteriole constriction, followed by vascular proliferation of abnormal vessels, occurs. In most cases, the abnormal vessels gradually regress and normal vascularization occurs. Sometimes, however, the abnormal vascularization continues into the vitreous cavity, causing abnormalities of the retina, optic disk, and macula.

When visual impairment is present, the child usually manifests myopia. Total loss of vision can occur in the child who experiences a retinal detachment.

Diagnostic Tests
Ophthalmologic examination is indicated.

All infants under 1,500 g (3 lb, 7 oz) at birth and born before 32 weeks' gestation, as well as infants born after 32 weeks' gestation with other risks of ROP who are 1,500 to 2,000 g (3 lb, 7 oz to 4 lb, 3 oz), are assessed frequently by an experienced ophthalmologist.

The disease does not manifest itself before 4 to 6 weeks after birth, so regular eye examinations are needed until the risk is discounted.

For infants with signs of disease, eye examinations continue every 1 to 2 weeks.

Clinical Therapy
Laser therapy

Surgical procedures such as a scleral buckle procedure and vitrectomy for retinal detachments

Treatment of associated visual problems such as strabismus, amblyopia, and myopia to promote maximal development

See Table 14–3.

Nursing Management
Assessment
Assess for risk factors such as prematurity, low birth weight, and oxygen therapy with assisted ventilation.

Monitor respiratory status.

Monitor ventilatory equipment for performance and proper settings.

Table 14–3   Assessment and Treatment for Retinopathy of Prematurity (ROP)

Initial Assessment	Follow-Up Assessment
Who? All infants less than 1,500 g or less than 28 weeks' gestation; babies 1,500–2,000 g who have other risk factors	Every 2–3 weeks if vasculature is immature and extends to zone II but no retinopathy is present; Stage 1 or 2 ROP Zone III; or regressing ROP in Zone III. Every 2 weeks if ROP is Stage 1, Zone II, or regressing ROP in Zone II.
When? 4–9 weeks postnatal age or 31–36 weeks of postconceptual age	Every 2 weeks if ROP is Stage 1, Zone II or regressing ROP in Zone II.
What? Pupil dilation using binocular indirect ophthalmoscopy by an ophthalmologist experienced in ROP; one examination is satisfactory if full retinal vascularization is seen bilaterally	Every 1–2 weeks if no ROP but having incomplete vasculature in zone I; Stage 2 ROP, Zone II; regressing ROP, Zone I. Every week for infants with ROP in Stage 1 or 2; Zone I, Stage 3 ROP.

Source: Data from American Academy of Pediatrics, 2006.

Implementation
Refer to ophthalmologist as needed.

Provide kinesthetic, tactile, and auditory stimulation during play and in daily care.

Evaluate the environment for potential safety hazards based on age of child and degree of visual impairment.

Evaluate growth and development during all regular examinations as the child grows.

Patient and Family Education
Encourage parents of newborns at risk to return for scheduled appointments with ophthalmologist and developmental monitoring.

Help parents plan early, regular social activities with other children.

Refer parents to organizations, early intervention programs, and other parents of children with visual impairments.

Partner with parents during ongoing interventions to meet developmental, educational, and safety needs of the child with visual impairment.

See further suggestions for working with the child with visual impairment in Visual Impairment section.

Visual Impairment
Clinical Manifestations
Low vision, or the inability to correct vision to a normal level, is present in 1.2 to 1.4 children per 100. About 2% to 3% of children have visual impairment or blindness (Centers for Disease Control and Prevention, 2004).

Eyes may appear crossed or watery, and the lids may be crusty.

Verbal children may complain of itching; dizziness; headache; or blurred, double, or poor vision.

See Table 14–4 for further signs of visual impairment in children.

Diagnostic Tests
Vision screening, followed by referral to an eye specialist for full examination for any abnormalities

Responses to visual stimuli, symmetry of eye movements, location of corneal light reflex, cover-uncover testing, visual field testing, and funduscopic examination of retina

Clinical Therapy
Surgery

Medication

Supportive aids such as glasses or contact lenses

Management by an interdisciplinary team of specialists to treat condition and maximize development

Nursing Management
Visual screening appropriate for age at each health promotion examination

Visual acuity programs in schools

Table 14–4   Signs of Visual Impairment

Infants	Toddlers and Older Children
May be unable to follow lights or objects	May rub, shut, or cover eyes
Do not make eye contact	Tilt or thrust head forward
Have a dull, vacant stare	Blink frequently
Do not imitate facial expressions	Hold objects close
	Bump into objects
	Squint

Developmental screening; abnormalities may indicate visual impairment.

Teach safety, and encourage protective eyewear in activities such as sports (e.g., hockey, handball, football).

Work with school personnel to establish guidelines for protective eyewear for chemistry and other science or industrial education courses.

Keep laser pointers away from children because they can cause retinal damage, especially when stared at for 10 seconds or longer.

For the child with visual impairment, nursing care focuses on encouraging the child's use of all senses, promoting socialization, helping parents to meet the child's developmental and educational needs, and providing emotional support to parents.

Announce another person's presence to the child when approaching.

When walking with a blind child, walk slightly ahead of the child so he or she can sense your movements.

Let the child hold the seeing person's arm rather than the reverse.

Identify the contents of meals and encourage the child to feed himself or herself.

Orient the child to new settings by explaining and allowing the child to feel objects.

Patient and Family Education

Stroke, rock, and hug infants and children who are visually impaired. Sing and talk to them. Infants with visual impairment appreciate and use touch and verbal interactions more, both in interactions with others and when exploring new objects. These infants do not make eye contact and have rather blank expressions. Encourage parents to plan for interactions between the child and a variety of other children.

Teach parents to read body language and vocalization as expressions of emotion. Facial expressions give a great deal of information, but infants and children with poor vision do not have the ability to learn by visual imitation. Show parents how to use tactile means to teach appropriate facial expressions. For example, a touch on the arm can be soft and stroking to indicate a smile, but firmer to indicate dismay or frown.

Explain to parents that discipline and rewards for children with poor vision should be the same as those for other children in the family. The child should be given age-appropriate tasks.

Encourage contact with peers as the child grows older. Teach the child to look directly at persons who are talking to him or her. Play, sports, and other activities can be modified to give the visually impaired child the same social experiences as a sighted child.

Foster physical activity for visually impaired children by encouraging involvement in early intervention programs; recommending programs that increase cardiovascular strength, endurance, upper body strength, and flexibility; and facilitating participation in and reward for sports and athletics. Ensure safety to prevent injury around the home, at school, and in other settings.

Provide parents with information about educational options before their child reaches school age. Education should take place in a setting that allows the child to have contact with other children and to participate in social activities. As the child enters middle and high school, it may be challenging to move to new schools or communities unfamiliar to the child. Help the parents to plan activities that will enable the youth to meet new friends.

The child may be mainstreamed with a tutor, be partially mainstreamed in a resource room, attend special classes, or be tutored at home. If the child is to attend public school, suggest to parents that they contact the school well before enrollment to ensure that school staff plans for the individualized educational needs of the child.

Make sure that items such as large-print books, Braille materials, audio equipment, or a visual reading device is available. Ensure that frequent eye examinations are performed, and assist with proper use and care of prescribed glasses or contact lenses, as necessary.

Injuries of the Eye

Sports, darts, fireworks, air-powered BB guns, paint balls, blunt and sharp objects, chemical and thermal burns, physical irritants, and abuse are common causes of eye trauma in children (Kliegman, Behrman, Jenson, et al., 2007).

Teach about protective eyewear for sports and other hazardous activities.

Inquire about tetanus immunization history for all eye injuries; if a booster has not been administered in 5 years or more or if basic tetanus series is not completed, administer tetanus-diphtheria-acellular pertussis booster (Tdap).

Table 14–5   Clinical Manifestations and Emergency Treatment of Eye Injuries

Condition and Etiology	Clinical Manifestations
Subconjunctival hemorrhage (caused by coughing, mild trauma, or increased physical activity)	Reddened area in conjunctiva
Periorbital ecchymosis	"Black eye," or bruising of the skin around the eye
Foreign body on conjunctiva	Intense pain or feeling of something in the eye
Corneal abrasion	Intense pain and redness
Burns (alkaline burns readily penetrate cornea and are more serious than acid burns)	Pain and/or complaints of "blindness" or vision loss
Penetrating and perforating injuries	Pain
Eye injuries caused by severe blows to head and eye (blunt trauma can seriously injure all eye structures, including orbit, which can be fractured)	Pain and redness

See Table 14–5 for further information on clinical manifestations of eye injuries.

Ice application is used for subconjunctival hemorrhage; corneal abrasions must be examined and treated by an ophthalmologist; chemical burns are immediately treated with irrigation followed by transfer to emergency facility; emergency care is always needed for penetrating injuries and blows to the eye.

DISORDERS OF THE EAR

Otitis Media
Clinical Manifestations

Otitis media is common, with approximately 70% of infants having at least one case in the first year of life, and 93% affected by age 7 years; peak incidence occurs from 6 to 20 months of age (Bernius & Perlin, 2006). The short, horizontal eustachian tube of young children puts them at risk for this infection.

Risk factors include young age (6–12 months), males, attendance at childcare centers, having allergies, exposure to tobacco smoke, and extensive pacifier use; winter months and conditions such as cleft lip and palate or Down syndrome also predispose children; breastfeeding is protective against otitis media.

Acute otitis media (AOM) is diagnosed when the child has acute onset of ear pain, marked redness of the tympanic membrane on otoscopy, and middle ear effusion; recurrent AOM is characterized by repeated episodes of AOM, such as three in 6 months, or four in 12 months.

Otitis media with effusion (OME) is evidence of fluid in the middle ear without inflammation.

Pulling at the ear is a sign of ear pain.

Diarrhea, vomiting, and fever are typical of otitis media.

Irritability with night awakenings and crying is common due to increased pressure when prone or supine.

Diagnostic Tests
Diagnosis of otitis media is based on otoscopic examination, often accompanied by pneumatic otoscopy and/or tympanography.

AOM is diagnosed by a history of acute and rapid onset, irritability, malaise, and poor feeding. On otoscopy, there is a bulging tympanic membrane, air fluid behind the membrane, decreased mobility, erythema, loss of light reflex, or change in landmarks (Subcommittee on Management of Acute Otitis Media, 2004).

OME is diagnosed by decreased response to sounds, decreased tympanic membrane mobility with pneumatic otoscopy and tympanography, and loss of landmarks.

Clinical Therapy
AOM treatment is delayed 48 to 72 hours in children aged 6 months to 2 years with nonsevere illness at presentation **and** uncertain diagnosis or in children 2 years and older without severe symptoms **or** with uncertain diagnosis; many children improve without specific treatment.

When needed, AOM is treated with antibiotic therapy for 10 days in children younger than age 6 years and 5 to 7 days for children 6 years and older.

Ibuprofen, acetaminophen, topical anesthetic eardrops, or herbal eardrops (a naturopathic herbal extract of *Allium sativum, Verbascum thapsus, Calendula flores*, and *Hypericum perforatum, lavender,* and *vitamin E*) may be used for pain relief.

OME is not treated with antibiotics but is evaluated periodically to be sure there is not an additional AOM that needs treatment; improvement usually occurs within 3 months.

Because OME is more commonly associated with hearing loss and cochlear damage, follow-up with audiology is essential; if hearing is abnormal, speech testing should be performed (Otitis Media with Effusion, 2004).

If infections recur despite antibiotic treatment for AOM or if OME continues 4 months or more with persistent hearing loss present, myringotomy (surgical incision of the tympanic membrane) may be performed, and tympanostomy tubes (pressure-equalizing tubes) may be inserted to drain fluid from the middle ear.

Nursing Management

Assessment

The tympanic membrane is assessed by otoscopy at each health promotion visit and during examinations for illness; examine the color, transparency, mobility, presence of landmarks, and light reflex.

Ask parents if the child has had a fever, been fussy, or been pulling at the ears. Inquire about the family's methods of pain relief for the child.

Observe for signs of impaired hearing, observing for the child's ability to hear whispered or soft sounds.

Implementation

Emphasize preventive measures to decrease risk factors for otitis media; prevention includes avoiding exposure to secondhand smoke, not placing babies to sleep with a pacifier, encouraging breastfeeding, and keeping immunizations up to date.

Explain treatment goals and plans; many parents may not understand why antibiotics are not used for every infection. When antibiotics and analgesics are prescribed, perform needed teaching.

Prepare for day surgery if myringotomy and tubes are the treatment choice.

Continue to monitor hearing, speech, and developmental milestones.

Hearing Impairment

About 1 million children in the United States have some form of hearing impairment (Yaeger, McCallum, Lewis, et al., 2006).

Clinical Manifestations

Conductive hearing loss occurs when conditions in the external auditory canal or tympanic membrane prevent sound from reaching the middle ear; it usually develops over time and can be treated. *Sensorineural hearing loss* occurs when the hair cells in the cochlea or along the vestibulocochlear (acoustic) nerve (cranial nerve VIII) are damaged. This leads to permanent hearing loss. A *mixed hearing loss* indicates a hearing loss having a combination of conductive and sensorineural causes.

Lack of normal speech or language, developmental delays occur; findings are related to degree of hearing impairment (Table 14–6).

See Table 14–7 for behavioral signs typical of hearing impairment.

Diagnostic Tests

Audiologic testing should be conducted for all newborn infants and regularly through childhood.

Otoscopic examination and tympanogram should be performed during health promotion visits.

Clinical Therapy

Removal of impediments in conductive loss

Hearing aid, bone conduction hearing aid, surgical placement of cochlear implants

Speech therapy and instructions in lipreading, signing, cueing, and fingerspelling

See Table 14–8 for communication techniques.

Table 14–6   Severity of Hearing Loss

Type of Loss	Decibel Level (dB)	Hearing Ability
Slight/mild	20–40	Some speech sounds are difficult to perceive, particularly unvoiced consonant sounds.
Moderate	41–60	Most normal conversational speech sounds are missed.
Severe	61–80	Speech sounds cannot be heard at a normal conversational level.
Profound	81–90	No speech sounds can be heard.
Deaf	>90	No sound at all can be heard.

Source: Data from American Speech-Language-Hearing Association, 2008.

Table 14–7 Behaviors Suggestive of Hearing Impairment

Age	Behavior
Infant	Has a diminished or absent startle reflex to loud sound
	Does not awaken when environment is very noisy
	Awakens only to touch
	Does not turn head to sound at 3–4 months
	Does not localize sound at 6–10 months
	Babbles little or not at all
Toddler and preschooler	Speaks unintelligibly, in a monotone, or not at all
	Communicates needs through gestures
	Appears developmentally delayed
	Appears emotionally immature, yells inappropriately
	Does not respond to doorbell or telephone
	Appears more interested in objects than people and prefers to play alone
	Focuses on facial expressions rather than verbal communications
School-age child and adolescent	Asks to have statements repeated
	Answers questions inappropriately, except when able to view speaker's face
	Daydreams and is inattentive
	Performs poorly at school or is truant
	Has speech abnormalities or speaks in a monotone
	Sits close to or turns television or radio up loudly
	Prefers to play alone

Nursing Management

Assessment

Conduct newborn hearing tests soon after birth; make observations of the infant's responses to sound.

Assess hearing at every well-child visit by observations of development, audiography, and tympanography.

Ask parents if they have concerns about their child's hearing; they are often the first to diagnose a hearing impairment.

Language milestones should be evaluated in the older infant and child with hearing impairment.

Evaluate hearing by audiography during screening programs in schools, and refer children who do not pass the screening test.

Monitor developmental milestones frequently in children with hearing impairment.

Table 14–8 Communication Techniques for Children Who Are Hearing Impaired

Technique	Description
Cued speech	Supplement to lipreading; eight hand shapes represent groups of consonant sounds, and four positions about the face represent groups of vowel sounds; based on the sounds the letters make, not the letters themselves; child can "see-hear" every spoken syllable a hearing person hears.
Oral approach	Uses only spoken language for face-to-face communication; avoids use of formal signs; uses hearing aids and residual hearing.
Total communication	Uses speech and sign, fingerspelling, lipreading, and residual hearing simultaneously; child selects communication technique depending on the situation.
Sign language	A language that allows the user to communicate quickly and accurately with others who understand signs. The signs, or hand movements, represent words or concepts. When a sign is not available, the word can be spelled out using signs. American Sign Language is most often used; British Sign Language is common in Europe.

Implementation

Encourage prevention of hearing loss due to exposure to loud noises such as from music and power and farm equipment; music should be turned down and ear protection worn for other activities.

Parents often need help to decide on the best method for hearing and language enhancement for the child.

Refer the parents to an early-intervention program as soon as the diagnosis of hearing impairment is made so as to foster the child's development.

Facilitate the child's ability to receive spoken language and to send information, help parents to meet the child's schooling needs, and provide emotional support to parents.

If a cochlear implant is planned, the child needs surgical care and follow-up to monitor results and integrate sound gradually into the child's life.

Patient and Family Education

Provide parents with information about adjustments that may have to be made for the hearing-impaired child who attends public school. By sitting at the front of the classroom, the child can hear and see more clearly. The teacher should always face the child when speaking, and background noise should be reduced.

Tell parents that children who are hearing impaired have the same intelligence quotient distribution as children without hearing impairment. However, communication and learning can be difficult, and extra support is needed.

Children with hearing impairment should reach their intellectual potential, although development in certain areas may take place more slowly than it does in children with no hearing impairment.

Teach care of hearing aids or other adaptive devices.

Teach the family about the community services available for medical, nursing, psychologic, and financial assistance. Link the family with the deaf or hearing-impaired community and resources.

Injuries of the Ear
Clinical Manifestations

Lacerations, infections, and hematomas may occur in the external ear structures, especially the pinna; children may place foreign objects in the ear, and insects may enter the ear canal. Rupture of the tympanic membrane may result from head injuries, blows to the ear, or insertion of objects into the ear canal. Serous drainage from the ear can indicate a basilar skull fracture due to accidents or child abuse (shaken child syndrome).

Earache, decreased hearing, imbalance problems, persistent bleeding, or other discharge may also occur (see Table 14–9 for emergency treatment of ear injuries).

Foreign bodies may need to be removed from the ears of young children. Ear is visualized with otoscope; objects may be removed with forceps, suction tip, hook, or irrigation (irrigation is avoided for materials that can absorb water because the object will swell, making removal even more difficult).

DISORDERS OF THE NOSE, MOUTH, AND THROAT

Epistaxis
Clinical Manifestations

Bleeding from the nose, unilateral or bilateral

Vomiting from swallowing large amounts of blood

Low hematocrit resulting from extended bleeding

Table 14–9 Emergency Treatment of Ear Injuries

Injury	Treatment
Pinna	
Minor cuts or abrasions	Wash thoroughly with soap and water and rinse well; leave exposed to air if possible or apply adhesive bandage; monitor for infection.
Hematomas	Needle aspiration should be performed and pressure dressing applied; undrained hematomas may become fibrotic; "cauliflower ear" deformity may develop.
Cellulitis or abscesses	Apply moist heat intermittently; make sure that prescribed antibiotic is taken; minor surgery may be performed for an abscess.
Deep lacerations	Apply pressure to stop bleeding; transport to physician's office or emergency department for suturing.
Ear canal	
Foreign bodies	Have child lie on back and turn head over edge of bed, with affected side down; wiggle earlobe, and have child shake head; foreign object may fall out as result of gravity; if object remains in ear, call physician; do not try to remove foreign body with tweezers because this may push the object further into the ear.
Insects	Shine flashlight into ear to try to attract insect; instilling a few drops of mineral oil, olive oil, or alcohol kills insect, and irrigating ear canal gently may remove dead insect.
Tympanic membrane	
Ruptures	Call physician if child has persistent ear pain after blow, blast injury, or insertion of foreign object; cover external ear loosely with piece of sterile cotton or gauze; if tympanic membrane has been ruptured, systemic antibiotics are prescribed.

Clinical Therapy

For anterior bleeding, child should sit upright quietly; the head should be tilted forward to prevent blood from trickling down the throat, which can lead to vomiting.

The nares should be squeezed just below the nasal bone and held for 10 to 15 minutes while the child breathes through the mouth; an ice bag can be applied to the nose or back of the neck.

If the bleeding does not stop, a cotton ball or swab soaked with phenylephrine (Neo-Synephrine), epinephrine, thrombin, or lidocaine may be inserted into the affected nostril to promote topical vasoconstriction or anesthesia.

Once the bleeding has stopped, the nostril may have to be cauterized with silver nitrate or electrocautery; if the bleeding cannot be stopped, absorbable packing may be used.

Posterior bleeding must also be stopped by packing, and the child must be monitored carefully; arterial ligation is occasionally needed.

Repeated or severe nosebleeds need further evaluation.

Nursing Management

Assess the child's hematocrit or hemoglobin if significant bleeding has occurred.

Children with frequent epistaxis should have a complete history taken and physical examination performed to rule out systemic disease.

Have the child avoid bending over, stooping, strenuous exercise, hot drinks, and hot baths or showers for 3 to 4 days after epistaxis.

Have the child sleep with the head elevated on two or three pillows; humidify the air with a vaporizer to prevent recurrence.

Nasopharyngitis

Known as the common cold or upper respiratory infection

Infection and inflammation of the nose and throat by one of more than 200 viruses or bacteria

Red nasal mucosa with clear nasal discharge and an infected throat with enlarged tonsils may be apparent; vesicles may be present on the soft palate and in the pharynx.

Lethargy, irritability, poor feeding, fever, and muscle aches are common.

For infants who cannot breathe through the mouth, normal saline nose drops can be administered every 3 to 4 hours, especially before feeding.

For infants older than 9 months of age, nasal stuffiness can be treated with normal saline nose drops followed by bulb syringe suction.

Decongestant nose drops and sprays should not be used for more than 4 or 5 days or more often than recommended.

Room humidification may help prevent drying of nasal secretions.

Antipyretics such as acetaminophen or ibuprofen reduce fever and make the child more comfortable; aspirin is not recommended because of its association with Reye syndrome.

Parents should NOT use cough and cold products in children under 2 years unless specifically directed to do so by the healthcare provider.

Ensure adequate intake of fluid to liquefy secretions.

Proper hand hygiene and disposal of tissues help to decrease the spread of the infection.

Sinusitis

Sinusitis is inflammation of one or more of the paranasal sinuses characterized by purulent nasal drainage or other symptoms; there is often accompanying facial pain, headache, and fever.

A history of recent upper respiratory infection is common, persistent cough from postnasal drip can occur, and nasal discharge or swelling can be apparent. Malodorous breath, fever, mouth breathing, hyponasal speech, and cervical lymphadenopathy may be present (Bernius & Perlin, 2006).

Young children may be anorexic or have difficulty feeding; older children may complain of headache.

Most sinusitis is treated with antibiotics, and recurrent cases are referred for further care by an otolaryngologist and allergy specialist.

Pharyngitis

Acute pharyngitis is an infection that primarily affects the pharynx, including the tonsils, and is caused by a virus or bacteria (see Table 14–10 for common symptoms of viral and bacterial pharyngitis).

Diagnosis is made by assessment; throat cultures are taken in cases of suspected bacterial infection and with history of exposure to strep throat.

Strep throat should be treated with oral penicillin for 10 days or by long-acting penicillin given in one injection; erythromycin, azithromycin, and clarithromycin are also sometimes prescribed.

Teach parents the importance of completing the entire course of antibiotics if prescribed for bacterial pharyngitis. After the child is on the medication for approximately 2 days, have the parents replace the child's toothbrush with a new one to avoid reinfection by bacteria that can survive on the moist brush.

Viral pharyngitis is treated symptomatically with acetaminophen, cool, nonacidic fluids and soft foods, ice chips, or frozen juice pops. Humidification, chewing gum, and gargling with warm salt water (5 g to 250 mL water; 0.25 teaspoon to 8 oz water) soothe an irritated throat.

Table 14–10 **Clinical Manifestations of Viral Pharyngitis and Strep Throat (Group A Beta-Hemolytic Streptococcus)[a]**

Viral Pharyngitis	Strep Throat
Nasal congestion	Abrupt onset
Mild sore throat	Tonsillar exudate[b]
Conjunctivitis	Painful cervical lymphadenopathy[b]
Cough	Anorexia, nausea, vomiting, abdominal pain
Hoarseness	Severe sore throat
Mild pharyngeal redness	Headache, malaise
Minimal tonsillar exudate	Fever $>38.3°C$ (101°F)
Mildly tender anterior cervical lymphadenopathy	Petechial mottling of soft palate
Fever $\leq 38.3°C$ (101°F)	

[a]Children 6 months to 3 years of age may have streptococcus with symptoms that resemble those of viral pharyngitis. Children with scarlet fever have the symptoms of strep throat plus a sandpaper-textured erythematous generalized rash and pallor around the lips.
[b]Classic signs of strep throat.

Tonsillitis

Tonsillitis is an infection or inflammation (hypertrophy) of the palatine tonsils caused by virus or bacteria.

Symptoms and signs include frequent throat infections with breathing and swallowing difficulties, persistent redness of the anterior pillars, enlargement of the cervical lymph nodes, and dry and irritated mucous membranes.

Diagnosis is made on the basis of visual inspection and clinical manifestations; tonsils appear large and inflamed.

Symptomatic treatment for tonsillitis is the same as for pharyngitis.

Surgical removal of tonsils (tonsillectomy) is often recommended when children have recurrent throat infections (approximately three per year for 3 years), chronic tonsillitis, obstructive sleep apnea, or malformations causing nasal speech or a facial growth abnormality.

Care after tonsillectomy includes the following:
■ Have the child drink adequate cool fluids or chew gum, as this reduces spasms in the muscles surrounding the throat.

- Give acetaminophen elixir as ordered (avoid aspirin and ibuprofen to decrease chance of bleeding).
- Apply an ice collar around the child's neck.
- Have the child gargle with a solution of 2.5 g (0.5 teaspoon) each of baking soda and salt in 8 oz of water.
- Have the child rinse the mouth well with viscous lidocaine and then swallow the solution.

Teach parents signs of complications such as hemorrhage or infection and how to seek emergency care for such conditions.

Mouth Ulcers

Mouth ulcers occur in a number of disease states and because of trauma.

Nurses examine mouth ulcers for size, location, drainage, and pain; for those at risk, such as children on chemotherapy, regular careful examinations of the oral mucosa are an important part of care.

Ensure that children have good oral care, including brushing teeth with a soft-bristle brush or by use of mouth sponges.

Rinse the mouth after all meals and snacks.

Teach the family correct administration of oral medications and topical preparations designed to treat infection or provide comfort.

When oral mucosa ulcers are predicted, such as with chemotherapy or in acquired immunodeficiency syndrome, begin oral protocols before lesions occur to decrease their appearance and severity (Shetty, 2006).

Encourage a diet that has only mild foods, avoiding spices and very sweet, sour, and acidic items; cold foods may be better accepted.

Monitor hydration status to ensure adequate fluid intake.

Teach parents the correct administration of acetaminophen or other analgesic treatment.

Use standard precautions to protect the child from infections and prevent their flora from being transferred to other children or family members.

Encourage parents to keep children with herpes gingivostomatitis out of contact with other children if active lesions or drooling are present (Blevins, 2003).

Mouth and Dental Emergencies

Teach the child and family to use mouth guards to protect from injury in sports.

When a tooth is removed during an injury, prompt treatment may influence the chance that it can be reimplanted. If the child's condition is stable, try to reimplant the tooth and then transfer the child to an emergency dental facility.

- Handle the tooth only by the crown (its top).
- Gently rinse the tooth with a stream of sterile saline. Do not place it under running water.
- Insert into the socket.
- Have the child provide gentle pressure by biting a piece of gauze or a tea bag.
- If child is unstable or has other injuries, enlist emergency medical transportation (call 911); transport the tooth with the child.
- If the tooth cannot be inserted into the child's mouth, place it in milk, saline, saliva, or water; if a dental aid kit is available, it may contain a transport liquid such as Viaspan or *Hank's Balanced Salt Solution* (Krause-Parello, 2005).

15 ALTERATIONS IN RESPIRATORY FUNCTION

URGENT RESPIRATORY THREATS: RESPIRATORY DISTRESS AND RESPIRATORY FAILURE

Assessment of the child's respiratory signs and symptoms is essential so care can be initiated to prevent respiratory distress from progressing to respiratory failure. Assess the following:

Respiratory rate (see chapter 1) and respiratory effort

Heart rate and quality of the pulse

Color

Cough

Behavior change

Signs of dehydration

Respiratory failure occurs when effective gas exchange can no longer be maintained due to an acute or chronic respiratory or neuromuscular condition. Hypoventilation occurs, leading to hypoxia, reflected in the child's behavior and vital signs. As respiratory distress progresses, hypoxemia and hypercarbia develop. Respiratory efforts waste more oxygen than is obtained. Without intervention, the oxygen deficit becomes overwhelming, and central nervous system changes are seen.

Clinical Manifestations

Signs of respiratory distress include tachypnea, retractions (use of accessory muscles), nasal flaring, inspiratory stridor, and expiratory grunting.

Signs of respiratory failure include the following:

Early: restlessness, tachypnea, tachycardia, and diaphoresis

Early decompensation: nasal flaring, retractions, grunting, wheezing, anxiety and irritability, mood changes, headache, hypertension, and confusion

Imminent respiratory arrest: dyspnea, bradycardia, cyanosis, stupor, and coma

Respiratory failure may develop gradually when the child has a chronic respiratory or neuromuscular condition. Be alert for subtle changes in respiratory signs and behavior.

Diagnostic Tests

Pulse oximetry and arterial blood gases assess respiratory distress and respiratory failure. See chapter 5 for arterial blood gas normal values. Signs of respiratory failure include hypercarbia in the presence of acidosis and hypoxemia unresponsive to supplemental oxygen.

Clinical Therapy

Reversal of severe hypoxemia is managed with oxygen, mechanical ventilation, and continuous positive end-expiratory pressure (CPAP) to increase functional residual capacity. Medical management is focused on treating the cause of respiratory failure. An endotracheal tube is used to stabilize the airway as necessary.

Nursing Management

Assessment

Perform the respiratory assessment. Attach a cardiorespiratory monitor and pulse oximeter. Frequently monitor the child's vital signs, respiratory status, and level of responsiveness.

If the child has an endotracheal tube or tracheostomy tube, assess for secretions, which may further obstruct the airway.

Implementation

Elevate the head of the bed, and keep the head in midline to help maintain the airway. Administer oxygen as ordered. Keep emergency equipment readily available.

Suction airway secretions as needed, and provide endotracheal/tracheostomy tube care if present. Provide good skin care around the tube to prevent skin breakdown under pressure points.

Provide support to parents and children, who will be stressed by this life-threatening disorder.

RESPIRATORY CONDITIONS

Apparent Life-Threatening Event

An episode of central or obstructive apnea occurring in a term infant who is younger than age 4 months. Potential causes include respiratory disorders, gastroesophageal reflux, seizures or breath-holding spells, cardiac arrhythmias, obstructive sleep apnea, a small mandible leading to airway obstruction, metabolic and endocrine problems, and child maltreatment.

Clinical Manifestations

Apnea, color change (cyanosis, pallor, or occasionally ruddiness), limp muscle tone, choking, gagging, unresponsiveness. No signs present at time of examination.

Episodes may occur during sleep, wakefulness, or feeding.

Diagnostic Tests

Tests determined from history and physical examination findings (Brand, Altman, Purtill, et al., 2005). The focus of the physical examination is to detect signs of injury, infection, neurologic abnormalities, or features suggestive of a genetic or metabolic syndrome. Potential testing includes a complete blood count, serum metabolic panel, lactate level, electrocardiogram, computed tomography (CT) scan of the head, electroencephalogram, or polysomnogram. No cause is found for half of ALTE cases (Fu & Moon, 2007).

Clinical Therapy

Observation and treatment of the underlying cause, if one is found. Physical stimulation or emergency resuscitation is usually required to revive the infant.

Nursing Management

Assessment

Collect detailed history about the characteristics and duration of the episode; relationship with feeding; sleep position, recent infections, medications, seizure activity; birth history or perinatal insults; any prior episodes; family history of infant deaths, apnea, or cardiac problems.

Assess respiratory function. Attach a cardiorespiratory monitor and pulse oximeter for continuous monitoring.

Implementation

Explain tests and treatment to increase parents' understanding of the situation and to reduce their fear and anxiety.

Encourage parents to hold infant and to participate in care. Encourage the mother to continue breastfeeding. Keep emergency resuscitation equipment and drugs accessible.

Teach parents how to use an apnea monitor if prescribed, how to respond to an apneic episode, and techniques for choking intervention. Encourage parents to attend a cardiopulmonary resuscitation class.

ASTHMA

A chronic inflammatory airway disorder with acute exacerbations or persistent symptoms, caused by the interplay of multiple factors (environmental exposures, viral illnesses, allergens, and a genetic predisposition) that occur at a crucial time in the immune system development. Most children experience their first symptoms before 5 years of age.

The inflammation of an asthma flare (sudden onset of breathing difficulty with cough, wheeze, or breathlessness) leads to mucous formation, mucosal swelling, airway muscle contraction, and airway obstruction. Asthma flare triggers include exercise, infectious agents, allergens, fragrances, food additives, pollutants, weather changes, exercise, and emotions. Decreased perfusion of the alveolar capillaries leads to hypoxemia. Repeated episodes lead to chronic inflammatory changes and airway remodeling that are not fully responsive to current therapy (Brashers, 2006).

Clinical Manifestations

Coughing, expiratory wheeze, shortness of breath, chest tightness, respiratory fatigue, rapid and labored breathing, nasal flaring, intercostal retractions, decreased air movement, and anxiety

Head bobbing when accessory muscles (sternocleidomastoids) are used to breathe

Wheezing may not be heard with poor airflow due to severe obstruction.

Agitation or lethargic irritability due to hypoxia and cumulative effect of medications

Diagnostic Tests

A spirometer or pulmonary function test to measure expiratory flow volume and severity of airway obstruction

A chest radiograph if problems such as a foreign body or pneumonia could be present

Skin testing may be used to identify allergens that trigger asthma.

Clinical Therapy

Pharmacologic therapies are matched to the severity of asthma (intermittent or mild, moderate, or severe persistent) for long-term management of asthma. Control of asthma symptoms long term using the least amount of medication is the goal. A stepwise approach to medication therapy is now recommended that matches the child's asthma severity, adding or changing specific medications if the severity progresses (National Asthma Education and Prevention Program, 2007, p. 284). See Table 15–1 for the national treatment guidelines for children age 5 years and older. A similar guideline exists for children younger than 5 years available at http://www.nhlbi.nih.gov/guidelines/asthma/asthgdln.htm. See medications used in Table 15–2.

Signs of good asthma control for children include the following (National Asthma Education and Prevention Program, 2007, pp. 309, 310, 345):

- Symptoms 2 or fewer days a week
- Nighttime awakenings no more than once a month (twice a month in 12 years and older)
- No interference with normal activity, school, or exercise
- Use of short acting beta$_2$-agonist used for symptom control 2 or fewer days a week
- Greater than 80% of predicted peak flow (in children 5 years and older)
- No more than 1 asthma flare a year requiring oral system corticosteroids

Children should have a detailed written asthma action plan for managing asthma at school and at home.

Nursing Management
Assessment
Assess the ABCs—airway, breathing, and circulation—to make sure that the child's condition is not life-threatening.

Assess the respiratory system for rate, retractions, quality of breath sounds, presence or absence of wheezing, cough or stridor, color, and heart rate. Assess the child's anxiety.

Attach a pulse oximeter to monitor oxygen saturation. Assess peak expiratory flow rate, skin turgor, intake and output, and urine specific gravity. Then complete the assessment to identify other associated problems.

Implementation
Maintain the airway; provide supplemental humidified oxygen by cannula or face mask. Position child in semi-Fowler or upright position.

Administer aerosol medications. Monitor for side effects of medications.

Table 15-1 Classification of Asthma Severity in Children 5 to 11 Years of Age and 12 Years to Adulthood

Components of Severity		Classification of Asthma Severity (5 to 11 Years of Age and 12 Years to Adulthood)			
		Intermittent	Persistent		
			Mild	Moderate	Severe
Impairment	Symptoms	2 or fewer days a week	Greater than 2 days a week, but not daily	Daily	Throughout the day
	Nighttime Awakenings	2 times or less per month	3 to 4 times a month	Greater than 1 time a week, but not nightly	Often 7 times a week
	Short-acting beta$_2$ agonist use for symptom control (not prevention of exercise-induced bronchospasm)	2 or fewer days a week	Greater than 2 times a week, but not daily	Daily	Several times a day
	Interference with normal activity	None	Minor limitation	Some limitation	Extremely limited
	Lung function (5 to 11 years)	Normal FEV$_1$ between exacerbations; FEV$_1$ greater than 80% predicted; FEV$_1$/FVC greater than 85%	FEV$_1$ equals greater than 80% predicted; FEV$_1$/FVC greater than 80%	FEV$_1$ equals 60% to 80% predicted; FEV$_1$/FVC equals 70% to 80%	FEV$_1$ less than 60% predicted; FEV$_1$/FVC less than 75%
	Lung function (12 years to adulthood); Normal FEV$_1$/FVC: 8–19 yr 85%	Normal FEV$_1$ between exacerbations; FEV$_1$ greater than 80% predicted; FEV$_1$/FVC normal	FEV$_1$ equals greater than 80% predicted; FEV$_1$/FVC normal	FEV$_1$ equals 60% to 80% predicted; FEV$_1$/FVC reduced 5%	FEV$_1$ less than 60% predicted; FEV$_1$/FVC reduced more than 5%

Risk	0 to 1 time a year	← 2 or more times a year →		
Exacerbations requiring oral systemic corticosteroids		← Consider severity and interval since last exacerbation → Frequency and severity may fluctuate over time for patients in any severity category.		
Recommended step for initiating therapy (5 to 11 years)	Step 1	Step 2	Step 3, medium dose inhaled corticosteroid option	Step 3, medium dose inhaled dose corticosteroid option, or Step 4
			Consider short course of oral system corticosteroids	Consider short course of oral system corticosteroids
Recommended step for initiating therapy (12 years to adulthood)	Step 1	Step 2	Step 3	Step 4 or 5
			Consider short course of oral system corticosteroids	Consider short course of oral system corticosteroids

For both age groups, evaluate level of asthma control achieved in 2–6 weeks and adjust therapy accordingly.

FEV_1 = forced expiratory volume in 1 second; FVC = forced vital capacity

Source: Adapted from *Expert Panel Report 3: Guidelines for the Diagnosis and Management of Asthma* (pp. 308, 344), by National Asthma Education and Prevention Program, 2007, Bethesda, MD: National Heart Lung and Blood Institute, National Institutes of Health, retrieved July 8, 2008, from http://www.nhlbi.nih.gov/guidelines/asthma/asthgdln.htm.

Alterations in Respiratory Function **213**

Table 15–2   Quick Relief and Daily Control Medications Used to Treat Asthma

Quick Relief Medication	Nursing Management
Short-acting Beta₂-agonists (SABA) Albuterol, Levalbuterol, Pirbuterol *Metered-dose inhaler or nebulizer*	Use before inhaled steroid, wait 1–2 minutes between puffs. Hold breath 10 seconds after inspiring. Wait 15 minutes to give inhaled steroid. Rinse mouth; avoid swallowing medication. Use a spacer. Monitor for side effects (tachycardia, nervousness, nausea and vomiting, headaches). Use more than 2 days a week indicates a loss of control and need for additional therapy.
Corticosteroids Methylprednisolone Prednisone Prednisolone: *Oral*	Continue short-term therapy until child achieves 80% peak expiratory flow personal best or symptoms resolve. Give with food. Give oral dose in early morning to mimic normal peak corticosteroid blood level. Assess for long-term therapy adverse effects: decreased growth, unstable blood sugar, immunosuppression.
Anticholinergic Ipratropium: *Metered-dose inhaler or nebulizer*	Not for primary emergency treatment because of its delayed onset. Rinse bitter taste from mouth. Monitor for side effects (increased wheezing, cough, nervousness, dry mouth, tachycardia, dizziness, headache, palpitations). Prevent medication contact with eyes.

Daily Control Medications	Nursing Management
Long-acting Beta₂-agonists (LABA) For children should only be used in combination with inhaled corticosteroids (Aungst, 2008) *Dry powder inhaler*	Do not use for acute asthma flares. Take pre-exercise dose 30 to 60 minutes before activity, unless already using twice-daily doses 12 hours apart. Caution against extra dose; side effects (tachycardia, tremor, irritability, insomnia) last 8 to 12 hours. Report failure to respond to usual dose; may indicate need for stepped-up therapy.

Table 15-2 Quick Relief and Daily Control Medications Used to Treat Asthma (Continued)

Daily Control Medications	Nursing Management
Inhaled corticosteroids (ICS) Bechlomethasone Budesonide Flunisolide Fluticasone Mometasone Triamcinolone *Metered-dose inhaler or nebulizer*	Administer with spacer or holding chamber. Rinse mouth and gargle afterward to remove drug from oropharynx. Separate parts and clean inhaler daily. Monitor growth. Prevent eye exposure. Monitor for side effects (headache, gastrointestinal upset, dizziness, infection).
Methylxanthines Theophylline *Oral*	Tablet should not be crushed or chewed. Used for long-term control; works best when a therapeutic serum level, 10–20 mcg/L is maintained; give same time each day. Requires serum level checks and dose adjustment. Limit caffeine intake. Monitor for side effects (tachycardia, dysrhythmias, restlessness, tremors, seizures, insomnia, hypotension, severe headaches, vomiting, and diarrhea).
Mast cell inhibitors Cromolyn sodium Nedocromil: *Metered-dose inhaler or nebulizer*	Not used at time of symptom development or acute exacerbation. Must be used up to 4 times a day to be effective. Therapeutic response seen in 2 weeks; maximum benefit may not be seen for 4 to 6 weeks. Monitor for adverse reactions (wheezing, bronchospasm, throat irritation, nasal congestion, anaphylaxis) and report immediately.
Leukotriene receptor anatagonist (LTRA) Montelukast, Zafirlukast *Oral*	Available in granules for infants and chewable tablets for young children. Administer in evening, with food or without. Chew the chewable montelukast tablet; do not swallow whole; mix granules in applesauce or ice cream, not liquid. Administer zafirlukast 1 hour before or 2 hours after meal. Report fever, acute asthma flares, flulike symptoms, severe headaches, or lethargy. Take as prescribed; do not withdraw abruptly.

Table 15-2 Quick Relief and Daily Control Medications Used to Treat Asthma (Continued)

Daily Control Medications	Nursing Management
Immunotherapy Omalizumab	Approved for children 12 years and older with moderate or severe persistent asthma. Injections required every 2 to 4 weeks based on serum IgE levels.
Other Hyposensitization (allergy shots), subcutaneous	May be of value for child with allergies that can be addressed by immune therapy.

Source: Data from "Childhood Asthma: Part Two: Management Update," by N. C. Banasiak, 2007, *Journal of Pediatric Health Care, 21*(3), 184–191; *Prentice Hall Pediatric Drug Guide with Nursing Implications*, by R. Bindler & L. Howry, 2005, Upper Saddle River, NJ: Pearson Prentice Hall; "Inhaled Corticosteroids for Asthma," by E. W. Fon & R. H. Lewin, 2007, *Pediatrics in Review, 28*(6), e30–e35;. *Expert Panel Report 3: Guidelines for the Diagnosis and Management of Asthma* (pp. 311–318), by National Asthma Education and Prevention Program, 2007, Bethesda, MD: National Heart Lung and Blood Institute, retrieved August 30, 2007, from http://www.nhlib.nih.gov/guidelines/asthma/index.htm. Aungst, H. (2008, December 15). Asthma medications: What you need to know. Retrieved January 19, 2009 from http://contemporarypediatrics.modernmedicine.com/contpeds/article/articleDetail.jsp?id=572484.

Restore and maintain an adequate fluid balance to help thin mucus. Avoid giving iced beverages, which can precipitate bronchospasms. IV hydration is needed by some children. Prevent overhydration.

Group tasks to promote rest for the child exhausted by labored breathing and hypoxia.

Reduce stress. Keep the parent and child informed about procedures.

Patient and Family Education

Identify knowledge of the condition.

- Review why asthma occurs and that it is not an episodic illness. Assess parents' understanding of the physiologic process and its chronic and progressive nature.
- Help parents explore and understand how asthma affects their child.
- Identify asthma triggers and assess parents' understanding of how to prevent, avoid, or minimize their e`ffect in a timely manner.
- The use of a peak expiratory flow meter can help to identify when a flare is beginning.
- Help parents understand the need for daily management to have control over asthma.
- Ensure that the family knows when and where to seek emergency medical help. Describe actions the family can take before seeking medical assistance.

Review medication therapy:

- Make sure the parents know the difference between daily control medications and quick relief medications.
- Regularly evaluate the child's inhaler and nebulizer technique.
- Suggest diversions to help the child cooperate during the 8- to 10-minute nebulizer treatment.
- Provide a written action plan with daily management and steps for an asthma episode.

Review other care issues:

- Review plans for treatment at school or child care. Supply medications for school or child care and for home. Teach teachers to recognize respiratory distress and reduce the child's fear of going to the nurse for quick relief medications.
- Medical identification bracelet or medallion is worn by child.
- Reduce triggers in the home, such as pets, smoking in home, wood smoke, controlling dust mites in child's bedroom, and control of cockroaches.
- Encourage regular health promotion and maintenance care and routine immunizations, including influenza. Promote exercise and physical fitness.

BACTERIAL TRACHEITIS

A secondary infection of the upper trachea following viral laryngotracheitis, caused by *Staphylococcus aureus*, alpha-hemolytic streptococcus, group A streptococcus, *Moraxella catarrhalis*, or *Haemophilus influenzae*. The subglottis becomes edematous and ulcerated. Thick mucopurulent exudate may obstruct the trachea and main bronchi.

Clinical Manifestations

Viral upper respiratory infection, croupy cough, and stridor

Progression to high fever of more than 39°C (102.2°F), respiratory distress, and a toxic appearance; no drooling is present.

Diagnostic Tests

Blood cultures are performed after the child is found unresponsive to usual laryngotracheobronchitis (LTB) management. Endoscopic examination of the subglottic area may be performed to obtain a culture.

Clinical Therapy

When misdiagnosed as LTB and treated with nebulized epinephrine, the child's condition worsens.

Antibiotics for 10 to 14 days. Supplemental oxygen and intubation for 3 to 11 days.

Nursing Management

Until intubated, the child is never left unattended or transported away from equipment or personnel who can perform emergency airway interventions. Secure the airway before any anxiety-provoking procedures, such as venipuncture.

The intubated child is cared for in the intensive care unit. Assess airway patency frequently. Suction the endotracheal tube as needed, and provide humidified air or oxygen. Children often prefer to lie flat to conserve energy. Administer prescribed antibiotics and IV fluids.

Support parents as they cope with the sudden onset of a life-threatening illness. Keep parents informed, and permit them to stay and help keep the child calm.

BRONCHIOLITIS AND RESPIRATORY SYNCYTIAL VIRUS (RSV)

An inflammation and obstruction of the bronchioles caused by bacteria, mycoplasmas, and other viruses; RSV is the most common cause. Infection is most severe in children under age 24 months with chronic lung disease or significant congenital heart disease, and preterm infants under 35 weeks' gestation (Fowlkes & Fry, 2006).

Clinical Manifestations

May have mild symptoms: nasal stuffiness, cough (not usually noted in infants), low-grade fever, poor appetite, and vomiting and diarrhea that could lead to dehydration.

With a severe infection: respiratory rate over 70 breaths/min, grunting, increased wheezing, retractions, nasal flaring, irritability, lethargy, poor fluid intake, and a distended abdomen from overexpanded lungs. Hypoxia develops, leading to cyanosis and decreased mental status. Breath sounds diminish as airflow decreases. Noisy lungs indicate the ability to move air in and out of the lungs.

Airway hyperresponsiveness may persist for weeks after the virus has resolved.

Diagnostic Tests

Laboratory tests include immunofluorescent or enzyme immunoassay techniques from a posterior nasopharyngeal specimen. Viral cell culture may also be performed. Chest radiographs show hyperinflation, patchy atelectasis, and other signs of inflammation.

Clinical Therapy

Cardiorespiratory monitor and pulse oximeter; children with apnea or respiratory failure are cared for in the intensive care unit.

Humidified oxygen therapy by hood or face tent, mask, or nasal cannula

Intubation and mechanical ventilation (positive end-expiratory pressure (PEEP/CPAP)

Hydration with IV or oral fluids

Postural drainage and chest physiotherapy

Medications may include nonaspirin antipyretics; antibiotics only for secondary bacterial infection; neither inhaled bronchodilators or dexamethosone have demonstrated clinical value (AAP Subcommittee, 2006; Corneli, Zorc, Mahajan, et al., 2007). Ribavirin only for life-threatening cases, such as infants with complicated congenital heart disease or immunosuppression (AAP Subcommittee, 2006).

To prevent RSV infection, give 5 monthly injections of palivizumab (Synagis) beginning in October or November to high-risk infants and children (prematurity of less than 32 weeks' gestation, chronic lung disease, complicated congenital heart disease, and immunocompromised) (American Academy of Pediatrics, 2006, pp. 563–565).

Nursing Management

Assessment

Assess airway and respiratory function frequently to identify worsening respiratory symptoms. An oxygen saturation level below 90% indicates severe disease.

Weigh the child daily. Assess hydration status.

Signs of life-threatening illness in the infant include central cyanosis, respiratory rate over 70 breaths/min, listlessness, very diminished breath sounds, and apneic spells.

Implementation

Administer oxygen and pulmonary care therapies. Keep nasal passages clear. Elevate the head of the bed.

Provide small, frequent feedings. Nasogastric feedings may be needed when the risk of aspiration is high. An IV is used to rehydrate and maintain fluid balance until sufficient oral intake.

Administer medications to control fever and promote comfort as needed. Decrease stress and anxiety to promote rest. Partner with parents to comfort the child and provide care.

Patient and Family Education

When the child with less serious bronchiolitis is cared for at home, advise parents to call the healthcare provider if any of the following occur:

- Respiratory symptoms interfere with sleep or eating.
- Breathing is rapid or difficult.
- Symptoms persist in a child who is younger than 1 year old, has heart or lung disease, or was premature.
- The child acts sicker—appears tired, less playful, and less interested in food, or the parents feel the child is not improving.

BRONCHITIS

An inflammation of the trachea and bronchi caused most often by a virus—may result from bacterial invasion or in response to an allergen or irritant. Occurs most often in the winter.

The classic symptom is a coarse, hacking cough that increases in severity at night. Coughing leads to painful chest and ribs. Crackles and wheezing on auscultation.

Treatment is supportive unless bacterial infection occurs.

Nursing Management

Support respiratory function through rest, humidification, hydration, and symptomatic treatment. Encourage parents who smoke to quit or refrain from smoking in the child's presence.

BRONCHOPULMONARY DYSPLASIA (BPD) (CHRONIC LUNG DISEASE)

A chronic lung disease; the persistence of lung disease following premature birth and respiratory support (positive pressure ventilation and oxygen) provided in the neonatal period. BPD occurs in approximately a third of newborns with a birth weight less than 1000 g (Walsh, Szefler, Davis, et al., 2006). Infants with neonatal pneumonia, meconium aspiration syndrome, fluid overload, and lung hypoplasia may also develop BPD (Capper-Michel, 2004).

Clinical Manifestations

Persistent signs of respiratory distress: tachypnea, wheezing, crackles, irritability, nasal flaring, grunting, retractions, pulmonary edema, and failure to thrive.

Intermittent bronchospasms and mucous plugging lead to persistent air trapping. Persistent air trapping leads to a barrel-shaped chest.

Episodes of sudden respiratory deterioration with cyanosis or dusky color, agitation, and limited expiratory airflow may occur.

Diagnostic Tests

A chest radiograph often shows hyperexpansion, atelectasis, and interstitial thickening (Capper-Michel, 2004).

Clinical Therapy

Treatment to support respiratory function and maturation of the lungs. Supplemental oxygen with humidity to keep the SaO_2 at more than 90% to 92%, even during sleep and feeding. A tracheostomy for long-term airway management. Chest physiotherapy to help clear the airways. Infants are weaned from mechanical ventilation.

Increased calories to support growth. Gastrostomy or nasogastric feeding to supplement calories. Restrict fluids to prevent pulmonary edema.

Medications used include diuretics, bronchodilators, anti-inflammatories, and inhaled corticosteroids. See Table 15–3.

Oxygen and medications are gradually reduced as the child improves. Monitor electrolytes monthly.

Long-term sequelae include asthma and respiratory infections, frequent rehospitalization. BPD is a risk factor for cerebral palsy and difficulties with motor and cognitive skills (Ehrenkranz, Walsh, Vohr, et al., 2005).

Nursing Management

Assessment

Assess airway and respiratory function, vital signs, color, and behavior changes to identify signs of worsening symptoms even when oxygen is provided. Attach a cardiorespiratory monitor and pulse oximeter.

Monitor the tracheostomy for obstruction, and suction as needed.

Observe for signs of infection.

Monitor growth and evaluate development regularly. Coordinate periodic hearing and vision testing.

Implementation

When the infant is hospitalized, group tasks to reduce stimulation that increases respiratory effort. Position the infant to facilitate breathing. Provide tracheostomy care. Provide humidified oxygen if ordered.

Table 15–3   Medications Used to Treat Bronchopulmonary Dysplasia

Medication	Nursing Management
Bronchodilators (beta$_2$-adrenergic agonists, anticholinergics, theophylline, albuterol nebulizer)	Monitor vital signs and potential signs of toxicity. Give medications at same time each day. Encourage fluid intake.
Antiinflammatory agents (corticosteroids, inhaled cromolyn, becholmethasone)	Ensure parents use proper technique for inhaler and spacer. Rinse mouth to remove residual medication and to prevent candidiasis. Clean inhaler daily; rinse and dry parts.
Diuretics (furosemide, chlorothiazide, spironolactone)	Follow guidelines for allowable fluid intake. Monitor electrolyte levels. Teach families about sodium and potassium-rich foods to eat or avoid, depending upon diuretic prescribed.
Potassium chloride	Monitor serum potassium level. Teach about potassium-rich foods to avoid or use in moderation.
Antibiotics	Give at scheduled time, and give all doses.
Palivizumab, Synargis	Teach importance of monthly injections beginning in the fall.

Manage fluids, as excess fluids can lead to pulmonary edema. Supplement calories as needed. Administer medications. Manage fever to help reduce energy needs.

For home care, make referrals for needed oxygen, respiratory supplies, medications, an early-intervention program, home health nursing, and follow-up care. Help families plan a schedule for needed care and to identify other family members who can learn to care for the infant.

A formula supplemented with carbohydrates and medium-chain triglycerides may be given to promote weight gain.

Patient and Family Education

Teach family members to identify signs of respiratory compromise needing rapid intervention. Infants can become very ill rapidly and need rehospitalization. Assist parents to develop an emergency care plan.

Educate parents to balance fluid restrictions with nutritional requirements so that growth is supported and pulmonary edema is prevented. Teach procedures for nasogastric or gastrostomy feedings.

Promote the infant's normal development through rest, nutrition, stimulation, and family support.

Emphasize the need for frequent health promotion visits and immunizations. Encourage RSV prophylaxis.

CYSTIC FIBROSIS

An inherited autosomal recessive disorder of the exocrine glands that results in physiologic alterations in the respiratory, gastrointestinal, and reproductive systems. A defective cystic fibrosis transmembrane conductance regulator protein impairs chloride-ion transport across the exocrine and epithelial cells, causing decreased chloride secretion and increased sodium absorption affecting the sweat ducts, airway, pancreatic duct, intestine, biliary tree, and vas deferens. This causes the body to produce unusually thick, sticky mucus that clogs the lungs, leading to infections, and obstructs the pancreas, stopping natural enzymes that enable the body to digest and absorb food (Cystic Fibrosis Foundation, 2007a; Strausbaugh & Davis, 2007). Damage to the pancreas may interfere with insulin secretion, leading to cystic fibrosis–related diabetes mellitus. Excessive electrolyte loss through perspiration, saliva, and mucus secretion place children at risk for dehydration.

Clinical Manifestations

Meconium ileus may be the first sign in newborns with cystic fibrosis.

Steatorrhea and frothy, foul-smelling, and floating stools. Constipation is common, and intestinal obstruction may occur in older children.

Skin has salty taste.

Chronic moist, productive cough and frequent infections occur. Nasal polyps are often present.

Frontal headaches, facial tenderness, purulent nasal discharge, and postnasal discharge occur with chronic sinus infections.

Voracious appetite and difficulty maintaining and gaining weight occur because of food malabsorption and an increased metabolic rate due to frequent infections.

Clubbing of the distal extremities.

Children with mild disease may be adolescents or young adults before symptoms appear.

Adolescents have chronic chest pain, related to regular use of accessory muscles.

Diagnostic Tests

Newborn meconium ileus, malabsorption or failure to thrive, chronic recurrent respiratory infections, fecal impaction, and intussusception often trigger diagnostic testing.

Newborn screening: testing of dried blood samples can detect high immunoreactive trypsinogen (IRT) concentrations found in infants with cystic fibrosis. A chromosome mutation analysis is then performed to detect a defective gene.

A sweat chloride test by pilocarpine iontophoresis is often used to confirm the diagnosis. A chloride level greater than 60 mEq/L is diagnostic with other signs (meconium ileus, high IRT concentration, or positive family history).

Spirometry tests to monitor pulmonary function. Sputum culture and sensitivity for suspected infections.

Clinical Therapy

Treatment is focused on controlling infection and inflammation and on reducing mucus accumulation to slow the progression of airway damage. Numerous medications are used. See Table 15–4. Bronchial hygiene therapy (chest physiotherapy, positive expiratory pressure,

Table 15–4   Medications Used to Treat Cystic Fibrosis

Medications	Actions
Beta₂-adrenergic receptor agonist bronchodilators aerosol	Use before chest physiotherapy and with symptoms to open large and small airways.
Dornase alpha (DNAse or Pulmozyme) aerosol	Liquefies and thins pulmonary secretions. Decreases risk of developing pulmonary infections (Flume, O'Sullivan, Robinson, et al., 2007).
Hypertonic saline (7%) aerosol	Use after a bronchodilator. Improves mucus clearance by hydrating the airway; leads to fewer infections (Elkins, Robinson, Rose, et al., 2006).
Montelukast oral	Helps reduce airway inflammation, but insufficient evidence for routine use (Flume, O'Sullivan, Robinson, et al., 2007).

Table 15–4 Medications Used to Treat Cystic Fibrosis (Continued)

Medications	Actions
Ibuprofen	Administered twice daily to slow the rate of pulmonary function decline (Flume, O'Sullivan, Robinson, et al., 2007).
Tobramycin aerosol	Aminoglycoside antibiotic for chronic *Pseudomonas aeruginosa* infection; suppresses bacterial growth. Given in alternating 28-day cycles (Bell, 2006b).
Azithromycin oral	An azalide antibiotic; reduces the risk of pulmonary exacerbation in children with or without chronic *Pseudomonas aeruginosa* (Clement, Tamalet, Leroux, et al., 2006).
Antibiotics oral, IV	Treats infections; selection based upon culture and sensitivities. Higher doses than normal and prolonged courses may be needed.
Pancreatic enzyme supplements (Cotazym-S, Pancrease, Viokase)	Assists in digestion of nutrients, decreasing fat and bulk. Given prior to meals and snacks.
Multivitamins and vitamin E in water-soluble form, vitamins A, D, and K given when deficient; iron supplementation	Cystic fibrosis interferes with vitamin production; water-soluble supplements are better absorbed (vitamins A, D, E, and K are naturally fat soluble); iron deficiency results from malabsorption syndrome.
Ursodeoxycholate	May slow progression of hepatic lesion in cystic fibrosis. Given when patient has elevated liver enzymes or evidence of portal hypertension.
Lactulose	May abort early distal intestinal obstruction syndrome and prevent recurrences.
Growth hormone subcutaneous	May improve height and weight and bone mineral density in prepubertal children; still experimental (Hardin, Adams-Huet, Brown, et al., 2006).

flutter valve, or high-frequency chest wall oscillation) one to three times daily reduces mucous accumulation.

A well-balanced high-calorie diet is recommended to support growth and meet energy needs. Supplemental nasogastric or gastrostomy feedings help when the child's weight is 85% to 90% of ideal weight. Children with adequate nutrition have a longer life expectancy. Cystic fibrosis–related diabetes is challenging to manage because the large caloric intake must be balanced by insulin dosage.

The disease is ultimately terminal. Double-lung transplantation is sometimes performed, and approximately 50% of cases survive for the first 5 years. However, little improvement in survival and long-term outcomes has occurred over the past 20 years (Visner & Goldfarb, 2007).

Nursing Management
Assessment
Assess respiratory status, noting crackles, wheezes, cyanosis, and clubbing. Ask about the cough character and frequency and sputum characteristics. Compare to baseline data; changes in the cough may indicate a new infection. Obtain oxygen saturation and spirometry readings if changes in respiratory status are suspected.

Evaluate the child's growth pattern, plotting the weight and height on a growth curve. Inquire about the child's appetite, food intake, and use of nutritional supplements, pancreatic enzymes, and vitamins. Growth delay and delayed appearance of secondary sex characteristics are often due to nutrition status.

Assess the child's stooling pattern. Identify any problems with abdominal pain or bloating and if these problems are related to eating, stooling, or other activities. Palpate the abdomen for liver size, fecal masses, and evidence of pain.

Assess hearing periodically, as tobramycin is associated with hearing loss.

Identify how the child's illness affects day-to-day functioning, conflicts with family activities, and how the family has adapted to the child's need for care. Ask how the child or adolescent feels about the daily care routine.

Implementation
Periodic hospitalization required for a severe infection or for a pulmonary and nutritional "tune-up." Place the child in a single room with standard precautions to reduce risk for transfer of *Pseudomonas* and

Burkholderia cepacia. Respect and support the parents who need to take advantage of the respite from daily care.

Chest physiotherapy is performed one to three times per day before meals to facilitate removal of secretions from the lungs. A bronchodilator, hypertonic saline, and DNase are given by nebulizer to help thin respiratory secretions. Identify the chest physiotherapy regimen most acceptable to the child and family.

Antibiotics are necessary for an acute exacerbation by oral, inhalation, and IV routes. With an increased clearance of nearly all antibiotics, higher dosages and up to 14 days of treatment are needed. Monitor renal function, and test antibiotic serum drug levels to ensure therapeutic dosing.

Give pancreatic enzymes with all meals and snacks to promote absorption of dietary nutrients and water-soluble vitamin supplements. Fats and extra salt are needed in the diet. Increase calorie intake with snacks between meals and before bed. The goal is to achieve near-normal, well-formed stools and adequate weight gain. Make a referral to a nutritionist before discharge.

Assist the child and parents with issues relating to discipline; body image (stooling and odor, clubbing, barrel chest); frequent rehospitalization; the potential fatal nature of the illness; the child's feeling of being different from friends; and overall financial, social, and family concerns. Refer families to psychosocial counseling as needed.

Assist families with a newly diagnosed child to obtain necessary equipment. Make referrals to social services as needed for financial assistance.

Help adolescents establish appropriate educational and occupational goals for their future and to transition to adult healthcare services.

Initiate palliative care planning with adolescents and young adults as the disease progresses to respiratory failure.

Patient and Family Education
During hospitalization, review basic and new information about the disorder, respiratory care, medications, and nutrition.

Review the child's use of aerosol medications and airway clearance techniques.

Encourage a regular, vigorous exercise regimen and aerobic fitness.

During periods of exercise and increased sweating, encourage the child to drink more fluids and increase salt intake. Teach parents to recognize early symptoms of salt depletion (fatigue, weakness, abdominal pain, and vomiting) and to contact the child's healthcare provider if these symptoms occur.

Review dietary needs and methods to provide extra calories needed for growth and increased energy expenditures.

Teach adolescents to assume responsibility for daily disease management. Discuss ways to perform the daily care regimen and interact with peers at school. Provide information about potential infertility and guidelines for safe sexual practices. Discuss the need for contraception with adolescent females. Refer to genetic counseling.

LARYNGOTRACHEOBRONCHITIS, OR CROUP

A viral invasion of the upper airway that extends throughout the larynx, trachea, and bronchi common in children 6 months to 6 years of age, with a peak age of 2 to 3 years (Dykes, 2005). Viruses causing LTB include parainfluenza virus type I, II, or III; influenza A and B; adenovirus; RSV; and measles. Inflammation and edema narrow the subglottic area of the airway and cause respiratory distress.

Clinical Manifestations

Upper respiratory symptoms that progress to a cough and hoarseness

Low-grade fever, runny nose, tachypnea, inspiratory stridor, and a seal-like barking cough

Expiratory stridor, severe tachypnea, and retractions

Physical exhaustion can diminish the intensity of retractions, and stridor and breath sounds may actually diminish. Responsiveness decreases as hypoxemia increases.

Diagnostic Tests

Diagnosis is achieved through history and clinical signs. Pulse oximetry is used to detect hypoxemia. A radiograph of the upper airway may show a tapered, symmetric subglottic narrowing and rule out a foreign body.

Throat cultures or visual inspection of the inner mouth and throat are contraindicated, as they can cause laryngospasms and further compromise the airway.

Clinical Therapy

Management involves medications, and humidified supplemental oxygen when the saturated oxygen level is less than 92%. See Meds 15–5 for medications used to treat LTB. Airway obstruction is a

Meds 15–5   Medications Used for Laryngotracheobronchitis Treatment

Medication	Nursing Management
Alpha- and Beta$_2$-adrenergic agonist (racemic epinephrine): aerosolized through face mask	Provides temporary relief after 30 minutes, lasting about 2 hours; provides time for the corticosteroid to work.
	Monitor for tachycardia (160–200 beats/min) and hypertension; dizziness, headache, and nausea; may necessitate stopping medication.
Corticosteroids (e.g., dexamethasone): IM, PO, nebulized budesonide	Monitor for potential cardiovascular symptoms (hypertension).
	Child less frequently needs intubation; stridor resolves faster.

potential complication. Intubation is performed for imminent airway obstruction.

Nursing Management

Assessment

Assess the child's respiratory status, and continuously monitor for development of airway obstruction (absence of voice sounds, increasing degree of respiratory distress, inability to swallow, and acute onset of drooling). If any of these signs occur, get medical assistance immediately. *The quieter the child, the greater the cause for concern.*

Monitor the level of consciousness—for anxiety, lethargy, or stupor as hypoxia increases.

Implementation

Provide humidified supplemental oxygen if hypoxemia is present.

Allow the child to assume a position of comfort to help maintain the airway, usually sitting or lying with the head elevated. Administer medications.

Be immediately available to attend to the child's respiratory needs; the child will have difficulty communicating about worsening respiratory symptoms. Keep emergency equipment at bedside.

Encourage the child to drink cool, noncarbonated, nonacidic beverages to liquefy secretions and provide calories for energy and metabolism.

Teach parents about actions to take if symptoms recur at home.

PNEUMONIA

An inflammation or infection of the bronchioles and alveolar spaces of the lungs, caused by viral, bacterial, mycoplasmal, and fungal organisms—the incidence is higher among children under 5 years (Sandora & Harper, 2005). Noninfectious causes of pneumonia include aspiration of food or gastric acids, foreign bodies, and hydrocarbon ingestions (Sectish & Prober, 2007).

Clinical Manifestations

Mycoplasma pneumoniae: insidious onset, malaise, muscle aches, headache, fever, sore throat, rhinorrhea, dry and hacking cough that becomes productive, fine crackles, and anorexia.

Viral pneumonia: sudden or insidious onset, rhinitis, slight cough that may become productive, fever and chills, crackles, and wheezes.

Streptococcus pneumoniae: sudden onset, high fever, cough, shaking, chills, chest pain, nasal flaring, retractions, fine crackles, dullness on percussion, and fremitus.

Staphylococcus aureus: upper respiratory infection and abrupt change in condition, high fever, cough, shaking, chills, lethargy, chest pain, nasal flaring, retractions, fine crackles, dullness on percussion, and fremitus.

Chlamydia pneumoniae: insidious onset, minimal or absent fever, tachypnea, malaise, persistent cough, and pharyngitis.

Newborns and infants may have grunting, nasal flaring, irritability, lethargy, and a diminished appetite. Diminished breath sounds in the affected lobe may be noted.

Diagnostic Tests

History, physical signs and symptoms, and chest radiography help distinguish the type of pneumonia present. Children with recurrent pneumonia need to be evaluated for immunodeficiency syndromes, foreign-body aspiration, obstruction or compression of the airway, structural abnormality, cystic fibrosis, and asthma (Sectish & Prober, 2007).

Clinical Therapy

Airway management, fluids, fever management, pain management, and rest; some children need oxygen and IV fluids to maintain hydration.

Hospitalization is necessary with severe respiratory symptoms (toxic appearance, supplemental oxygen needed, inability to tolerate oral fluids and food).

Antibiotics are prescribed for mycoplasma and bacterial pneumonias or for secondary bacterial infection of viral pneumonia.

Nursing Management
Assessment
Assess the respiratory rate, heart rate, and temperature, and observe color for pallor or cyanosis. Attach a pulse oximeter to monitor the SpO_2 level. Assess hydration status. Assess pain associated with coughing.

Implementation
Promote deep breathing to fully aerate the lungs and to promote coughing to clear secretions and cellular debris. Teach the child and parent how to splint the chest for pain management.

Provide pain medication (acetaminophen or ibuprofen), which can help with temperature control and aid sleep. Give antibiotic medications as prescribed.

Maintain hydration with clear fluids. IV fluids are used when oral fluids are inadequate. Encourage soft foods when tolerated.

Patient and Family Education
Educate family members about medication administration and any side effects.

Teach family members to recognize signs of a worsening condition and needing immediate care, such as increased difficulty breathing and refusal to take fluids.

Encourage pneumococcal conjugate vaccine immunization. For children older than age 2 years with immunosuppression or chronic diseases, encourage immunization with the 23-valent pneumococcal vaccine.

TUBERCULOSIS
Tuberculosis (TB) is an infection caused by the organism *Mycobacterium tuberculosis,* transmitted through the air by droplets when a person with active infection coughs, sneezes, speaks, or sings. Inhaled bacilli are small enough to travel directly to the alveoli and replicate. An immune response is initiated, and macrophages try to

kill the bacillus. Surviving bacilli multiply within the macrophage that has walled it off in a granuloma. Latent TB infection (LTBI) occurs when the bacilli remain in the granuloma; when bacilli escape, active infection occurs. The risk of transitioning from LTBI to active TB is greatest during the first 2 years of life and during adolescence. Up to 40% of untreated infants with LTBI develop active TB within 2 to 12 months after initial infection (Reznick & Ozuah, 2005). Children under age 6 years have a greater risk for developing extrapulmonary TB (Peredo-Pinto & Jacobs, 2008; Feja & Saimain, 2005).

Clinical Manifestations

Latent TB is asymptomatic. Signs of active pulmonary TB include (Feja & Saimain, 2005):

Infants—persistent cough, weight loss or failure to gain weight, and fever. Wheezing, crackles, and decreased breath sounds may be present.

Children—fatigue, cough, anorexia, weight loss or growth delay, night sweats, chills, and a low-grade fever.

Adolescents—same as adults, fever, weight loss, productive cough, hemoptysis, and night sweats.

Signs are specific to the system invaded in cases of extrapulmonary TB.

Diagnostic Tests

Intradermal purified protein derivative (PPD); only children at high risk of exposure or with impaired immune status are routinely tested. A positive test means the child has been exposed to and infected with TB, and antibodies have been produced against the bacillus. An enzyme-linked immunosorbent assay QuantiFERON-TB Gold (QFT-G) can diagnose TB in 24 hours.

Confirmation of the diagnosis with cultures and acid-fast stains of blood, gastric aspirate, or sputum, and a chest radiograph. Pleural biopsy may also be performed for culture and tissue examination.

Clinical Therapy

Combinations of medications are used for treatment of active TB for 6 months (Table 15–6). For infants, children, and adolescents with latent TB, a single daily dose of isoniazid is given for 9 months. Direct observed drug therapy is recommended to reduce treatment failure and development of drug-resistant organisms. Active TB cases are reported to the public health department.

Table 15–6 Medications Commonly Used to Treat Latent and Active TB in Children

Medication	Nursing Management
Isoniazid (bactericidal)	Assess baseline weight, as well as ophthalmologic status, hematopoetic, bilirubin, and liver function studies.
	Give 1 hour before or 2 hours after meals; give with food if GI irritation. Tablets can be crushed.
	Interferes with hepatic metabolism of phenytoin; may cause toxicity.
	Monitor for signs of hypersensitivity, hepatotoxicity (anorexia, fever, malaise, nausea, vomiting, diarrhea, weight loss), dark urine, jaundice.
	Adolescent should avoid alcohol.
	Pyridoxine supplementation (vitamin B6) is recommended for children and adolescents with HIV infection, pregnancy, meat- and milk-deficient diets, nutritional deficiencies; infants exclusively breastfed.
Rifampin (bactericidal)	Obtain baseline bilirubin and liver function studies; this drug can alter the pharmacokinetics and serum concentrations of other drugs; assess renal and hematopoetic status studies.
	Assess for potential medication interaction with rifampin (e.g., diazepam, beta-adrenergics, barbiturates, analgesics, corticosteroids, digitalis, and others); oral contraceptives become ineffective.
	Give 1 hour before or 2 hours after meals; give with food if GI irritation occurs. Capsule contents can be sprinkled on applesauce or suspended in flavored syrup.
	Monitor for signs of jaundice and other side effects.
	Inform parents and child about orange-colored body fluids and contact lenses if used.
Pyrazinamide (bacteriostatic)	Obtain baseline liver function studies, and renal and hematopoetic status studies. Monitor for hepatotoxicity.
	Monitor blood glucose level in children with diabetes, as glycemic control may be affected.
	When used in combination with isoniazid and rifampin, a 6-month course of therapy is possible.
Ethambutol (bacteriostatic or bacteriocidal, depending upon dosage used)	Obtain baseline liver function studies and renal and hematopoetic status studies.
	Perform a baseline and monthly ophthalmologic exam; drug may cause optic neuritis, particularly when renal function is impaired.
	Give with meals if GI irritation occurs.
	Inform parents and child to report any vision changes.

Nursing Management
Assessment
Identify children at higher risk for exposure to TB (recent contact or family member with TB; positive PPD in family member; born in any country other than United States, Canada, Australia, New Zealand, or Western Europe; travel for longer than a week in any country other than those listed, with resident contact) (American Academy of Pediatrics, 2006, p. 684).

Monitor the health of infants and young children who have a PPD conversion. Assess for signs of active TB (weight loss, fever, fatigue, coughing).

Implementation
Implement airborne precautions when hospitalized. Provide supportive care when hospitalized.

Assist with the collection of blood, sputum, and gastric aspirate cultures.

Patient and Family Education
Emphasize keeping appointments for "directly observed drug therapy" and the importance of completing daily home administration of medications. Give medications on an empty stomach. Emphasize the importance of completing the full course of medications.

Encourage proper nutrition and rest to promote recovery.

The child can return to school or child care when effective therapy is instituted, adherence to therapy is documented, and clinical symptoms have diminished (American Academy of Pediatrics, 2006, p. 696). Facilitate PPD testing of family members and close contacts.

INJURIES OF THE RESPIRATORY SYSTEM
Aspirated Foreign Bodies (AFB)
Inhalation of any object (solid or liquid, food or nonfood) into the respiratory tract, causing partial or complete obstruction. Infants and young toddlers are at high risk because of increasing mobility and tendency to mouth objects, but aspiration occurs at all ages. Common aspirated items include the following:

- Foods such as nuts, popcorn, hard candy, meat bones, or small pieces of raw vegetables or hot dog
- Small, loose toy parts such as small wheels and bells
- Household objects and substances such as beads, safety pins, coins, buttons, balloon pieces, and colorful liquids (mouthwash, perfume) in enticing packages (small screw-bottle tops)

Most AFBs cause bronchial obstruction, often in the right lung. An object lodged in the trachea is life-threatening. AFBs may migrate from the bronchus to the trachea and cause severe symptoms.

Clinical Manifestations

Spasmodic coughing, gagging, dysphonia, stridor, wheezing without fever or other symptoms of illness; may be brief or last for hours.

Clutching the neck is the universal sign of choking, seen in older children.

Signs of increased respiratory effort such as dyspnea, tachypnea, nasal flaring, and retractions. Concentrated focus on breathing, an anxious expression, and tripod position with the neck extended.

Behavior changes such as irritability and decreased responsiveness as the child becomes hypoxic.

Diagnostic Tests

A chest radiograph or a forced expiratory film (shows hyperinflation and mediastinal shift on affected side) is indicated.

Clinical Therapy

Perform back blows and chest thrusts for an infant and abdominal thrusts for older children.

Administer oxygen.

Fluoroscopy and fiberoptic bronchoscopy are performed in the operating room to extract the foreign body; removal of visible foreign body with a laryngoscope and Magill forceps.

Treatment for pneumonia is initiated, if present.

Nursing Management

Assessment

Continuously assess the child, as a complete obstruction may occur. Monitor for increasing respiratory distress. Breath sound changes from noisy to decreasing to absent on the affected side can indicate that the object is moving and blocking a main stem bronchus.

Attach a cardiorespiratory monitor and pulse oximeter to assess increasing hypoxia.

Assess the family's level of distress and coping ability.

Implementation

Keep emergency resuscitation equipment immediately accessible.

Allow the child to select the position of comfort, such as sitting upright or a semi-Fowler position.

Avoid any procedure that increases the child's anxiety.

Provide a quiet environment and keep parents close to help reduce the child's anxiety.

Provide education about potential safety hazards in the home. Encourage the parents to learn CPR.

Pneumothorax

In pneumothorax, air enters the pleural space because of tears in the tracheobronchial tree, the esophagus, or the chest wall, resulting in lung collapse. Causes of pneumothorax include the following:

- Complication of mechanical ventilation or high peak inspiratory or end-expiratory pressure
- Gas trapping and alveolar hyperinflation in chronic lung conditions such as neonatal respiratory distress syndrome, status asthmaticus, and cystic fibrosis
- Blunt trauma to the chest

An open pneumothorax results from any penetrating injury that exposes the pleural space to atmospheric pressure.

A tension pneumothorax, a life-threatening emergency, results when air leaks into the chest on inhalation and cannot escape during exhalation. Building pressure compresses the chest contents, collapses the lung, and causes a mediastinal shift that impairs venous blood return to the heart and decreases cardiac output.

Clinical Manifestations

Restlessness, cyanosis, subcutaneous emphysema (air leakage in the tissue).

Open pneumothorax: a sucking sound may be heard as the air moves through the opening on the chest wall; restlessness, cyanosis, or air leakage into the tissue.

Closed pneumothorax: decreased or absent breath sounds on the injured side; respiratory distress.

Tension pneumothorax: increasing respiratory distress, absent breath sounds, cardiovascular instability, and a tracheal shift to the unaffected side.

Diagnostic Procedures

Physical signs are used to make the diagnosis. A chest radiograph reveals the lung collapse.

Clinical Therapy

Open pneumothorax: immediately cover the wound with an airtight seal.

Closed pneumothorax: thoracostomy and chest tube insertion attached to a closed drainage system that helps remove the air and reinflate the lung.

Tension pneumothorax: immediate needle thoracentesis allows air to escape and relieve the tension. A chest tube is inserted and attached to a closed drainage system.

Nursing Management

Assess for respiratory distress or change in respiratory function and monitor vital signs. Monitor the chest tube and drainage system. When the chest tube is removed, cover the site with an occlusive dressing, and monitor the child's respiratory status for signs of respiratory distress.

Pulmonary Contusion

Bruising damage after the energy from blunt trauma is transferred directly through the child's chest wall to the lung tissues. The capillaries bleed into the alveoli, and capillary rupture in the air sacs may occur. As blood and fluid from damaged tissues accumulate in the lower airways, pulmonary edema develops. Lower airway obstruction and atelectasis may result in impaired gas exchange, acute respiratory distress, and respiratory failure (Pitetti & Walker, 2005).

Clinical Manifestations

Initially, the child may appear asymptomatic.

Signs of respiratory distress often develop over several hours and include wheezing, hemoptysis, fever, and crackles. Agitation and lethargy can signal increasing hypoxia.

Diagnostic Tests

Careful observation is required during the first 12 hours after the injury to detect decreased perfusion related to ventilatory impairment. Chest radiographs or computed tomography are used for diagnosis, but it takes hours for signs to appear.

Clinical Therapy

Intubation and mechanical ventilation with positive end-expiratory pressure as the lung tissues heal; humidified oxygen; fluid restriction and diuretics to decrease edema in the interstitial pulmonary tissue; incentive spirometry; and pain management.

Nursing Management

Monitor respiratory function to detect signs of deterioration using level of consciousness as a key indicator. Inspect the thorax for symmetric chest wall movement. Observe for hemoptysis (fresh blood in the sputum), dyspnea, decreased breath sounds, wheezes, crackles, and a transient temperature elevation. Cyanosis in children is often a late indicator of respiratory distress. Carefully monitor for acute respiratory distress syndrome.

Provide physiologic support, such as oxygen therapy, positioning, incentive spirometry with pain management for coughing, and comfort measures. Carefully manage fluids to prevent large increases in pulmonary edema.

Smoke-Inhalation Injury

Exposure of the child's face and airway to fire or high heat leads to airway thermal injury and edema. Exposure to noxious chemicals and irritants results in mucosal airway damage, bronchospasm, depletion of alveolar surfactant, and mucous plugging from soot and sloughed airway mucosa.

When the child is trapped in a closed space, carbon monoxide exposure rapidly produces hypoxia. Confusion, myocardial depression, and ventricular arrhythmias result as the vital organs are deprived of oxygen.

Soot carried deep into the lungs combines with moisture in the lungs to produce acid chemicals that burn and cause loss of cilia, loss of surfactant, and edema. Gas exchange is disrupted, and sloughing lung tissue obstructs the airways. Microorganisms grow in damaged tissue. Acute respiratory distress syndrome, pneumonia, and pulmonary embolism may develop (Antoon & Donovan, 2007).

Clinical Manifestations

Burns of the face and neck, singed nasal hairs, soot around the mouth or nose, and hoarseness with stridor or voice change.

Respiratory distress may develop over a few hours with tachypnea, stridor, coughing, and wheezing. Respiratory distress may progress to respiratory failure.

If carbon monoxide poisoning is present, the child is confused or unconscious and has cardiac arrhythmias.

Diagnostic Tests

Diagnosis is based on history of the child being exposed to smoke in a closed area and signs of soot around the nose and mouth. Arterial blood gases and a carboxyhemoglobin level are obtained.

Clinical Therapy

Hospitalization and monitoring for progression of respiratory distress.

Initial treatment is 100% humidified oxygen administered through a nonrebreather mask.

If respiratory distress develops, an endotracheal tube, mechanical ventilation, and monitoring are provided in the intensive care unit.

Chest physiotherapy and suctioning to keep the airway clear.

All other fire-related injuries are treated.

Nursing Management

Monitor for development of respiratory distress, and check vital signs frequently. Attach a pulse oximeter. Auscultate the lungs for crackles, wheezes, and decreased breath sounds. Assess for level of consciousness and behavior changes that could indicate increasing hypoxia.

Provide oxygen as ordered. Position the child to promote respiratory function. If the child's condition deteriorates, assist with procedures to secure the child's airway and prepare the child for transfer to the intensive care unit. Assess the family's response to the life-threatening crisis and offer support with information about the child's condition.

16 Alterations in Cardiovascular Function

CONGENITAL HEART DISEASE

Congenital heart disease is a defect in the heart or great vessels or the persistence of a fetal structure after birth. Congenital heart defects are categorized by the pathophysiology and hemodynamics.

Defects Causing Increased Pulmonary Blood Flow

A connection between the left and right side of the heart (septal defect) or between the great arteries (patent ductus arteriosus [PDA]) allows blood to flow between the sides of the heart. The higher pressures on the left side shunt blood to the right side, increasing the volume of blood pumped to the lungs. Congestive heart failure (CHF), pulmonary vascular resistance, and right ventricular hypertrophy may develop.

Clinical Manifestations

Increased heart and respiratory rates and increased metabolic rate

Diaphoresis with feeding; poor weight gain

Signs of CHF (dyspnea, tachypnea, intercostal retractions, and periorbital edema); frequent respiratory infections

See Box 16–1 for heart defects in this classification.

Diagnostic Procedures

Chest radiograph, electrocardiogram (ECG), two-dimensional echocardiogram, transthoracic echocardiogram, cardiac catheterization, exercise testing, computed tomography, magnetic resonance imaging (MRI), and a hyperoxia test

A complete blood count, urinalysis, coagulation studies, platelet counts, and serum electrolytes before surgery

Clinical Therapy

Surgery or interventional cardiac catheterization may be performed early in infancy to prevent irreversible pulmonary vascular disease, or surgery may be postponed until the child is symptomatic or older. Indomethacin IV may be given to preterm infants when immediate PDA closure is needed. See Box 16–1.

Box 16–1 Heart Defects That Increase Pulmonary Blood Flow, Their Clinical Manifestations, and Clinical Therapy

Atrial Septal Defect (ASD)

An opening in the atrial septum permits left-to-right shunting of blood.

Asymptomatic if opening is small. A soft systolic ejection murmur in the pulmonic area with wide fixed splitting of S_2. CHF, easy tiring, and poor growth occur with a large ASD.

Surgery to close or patch the ASD or closure by a septal occluder during cardiac catheterization.

Atrioventricular (AV) Canal (Endocardial Cushion Defect)

A combination of defects in the atrial and ventricular septa and portions of tricuspid and mitral valves. The most complex malformation results in one AV valve and large septal defects between both atria and ventricles.

CHF, tachypnea, tachycardia, poor growth, recurrent respiratory infections, and repeated respiratory failure. A holosystolic murmur is loudest at left lower sternal border (mitral regurgitation). Accentuated S_1 and split S_2.

Surgery before age 6 months to reduce risk of pulmonary vascular disease. Patches are placed over septal defects, and valve tissue is used to form functioning valves. Mitral valve may be replaced.

Patent Ductus Arteriosus (PDA)

Persistent fetal circulation. Blood is shunted from the aorta through the PDA to the pulmonary arteries, increasing circulation to the pulmonary system.

CHF, intercostal retractions, hepatomegaly, and growth failure. Infant is at risk for frequent respiratory infections, pneumonia, and infective endocarditis. Continuous "machinery" murmur during systole and diastole, a thrill in the pulmonic area.

Surgical ligation of PDA or insertion of obstructive device during cardiac catheterization. IV indomethacin often stimulates PDA closure in premature infants.

Ventricular Septal Defect (VSD)

An opening in the ventricular septum allows blood to flow from the left ventricle directly into the pulmonary artery.

Small VSDs are asymptomatic. Large VSDs cause tachypnea, dyspnea, poor growth, reduced fluid intake, CHF, increased number of pulmonary infections, and pulmonary hypertension. A systolic murmur at the third or fourth left intercostal space at the sternal border.

Small VSDs often close spontaneously by 6 months of age. Surgical patching of VSD or closure by transcatheter device during cardiac catheterization.

Postpericardiotomy Syndrome

Pericardial and pleural inflammation may occur within a few weeks to a few months in up to 30% of patients after any surgery requiring an incision through the pericardium.

Signs include high fever up to 40°C (104°F) and severe chest pain that worsens with deep inspiration and in supine position. The condition lasts 2 to 3 weeks.

Mild cases are treated with bed rest and nonsteroidal anti-inflammatory drugs. Severe cases may need hospitalization, pericardiocentesis, diuretics, and corticosteroids (Park, 2008, p. 378).

Nursing Management of the Child Undergoing a Cardiac Catheterization

Assessment
Before the procedure: assess vital signs, hematocrit and hemoglobin, capillary refill, skin temperature and color, and strength of the pedal and popliteal pulses.

After the procedure: assess vital signs (check for arrhythmia), perfusion of leg below catheter site (pedal and popliteal pulses, skin temperature, color, capillary refill, and sensation), and intake and output. Assess the pressure dressing over the catheterization site every 15 minutes for 1 hour and then every 30 minutes for 1 hour. Monitor for bleeding (checking under buttocks for blood) and hematoma or thrombus formation at the catheterization site.

Implementation
Before the procedure:

- Keep the child NPO for several hours, except for medications. Give the ordered sedative to older children. Infants and young children are given deeper sedation to keep them still during the procedure.
- Provide age-appropriate information to prepare the child for the procedure. Explain the sensations that will be experienced.

After the procedure:

- Apply direct pressure over the catheterization site for 15 minutes after wires and catheters are removed. Place a pressure bandage for 6 hours.
- Keep the child on bed rest for 6 hours and avoid flexion of the hips. Then limit activity for 24 hours.
- Begin with clear liquids and progress to other fluids and food as tolerated. Monitor hydration status (contrast medium causes diuresis, and dehydration is a risk for the child treated with diuretics).

Patient and Family Education
Check several times in first 24 hours after catheterization for fever, bleeding or a bruise increasing in size at the catheterization site, loss of feeling in foot, or cooler foot on side of catheterization.

If the child is treated with diuretics, observe for dehydration (dry mucous membranes, no tears, sunken fontanel).

Notify physician immediately if any of these signs are noted within the first 24 hours after the catheterization.

Encourage fluids to help flush the dye out of the body.

Permit quiet play for 24 hours, then allow more active play.

See Box 16–2 for antibiotic prophylaxis guidelines.

Nursing Management Before Surgery

Monitor the infant for poor growth and signs of CHF as described in Congestive Heart Failure; see page 256.

Provide psychosocial support to the parents coping with the infant's diagnosis.

Provide nursing care as described for the infant with CHF.

Teach parents to care for the child at home until surgery, encouraging adequate nutrition, reducing exposure to infectious diseases, monthly prophylaxis for respiratory syncytial virus with palivizumab during the peak season, and other routine health promotion and maintenance visits.

Box 16–2 Cardiac Conditions Needing Infective Endocarditis Antibiotic Prophylaxis

---

Prosthetic cardiac valve or prosthetic material used for cardiac valve repair
Previous infective endocarditis
Congenital heart disease (CHD) with these specific parameters:
  • Unrepaired cyanotic CHD, including palliative shunts and conduits
  • Completely repaired congenital heart defect with prosthetic material or device, whether placed by surgery or by catheter intervention, during the first 6 months after the procedure
  • Repaired CHD with residual effects at the site or adjacent to the site of a prosthetic patch or prosthetic device (which inhibit endothelialization)
Cardiac transplantation recipients who develop cardiac valvulopathy

---

Source: From "Prevention of Infective Endocarditis: Guidelines from the American Heart Association Rheumatic Fever, Endocarditis, and Kawasaki Disease Committee, Council on Cardiovascular Disease in the Young, and the Council on Clinical Cardiology, Council on Cardiovascular Surgery and Anesthesia, and the Quality of Care and Outcomes Research Interdisciplinary Working Group," by W. Wilson, K. A. Taubert, M. Gewitz, P. B. Lockhart, L. M. Baddour, et al., 2007, *Circulation, 116*, 1736-1754.

Nursing Management at the Time of Surgery

Assessment

Before surgery: assess behavioral patterns, cardiac function, respiratory function, weight, and fluid status and for signs of acute illness.

After surgery: assess vital signs, temperature, breath sounds, respiratory effort, and surgical incision site for erythema or wound drainage. Auscultate the apical pulse. Use pulse oximetry to assess oxygen saturation. Monitor intake and output. Identify signs of surgical complications such as infection, arrhythmias, and impaired tissue perfusion. Assess the child's pain.

Implementation

Provide pain management with intravenous (IV) opioids 24 hours a day until the child is taking fluids. Then provide oral analgesics around the clock. Carefully lift and move the child to avoid stress on the incision and pain. Do not lift the child under the arms.

Encourage deep breaths and coughing, or perform spirometry exercises regularly. Chest physiotherapy is used for children younger than 3 years old.

Encourage oral fluids and nutrition when permitted. Oral fluids are rarely limited.

Inspect incision for infection. Administer antibiotics as ordered.

Encourage a gradual increase in activity with longer periods out of bed every day. Ensure adequate rest periods to promote healing.

Patient and Family Teaching

Sponge bathe the infant or use a tub bath with low water level to bathe the child. Clean the incision daily with gentle baby or pH-balanced soap. Keep the incision clean and dry.

Demonstrate methods to lift and move the child to prevent pain and stress on the incision.

Encourage a nutritious diet and snacks so previous growth deficits can be reversed.

Call the healthcare provider for signs of wound infection (redness, swelling, tenderness, or drainage around the incision), fever, a change in appetite or activity level, irritability, or an increased respiratory rate; or signs of postpericardiotomy syndrome (fever of more than 40.3°C [101°F], severe chest pain with inspiration, flulike symptoms up to 2 months after surgery).

Give appropriate dose of acetaminophen or ibuprofen for pain control.

Place a small blanket over the incision for protection while in the car safety seat.

Allow the child to gradually increase activity. No rough play, bike riding, or climbing for 6 weeks until the sternum incision has healed completely. Report increased fatigue or decreased activity tolerance to the physician.

Prepare parents for the child's potential response to hospitalization stress (nightmares, separation anxiety, and overdependence on parents).

When a complete correction of the cardiac defect has been performed, encourage parents to allow the child to live a normal and active life.

See Box 16–2 for antibiotic prophylaxis guidelines for infective endocarditis.

Defects That Cause Decreased Pulmonary Blood Flow and Mixed Defects

Defects causing decreased pulmonary blood flow often permit little or no blood to reach the lungs for oxygenation. When an atrial septal defect or ventricular septal defect exists, higher right-sided pressures shunt blood to the left side. Polycythemia develops to increase the hemoglobin to carry oxygen to the tissues and places the child at higher risk for the following:

- Impaired clotting and risk of bleeding with surgery
- Thromboembolism (cerebral or pulmonary)
- Brain abscesses
- Hypercyanotic episodes: a life-threatening condition associated with an abrupt decrease in systemic resistance and pulmonary blood flow combined with a sudden increase in cardiac output and venous return. Triggered by crying, feeding, exercise, warm bath, or straining with defecation. Hypoxemia worsens as increased respiratory effort further increases the cardiac output.

Mixed defects: the newborn is dependent on the mixing of the pulmonary and systemic circulation blood for survival, resulting in desaturated systemic blood flow and cyanosis. Increased pulmonary blood flow and obstruction of systemic flow cause pulmonary congestion.

Clinical Manifestations
Defects causing decreased pulmonary blood flow (see Box 16–3 for heart defects in this classification):

- Cyanosis when the ductus arteriosus closes, dyspnea, and a loud murmur

Pulmonic Stenosis

Narrowing of the pulmonic valve obstructs blood flow into the pulmonary artery. Increased preload and right ventricular hypertrophy results.

Dyspnea and fatigue on exertion. CHF and chest pain on exertion in severe cases. A loud systolic ejection murmur, widely split S_2, and thrill in the pulmonic area.

Dilation by balloon valvuloplasty during cardiac catheterization or surgical valvotomy when other defects are present.

Tetralogy of Fallot

A combination of pulmonic stenosis, right ventricular hypertrophy, ventricular septal defect, and overriding of aorta. An open foramen ovale or atrial septal defect in some cases.

Hypoxia and cyanosis occur as the ductus arteriosus closes. Polycythemia, hypercyanotic episodes, metabolic acidosis, poor growth, clubbing, and exercise intolerance may develop. Systolic murmur in the pulmonic area transmitted to suprasternal notch. A thrill in the pulmonic area.

Hypercyanotic episodes managed with knee–chest positioning, calming, oxygen, IV morphine, and IV propranolol. Surgical correction is performed before age 6 months if a hypercyanotic episode occurs. A palliative procedure may precede surgery to allow the infant to grow and improve outcome.

Pulmonary Atresia/Tricuspid Atresia

Pulmonary atresia: no communication between the right ventricle and the pulmonary artery. The right ventricle pushes blood back through the tricuspid valve for passage through the foramen ovale. The ductus arteriosus provides the only flow of blood to the pulmonary arteries.

Tricuspid atresia: no communication between the right atrium and ventricle. Blood flows through the foramen ovale as in pulmonary atresia.

Cyanosis at birth. Tachypnea, CHF, pulmonary edema, hepatomegaly, acidosis, hypoxic spells, clubbing, polycythemia, and growth delays. A continuous murmur from the patent ductus arteriosus in pulmonic area. A single S_2 in aortic area, and a harsh systolic murmur in the tricuspid area in pulmonary atresia.

Prostaglandin E_1 to maintain a patent ductus arteriosus. Digoxin and diuretics are used. The Rastelli balloon atrial septostomy is performed to increase the atrial opening. A Rastelli or modified Fontan procedure improves survival.

- Fatigue, clubbing of the fingers and toes, exertional dyspnea, tiring and diaphoresis with feeding, poor weight gain, and delayed developmental milestones
- Low oxygen saturation level because unoxygenated and oxygenated blood mixes; supplemental oxygen does not improve the oxygen saturation level or cyanosis.
- Hypercyanotic episodes: increased rate and depth of respirations; increased cyanosis, pallor, and poor tissue perfusion; increased heart rate; diaphoresis; irritability and crying; and loss of consciousness. The child may have a seizure or cerebrovascular accident and die.
- Exercise-induced dizziness and syncope in an older child

Mixed defects (see Box 16–4 for heart defects in this classification):
- Varying degrees of cyanosis
- Signs of CHF

Box 16–4   Mixed Heart Defects Causing Cyanosis, Their Clinical Manifestations, and Clinical Therapy

Transposition of the Great Arteries
The pulmonary artery is the outflow tract for the left ventricle, and the aorta is the outflow tract for the right ventricle, creating parallel circulations.

Cyanosis at birth, does not improve with oxygen; progresses to hypoxia, acidosis, and CHF. Tachypnea (60 respirations/minute) without retractions or other signs of dyspnea. Difficulty feeding and growth failure. A systolic murmur only if a ventricular septal defect (VSD) is present; loud S_2.

Prostaglandin E_1 (PGE_1) to maintain a patent ductus arteriosus until surgery (arterial switch) before 1 week of age. Balloon atrial septostomy may be first stage to permit mixing of systemic and pulmonary blood. Other defects repaired in stages as the infant grows.

Truncus Arteriosus
A single large vessel empties both ventricles and provides circulation for the pulmonary, systemic, and coronary circulations. A VSD may be present.

Cyanosis soon after birth, increased pulmonary blood flow with severe CHF, dyspnea, retractions, fatigue, poor feeding, poor growth, polycythemia, clubbing, bounding peripheral pulses, increased pulse pressure, frequent respiratory infections, and cardiomegaly. The VSD produces a harsh systolic murmur at the lower sternal border. A systolic click at apex and pulmonic area.

Rastelli procedure to close the VSD and create a passage to pulmonary arteries. Repeated surgery to enlarge pulmonary artery conduit. Digoxin and diuretics may be given.

Total Anomalous Pulmonary Venous Return

The pulmonary veins empty into right atrium or veins leading to the right atrium rather than into the left atrium. The foramen ovale must remain patent for blood to pass to the systemic circulation.

Mild cyanosis and frequent respiratory infections. Increased cyanosis if the pulmonary veins are obstructed and increased pulmonary blood flow, resulting in tachycardia, dyspnea, pulmonary edema, retractions, crackles, hepatomegaly, poor feedings, irritability, and failure to thrive. A palpable precordial bulge. Wide, fixed split S_2 with ejection murmur in the pulmonic area, gallop rhythm.

PGE_1 to maintain patent ductus arteriosus. Hypoxemia and CHF are treated. Balloon atrial septostomy initially, then surgery to reconnect or baffle the pulmonary veins to the left atrium.

Double-Outlet Right Ventricle

Both great arteries leave the right ventricle, increasing pulmonary blood flow and reducing systemic blood flow. The only outlet for the left ventricle is a large VSD.

Growth retardation, tachypnea, signs of CHF, cyanosis, clubbing. Loud S_2 and upper left sternal border systolic murmur, systolic thrill.

Digoxin and diuretics for CHF. Pulmonary artery banding or balloon atrial septostomy when symptomatic. An arterial switch or Senning procedure with an intraventricular tunnel between the VSD and the pulmonary artery.

Diagnostic Procedures

Chest radiograph, ECG, echocardiogram, cardiac catheterization, hematocrit and hemoglobin, and clotting time

Clinical Therapy

Corrective surgery in newborn or young infant. A palliative procedure initially to preserve life, let the infant grow, and improve the success of corrective surgery.

Prostaglandin E_1 (PGE_1) is given to reopen the ductus arteriosus if its closure causes life-threatening cyanosis.

Hemoglobin and hematocrit values are monitored for polycythemia or anemia. Red blood cell pheresis is performed if the blood viscosity is too high.

Hypercyanotic episodes are treated aggressively to decrease the pulmonary vascular resistance:

- Calm the child, give oxygen.
- Administer IV morphine, IV propranolol, and IV fluids. Give dopamine and phenylephrine (Neo-Synephrine). If the child is

anemic, packed red blood cells are given to improve tissue oxygen delivery.
- Use knee–chest position to increase the systemic vascular resistance.
- Immediate palliative or corrective surgery is often scheduled.
- Antibiotic prophylaxis is indicated to prevent infective endocarditis.

Nursing Management

Assessment

Before surgery:
- Closely monitor the infant's cardiovascular status when on PGE_1 therapy. Assess vital signs, heart rhythm, skin color, peripheral pulses, capillary refill time, pulse oximetry, and blood gases.
- For infants at risk for CHF, assess for tachycardia, tachypnea, crackles, frothy secretions, low urine output, and edema.

Before or between stages of surgery at health visits:
- Assess growth and plot on growth curve.
- Identify signs of progressive deterioration in cardiac status (increased cyanosis in the morning or at other high-risk times; note clubbing of the fingers and toes).
- Observe for headache, dizziness, excessive irritability, and paralysis associated with thromboembolitic complication.

After surgery:
- Assess vital signs, pulse oximetry, skin color, perfusion of the skin by capillary refill, and distal pulses. Note any signs of respiratory distress. Observe for early signs of hemorrhage (sudden, sustained increase in pulse and respirations and a decrease in peripheral perfusion).
- Monitor fluid intake and output.
- Assess for pain.

Implementation

Care of the newborn:
- Monitor and carefully maintain the central, umbilical, or peripheral IV lines in the newborn receiving continuous infusion of PGE_1. Observe for common side effects of prostaglandin treatment (cutaneous vasodilation, bradycardia, tachycardia, hypotension, seizure activity, fever, and apnea).
- Have emergency equipment for apnea and IV fluids for hypotension.

Hypercyanotic episode management:
- Immediately place the infant in knee–chest position and administer oxygen. Attempt to calm the infant.
- Administer morphine as ordered.

- Immediately notify the physician for further orders if the episode continues despite interventions.
- Avoid any unpleasant or anxiety-provoking procedures.

Home care of the child before surgery:
- Make referrals to community-based early-intervention programs to promote the child's development. Reduce parental anxiety about developmental delays by informing them that gains are usually seen after surgery.
- Children with mild cyanotic lesions do not need to adjust activity. The child with moderate to severe disease should be able to tolerate crying for a few minutes; but prevent prolonged crying.
- Do not let child travel to high-altitude locations without physician approval. Supplemental oxygen for airplane travel may be necessary.

Patient and Family Education

Teach parents to seek early medical care for acute illnesses (e.g., fever, vomiting, or diarrhea). Educate parents about the signs of infective endocarditis and the need for antibiotic prophylaxis.

Teach parents to observe for signs of worsening cyanosis that could signal a hypercyanotic episode. Assist them to develop an emergency care plan. Provide guidelines for initial management of the hypercyanotic episode.
- Call for an ambulance and try to calm the infant.
- Place in knee–chest position by holding the infant facing the chest, with one arm under the knees, and folding the legs upward toward the infant's chest. Use the other arm to support the infant's back.
- Give oxygen if available without further upsetting the infant.

After surgery:
- Monitor for postoperative bleeding (especially in the chest tube), as bleeding times are prolonged and platelet counts are low in children with polycythemia.
- Nursing care is the same as described for the child having surgery for increased pulmonary blood flow.

Defects Obstructing Systemic Blood Flow

Stenosis of a valve or great artery obstructs blood flow, increases pressure (afterload) on the ventricle, and decreases cardiac output to the pulmonic or systemic circulation.

Clinical Manifestations

Signs of low cardiac output: diminished pulses, poor color, delayed capillary refill time, and decreased urinary output

CHF and pulmonary edema in severe obstructions; in mild obstructions, leg cramps, and cooler feet than hands

Stronger pulses and higher BP in the arms than the legs

See Box 16–5 for heart defects in this classification.

Diagnostic Procedures

Chest radiograph, ECG, echocardiogram, cardiac catheterization, computed tomography or MRI, and stress testing may all be used, depending on the type of defect.

Clinical Therapy

PGE_1 and inotrope medications may be required to support the systemic circulation until the obstruction is relieved or ventricular function improves. Interventional cardiac catheterization (valvuloplasty or balloon dilation) and/or surgery may be performed, depending on the defect. See Box 16–5.

Nursing Management

Care for children with aortic stenosis and coarctation of the aorta is similar to those having defects that increase pulmonary blood flow.

Care for infants with hypoplastic left heart syndrome is similar to those having defects causing decreased pulmonary blood flow and mixed defects. There is no cure, and parents must make decisions very quickly about the best treatment while being faced with the potential death of their newborn. Share information about each treatment option and associated mortality, the intense care a surviving child needs, potential neurocognitive and neurodevelopmental outcomes, and unknown long-term survival. If parents choose comfort or palliative care, PGE_1 is discontinued, and the infant is given pain medication and comfort. Provide supportive care to the family.

Pulmonary Artery Hypertension

Pulmonary artery hypertension is a complication of congenital heart defects that increase pulmonary blood flow, pulmonary conditions, or congenital diaphragmatic hernia. The pulmonary vascular bed tries to reduce excessive pulmonary blood flow by vasoconstriction, leading to smooth muscle hypertrophy in the small pulmonary arteries. The pulmonary artery pressure increases to push blood across the constricted vascular bed, resulting in inflammation, hypertrophy of pulmonary vessels, fibrosis, a right-to-left shunt, and impaired right

Defects That Obstruct the Systemic Blood Flow, Their Clinical Manifestations, and Clinical Therapy

Aortic Stenosis (AS)

Narrowing of the aortic valve obstructs blood flow to systemic circulation.
Usually asymptomatic, but life-threatening AS and congestive heart failure (CHF) seen in some newborns. Normal blood pressure with a narrow pulse pressure; weak peripheral pulses; tolerates exercise; some have chest pain after exercise. Fainting and dizziness are serious signs. Systolic heart murmur and thrill in the aortic or pulmonic areas, transmission to neck, ejection click. Split S_2 with severe aortic stenosis.

Newborns with life-threatening aortic stenosis need prostaglandin E_1 (PGE_1) to maintain a patent ductus arteriosus until the aortic valve can be dilated by balloon valvuloplasty during cardiac catheterization. Surgical valvuloplasty or aortic valve replacement.

Coarctation of the Aorta

Narrowing, or constriction, in the descending aorta, often near the ductus arteriosus or left subclavian artery, obstructs the systemic blood outflow.
Asymptomatic initially, but constriction of aorta is progressive. Lower blood pressure in legs and higher blood pressure in arms, neck, and head. Bounding brachial and radial pulses and weak or absent femoral pulses. Loud, single S_2. Systolic ejection murmur at the upper right and middle or lower left sternal border. A thrill in the suprasternal notch.

Balloon dilation of coarctation and surgical resection with the subclavian artery.

Hypoplastic Left Heart Syndrome

Absence or stenosis of mitral and aortic valves, abnormally small left ventricle, a small aorta, and aortic or mitral stenosis or atresia.
With closure of ductus arteriosus, progressive cyanosis, tachycardia, tachypnea, dyspnea, retractions, and decreased peripheral pulses. Systolic murmur may be present. Poor peripheral perfusion, pulmonary edema, and CHF eventually lead to shock, acidosis, and death.

PGE_1 to maintain a patent ductus arteriosus. No supplemental oxygen. Treatment options are the Norwood procedure, heart transplantation (see Heart Transplantation section), or comfort and palliative care.

heart function. Hypoxemia and acidosis result and help maintain the vasoconstriction. The condition is progressive.

Clinical Manifestations

Infants—tachypnea, cyanosis, retractions, fatigue, difficulty feeding, weight loss, fluid and electrolyte imbalance

Older children—decreased exercise tolerance, exertional dyspnea, chest pain, and syncope

Clinical Therapy

Cardiac catheterization to assess the severity of PAH and to select treatment (Ogawa, 2007)

Congenital heart defect—surgery to correct an obstructive lesion or close a defect

Medications: bronchodilators, antibiotics, corticosteroids, and low-flow oxygen; short-term nitric oxide therapy. Sildenafil and bosetin (pulmonary vasodilators) are undergoing FDA studies evaluating use in children (Bernstein, 2007).

No cure. Heart transplant may be considered.

Nursing Management

Promote rest, monitor fluid intake and output, and administer medications and oxygen. Permit exercise that does not cause dyspnea. Give parents needed support and information.

Heart Transplantation

Heart transplantation indications in children are end-stage cardiac failure, complex congenital heart defects with ventricular failure, or end-stage cardiomyopathy (Gabrys, 2005). Rejection and infection are the major causes of mortality and morbidity.

Clinical Manifestations

Signs of rejection include low-grade fever, increasing resting heart rate, fatigue, abdominal pain, nausea, vomiting, and decreasing exercise intolerance (Gabrys, 2005).

Diagnostic Procedures

Endomyocardial biopsy to detect rejection; echocardiogram to assess cardiac function

Clinical Therapy

Tacrolimus or cyclosporine, azathioprine, and corticosteroids are given for immunosuppression. Lovastatin is given to reduce the serum cholesterol level; calcium channel blockers are given for hypertension.

Provide treatment for bacterial, fungal, and viral infections. Macrolide antibiotics are avoided as they elevate serum cyclosporine and tacrolimus levels (Gabrys, 2005).

Nursing Management

Encourage return to school, activities, and exercise. Encourage a diet and exercise program to reduce the child's risk for obesity and osteoporosis.

Promote positive self-esteem when side effects of immunosuppression occur (hair growth, gum hyperplasia, weight gain, short stature, moon facies, acne, and rashes).

No live virus immunizations are given. If immunizations are not given before transplant, notify schools to report cases of measles, mumps, rubella, and chickenpox to family so child can receive preventive treatment if necessary. Encourage hand washing and other methods to reduce the spread of infection.

Educate the parents and child to follow the immunosuppression regimen, to recognize the signs of rejection, and to seek treatment promptly.

CONGESTIVE HEART FAILURE (CHF)

Cardiac output is inadequate to support the body's circulatory and metabolic needs, and it may result from one of the following:
- A congenital heart defect that causes increased pulmonary blood flow or obstruction to the systemic outflow tract
- Problems with heart contractility
- Conditions that require high cardiac output: severe anemia, acidosis, or respiratory disease
- Acquired heart disease: cardiomyopathy, rheumatic heart disease, or Kawasaki syndrome

Clinical Manifestations

Pulmonary venous congestion leads to tachypnea, wheezing, crackles, retractions, cough, dyspnea on exertion, grunting, nasal flaring, skin color changes (mottling, pallor, or cyanosis), feeding difficulties, irritability, tiring with play, and exercise intolerance.

Systemic venous congestion leads to hepatomegaly, ascites, periorbital edema, peripheral edema, weight gain from retained fluids, and neck vein distention in children.

Impaired cardiac output leads to tachycardia, weak and thready pulses, hypotension, S_3 gallop rhythm, capillary refill time greater than 2 seconds, pallor, cool extremities, oliguria, fatigue, restlessness, and enlarged heart.

High metabolic rate leads to weight loss, failure to thrive or slow weight gain, and diaphoresis.

Diagnostic Tests

Chest radiograph, ECG, echocardiography, endocardial biopsy in rare cases

Clinical Therapy

Medications include diuretics, inotropic medications and afterload-reducing agents, digoxin, and beta-blockers (Table 16–1). Serum potassium is monitored with use of diuretics.

Supportive medical therapy includes airway management, ventilatory support, oxygen, rest, and fluid and dietary management.

Surgery or interventional catheterization is indicated to correct a congenital heart defect; cardiac transplantation is indicated for end-stage cardiomyopathy or complex congenital heart defects such as hypoplastic left heart syndrome.

Table 16–1 Medications Used in Treatment of Congestive Heart Failure

Drug	Nursing Management
Digoxin	Assess the heart rate for 1 minute prior to giving a dose to detect bradycardia (below a guideline in physician's order) or changes in heart rhythm or quality.
	Verify the dose with a second nurse.
	Monitor the child for digitoxicity.
Furosemide	Monitor vital signs, intake and output, and for fluid and electrolyte imbalances during rapid diuresis.
Thiazides: chlorothiazide (suspension), hydrochlorothiazide (tablets)	Monitor blood pressure and intake and output rates and patterns.
	Monitor lab values for hypokalemia. Assess for digitoxicity if present.
Spironolactone	Assess for signs of fluid and electrolyte imbalance, and digitoxicity
Angiotensin-converting enzyme inhibitor	Assess for common side effects such as cough, hyperkalemia, and worsening renal function.
Propranolol	Monitor vital signs and peripheral perfusion. Monitor intake and output ratio; daily weight.
	Dietary sodium is usually restricted.
Carvedilol	Monitor digoxin levels, as drug may increase plasma digoxin concentration.
	Monitor liver function periodically.

Source: Data from *Pediatric Drug Guide*, by R. M. Bindler, & L. B. Howry, B. A. 2005, Upper Saddle River, NJ: Prentice Hall Health; and *Nurses' Drug Guide 2009*, by B. A. Wilson, M. T. Shannon, & K. M. Shields, 2009, Upper Saddle River, NJ: Prentice Hall.

Nursing Management
Assessment

Obtain a detailed history of the onset of symptoms.

Assess vital signs: quality of pulses and respirations and color. Assess for signs of fluid overload; intake and output; serial abdominal measurements; signs of exercise intolerance; feeding difficulty; irritability, behavior changes; growth status; diaphoresis; and skin redness and breakdown. Inspect, palpate, and auscultate the chest and heart.

Conduct a family assessment for knowledge of the child's condition; correct medication dosing; identification of changes in child's condition needing care; ability to provide needed care; anxiety level and coping strategies; support system and respite care; and financial status.

Perform a developmental assessment.

Observe for changes in feeding habits (decreased intake, vomiting, sleeping through feedings, and increased diaphoresis) that may indicate deteriorating cardiac status.

Implementation

Administer and monitor prescribed medications. Read labels carefully and double-check doses.
- Give digoxin at the same times daily.
- Check the apical heart rate for a full minute before giving any dose. If bradycardia is present, call for advice before giving the drug.
- Monitor serum potassium level if diuretics are ordered; hypokalemia increases the risk for digoxin toxicity.
- Observe for signs of digoxin toxicity (tachycardia in young children or bradycardia in older children, nausea, vomiting, anorexia, dizziness, headache, weakness, fatigue, and arrhythmia). Certain antibiotics (macrolides, azithromycin, tetracyclines, and β-lactams) increase digoxin serum concentration.

Provide frequent skin care when edema is present.

Monitor the oxygen flow rate, ensure delivery device is working properly, and provide humidification. Position the child in semi-Fowler or a 45-degree angle.

Group assessments and interventions to provide uninterrupted rest each hour. Encourage quiet activities. Encourage development with appropriate toys, short periods of activity, singing, talking, and music.

Ensure adequate calories for the increased metabolic rate and growth, with a high-calorie formula. Supplement nutrition by transpyloric, nasogastric, or gastrostomy tube as needed.

Patient and Family Education

Teach parents feeding techniques. Burp infants frequently to permit rest and prevent vomiting. Encourage breastfeeding if mother chooses. Some ways to decrease the work of feeding, either with breast or bottle, include the following (Cook & Higgins, 2004):

- Hold the infant at a 45-degree angle to help to decrease venous return to the heart and reduce metabolic demand. If the parent gets fatigued, the infant can be shifted to an infant seat at a 45-degree angle.
- Limit feeding time to 20 to 40 minutes, so the infant does not become overtired.
- Permit the infant to set his or her own rhythm for feeding and resting.
- Follow the infant's cues for hunger, satiety, and tiring.

Provide emotional support to the family.

Teach family about medication administration and safety, toxic effects of digoxin and other medications, and signs of worsening condition.

ACQUIRED HEART DISORDERS

Cardiomyopathy

Dilated cardiomyopathy: as the ventricles stretch or dilate to accommodate increased blood volume, over time the heart muscle pumps blood less effectively, leading to CHF. Blood may pool in the heart, allowing clots to form, and increase embolism risk. Myocarditis and neuromuscular disorders, such as muscular dystrophy, are the most common causes (Towbin, Lowe, Colan, et al., 2006).

Hypertrophic cardiomyopathy: hypertrophy of the ventricular muscles or ventricular septum makes the ventricular walls rigid, reduces the size of the ventricular chamber, and obstructs blood flow. Many cases are autosomal dominant transmission (Le & Chrisant, 2006).

Clinical Manifestations

Dilated cardiomyopathy: CHF, with tachypnea, wheezing, and poor cardiac output.

Hypertrophic cardiomyopathy: exertional dyspnea, fatigue, dizziness, fainting, palpitations, and chest pain. Abnormal heart rhythms may cause sudden death.

Clinical Therapy

Dilated cardiomyopathy: anticoagulants, vasodilators, antiarrhythmics, diuretics and digoxin; heart transplant may be considered.

Hypertrophic cardiomyopathy: beta-blockers, calcium channel blockers, and antiarrhythmics are indicated. Digoxin is contraindicated and diuretics may be harmful (Park, 2008, p. 337).

An implantable cardioverter-defibrillator may prevent sudden death from arrhythmias.

Nursing Management

Nursing management is the same as for CHF and for cardiac arrhythmias.

Dyslipidemia

One or more lipids have an abnormal blood level (total cholesterol, low-density lipoproteins, triglycerides, and/or high-density lipoprotein) that increases the risk for coronary artery disease. Primary dyslipidemia is familial. Secondary dyslipidemia results from a diet rich in saturated fat and too little exercise, diseases such as diabetes, hypothyroidism, and drugs (e.g., such as corticosteroids, isotretinoin, and beta blockers) (Belay, Belamarich, & Racine, 2004).

Clinical Manifestations

Children and adolescents rarely have signs or symptoms.

Diagnostic Tests

A nonfasting serum lipid panel is recommended for all children older than age 2 years who have a family history of cardiovascular disease before age 55 years (parents or grandparents) or have a parent with dyslipidemia. If this lipid panel is borderline or high, a fasting lipid panel should be obtained (Jolliffe & Janssen, 2006). See chapter 5 for laboratory values.

Clinical Therapy

Dietary changes: total fat intake is 20% to 35% of daily calories; saturated fats are less than 7% of total caloric intake; and cholesterol intake is less than 200 mg per day for treatment of elevated LDL-C levels (Gidding, Dennison, Birch, et al., 2005). If the child is obese, weight loss is encouraged. Exercise and other lifestyle changes are made.

Statins, cholestyramine or colestipol, and niacin are indicated for children older than age 10 years.

Nursing Management

Obtain data on familial heart disease, hypertension, diabetes, and smoking to determine risk factors. Identify children who need to have serum lipids measured.

Assess the child's diet, and provide dietary teaching for the entire family to reduce risk. Promote exercise and limit sedentary activity.

Assess the child's history of exercise patterns and weight and body mass index percentiles. Discourage smoking by the child and family.

Hypertension

Hypertension in children and adolescents is defined as a systolic or diastolic blood pressure reading that is equal to or greater than 95th percentile for age, sex, and height. Secondary hypertension in children is most commonly due to coarctation of the aorta and kidney disease. Primary hypertension may be associated with a genetic or familial predisposition and obesity.

Clinical Manifestations

Children rarely have symptoms.

Diagnostic Procedures

Diagnosis is based on three readings of an elevated BP a week or more apart.

Urinalysis, serum creatinine, and serum electrolyte levels are indicated, followed by a urine culture and renal ultrasound if one is abnormal.

Echocardiogram to assess for coarctation of the aorta; a lipid panel is obtained to detect secondary causes of hypertension; polysomnography; drug screen.

Clinical Therapy

Nonpharmacologic therapy: weight reduction, increased exercise, and reduced dietary sodium and saturated fats (less than 10% of calories; three to five fruit servings daily; adequate intake of calcium and dietary fiber).

Discourage smoking, alcohol, and illicit drugs; promote increased exercise.

Medications used for children with persistent, severe hypertension: angiotensin-converting enzyme inhibitors, calcium channel blockers (Mitsnefes, 2006).

Nursing Management
Assessment
Take a complete history of the child with borderline hypertension, including family history, weight, diet, sodium intake, and exercise routines.

Assess the BP with the correct size cuff; have child sit quietly 5 minutes before taking the BP. Include at least one leg BP reading; the systolic reading in the leg is normally at least 10 to 20 mm Hg higher than the arm reading (Cromwell, Munn, & Zolkowski-Wynne, 2005). Compare readings to normal BP for age, height percentile, and gender (see chapter 1).

Implementation
Teach the importance of weight reduction and dietary changes. Provide substitute seasonings for salt, lists of salty foods to avoid, and encourage intake of low-fat dairy products and fruits.

Encourage increased activity and reduced time for television and computer games.

Provide suggestions for stress management.

Teach the correct administration of prescribed medications when used.

Infective Endocarditis
Infective endocarditis is an inflammation of the lining, valves, and arterial vessels of the heart caused by bacterial, enterococci, and fungal infections. The causal organism enters the bloodstream and lodges on damaged or abnormal endocardial tissue. Children at greater risk have complex congenital heart disease with implanted vascular grafts, patches, or prosthetic valves, or have conditions requiring indwelling venous catheters (Hoyer & Silberbach, 2005). It is also associated with IV drug use. Not all cases can be prevented.

Clinical Manifestations
A prolonged low-grade fever, fatigue, weakness, weight loss, joint and muscle aches, diaphoresis, a new or changing murmur, CHF, decreased oxygen saturation levels, dyspnea, hematuria, petechiae, and splenomegaly

Pulmonary symptoms or signs of septic pulmonary embolism with indwelling catheters

Diagnostic Procedures
Blood, urine, and cerebrospinal fluid cultures, erythrocyte sedimentation rate, C-reactive protein, complete blood cell count, ECG, transesophageal and transthoracic echocardiogram

Clinical Therapy

IV antibiotics (e.g., penicillin G, ceftriaxone, vancomycin, nafcillin, oxacillin, gentamicin, ciprofloxacin, cefazolin) are indicated for 2 to 8 weeks until the infective organism is eradicated. Serum levels of antibiotics are monitored to maintain a therapeutic range.

Surgery may be indicated to replace a heart valve or because of embolism risk.

See Box 16–2 for antibiotic prophylaxis guidelines for dental and invasive respiratory procedures. Oral amoxicillin (alternatively IV ampicillin, cefazolin, or ceftriaxone) is given 30 to 60 minutes before procedures (Wilson, Taubert, Gewitz, et al., 2007).

Nursing Management

Prevent infective endocarditis when possible.

- Educate parents of children and adolescents to ask for prophylaxis before professional teeth cleaning and other dental procedures and invasive respiratory procedures.
- Discourage body piercing and tattoos, which increase risk (Braverman, 2006).

Care of the child who has infective endocarditis:

- Monitor the vital signs, oxygen saturation, level of consciousness, intake and output, and level of comfort. Monitor for signs of CHF or embolism. Assess the parents' coping.
- Administer IV medications as ordered, and monitor serum antibiotic levels. Monitor for side effects of antibiotics and for infusion site infiltration.
- Use careful aseptic technique for all invasive procedures.
- Plan appropriate activities; the child is often lethargic and on bed rest.
- Arrange for home antibiotic infusion therapy and home schooling.
- Encourage social interactions with peers during recuperation.

Kawasaki Disease

Kawasaki disease is an acute febrile, systemic vascular inflammatory illness of unknown cause that affects the small and mid-sized arteries. It is the leading cause of acquired heart disease in children in the United States (Vetter, 2006). Coronary arterial damage may cause narrowing and infarcts or aneurysms (Milana & Chandran, 2006).

Clinical Manifestations

Acute stage—irritability, fever, conjunctival hyperemia, red throat, swollen hands and feet, rash on the trunk and perineal area, unilateral enlargement of the anterior cervical lymph nodes, diarrhea, and hepatic dysfunction, lasting 1 to 2 weeks

Subacute stage—cracking lips and fissures, skin desquamation on the tips of the fingers and toes, joint pain, cardiac disease, and thrombocytosis, lasting 2 to 4 weeks

Convalescent stage—6 to 8 weeks after disease onset; child appears normal, but lingering signs of inflammation may be present

Diagnostic Procedures

Diagnosis based on specific clinical findings when a fever higher than 39°C (102.2°F) is present for 5 days or longer (Vetter, 2006):

- Bilateral conjunctivitis without exudate
- Dry, swollen, cracked lips and a strawberry tongue
- Intense erythema and induration of the hands and feet, followed by desquamation
- An erythematous maculopapular rash on the trunk
- Acute cervical lymphadenopathy

Echocardiograms are indicated to monitor heart and coronary artery changes.

Clinical Therapy

IV immunoglobulin (2 g/kg given in a single infusion) and high doses of oral aspirin within 10 days of fever onset reduces arterial damage; a second dose of immunoglobulin is used if the fever persists. Corticosteroids are indicated if IV immunoglobulin is not effective.

Careful monitoring for cardiac disease (coronary artery aneurysm or stenosis) continues for several weeks or months. Coronary artery angioplasty or coronary artery bypass grafts may be needed for coronary artery stenosis.

Nursing Management

Assessment

Take the temperature every 4 hours and before each dose of aspirin. Carefully assess heart sounds and rhythm.

Assess the extremities for edema, redness, and desquamation every 8 hours. Assess for conjunctivitis and mucous membrane inflammation.

Monitor dietary and fluid intake and weigh the child daily.

Implementation

Administer aspirin and monitor for side effects.

Administer IV immunoglobulin as a blood product, regulating the slow infusion rate to 1 mL/min or less. Monitor for infusion reaction.

Keep the child's skin clean and dry, and lubricate the lips. Use cool compresses to make the feverish child more comfortable. Change the child's clothes and bed linens frequently.

Give frequent, small feedings of soft foods and liquids that are neither too hot nor too cold.

Use passive range-of-motion exercises to facilitate joint movement.

Plan rest periods and quiet, age-appropriate activities.

Patient and Family Education
Teach the parents to administer aspirin as ordered and to watch for side effects. Take the child's temperature daily and report any fever above 37.8°C (100°F) to the physician.

Limit strenuous activity when coronary artery aneurysms or stenosis exist. Emphasize the need for follow-up care to monitor for cardiac complications.

Postpone measles and varicella immunizations, if not already given, for 11 months after immunoglobulin administration. Give other vaccines per schedule, including influenza.

Rheumatic Fever
Rheumatic fever is an inflammatory connective tissue disorder that results from an autoimmune response to M strains of group A beta-hemolytic streptococci. The disorder may cause long-term damage to heart valves, and affects the joints, brain, and skin tissues.

Clinical Manifestations
Hallmark signs occur 1 to 3 weeks after an untreated streptococcal infection and include the following:

A new heart murmur possibly indicating inflammation of the mitral and aortic valves; chest pain due to pericardial inflammation

Two or more joints with pain, swelling, tenderness, erythema, and heat; may migrate to different joints (migratory polyarthritis)

Subcutaneous nodules along bony prominences or extensor tendons

Pink macules with blanching in the middle of the lesions, on the trunk and proximal extremities but not on the face (Erythema marginatum)

Aimless movements of the extremities and facial grimacing (Sydenham's chorea or St. Vitus dance)

Diagnostic Procedures

Diagnosis is based on evidence of a preceding streptococcal infection (positive throat culture or rapid streptococcal antigen test, or elevated or rising streptococcal antibody titer) and physical signs of carditis, joint pain, fever, erythema marginatum, subcutaneous nodules, and chorea.

Echocardiogram is indicated to monitor for cardiac damage.

Clinical Therapy

Antibiotics and aspirin; corticosteroids (for severe carditis with CHF)

Long-term antibiotic prophylaxis to reduce the risk of recurrent attacks; children with cardiac valve damage also need infective endocarditis prophylaxis.

Nursing Management

Prevention of rheumatic fever:

- Perform a throat culture for all sore throats, especially if family members or other contacts have had a streptococcal infection.
- Emphasize giving the entire 10-day course of antibiotics when a culture is positive.

During the acute inflammatory phase while hospitalized:

- Monitor vital signs and take temperature every 4 hours. Auscultate the heart for any new sounds. Observe for changes in skin, joints, or behavior.
- Keep child on bed rest while monitoring for carditis onset and for 4 weeks if carditis develops. Provide quiet activities; the child is often lethargic.
- Perform throat cultures on family members.
- Administer antibiotic and aspirin as ordered.
- Place the child's joints in neutral position and handle them carefully, as the child often has joint pain until receiving several aspirin doses.

During the recovery phase at home:

- Limit activities, especially if heart damage is suspected. Help parents plan quiet activities. Arrange rest periods after the child returns to school.

Patient and Family Education

- Emphasize the importance of taking a daily oral low-dose antibiotic or monthly long-acting antibiotic injection until adulthood. Emphasize the need for follow-up care.

- Educate about the need for infective endocarditis prophylaxis.
- Educate about the need to culture future sore throats, as they may be streptococcal even when the child is taking daily antibiotics; additional antibiotics will be needed for an infection.

CARDIAC ARRHYTHMIAS

Long QT Syndrome

Long QT syndrome is a rhythm disturbance of delayed ventricular repolarization caused by an autosomal dominant and autosomal recessive inheritance, or may result from hypokalemia, hypocalcemia, or hypomagnesemia (Doniger & Sharieff, 2006). It increases the risk for ventricular fibrillation and sudden death.

Clinical Manifestations

Syncope or seizure; the arrhythmia commonly occurs without warning and may result in death. Early signs include a heart rate too fast to count, irritability, lethargy, poor feeding, poor perfusion (cool, pale skin, increased capillary refill time), decreased responsiveness, and decreased BP.

Clinical Therapy

If the child is resuscitated or evaluated due to early signs, an ECG detects the arrhythmia.

Beta-blockers (e.g., propranolol) and class 1B antiarrhythmic agents (mexiletene and phenytoin; Balaji, 2004; Doniger & Sharieff, 2006) are indicated.

Several medications may trigger episodes (e.g., antihistamines, macrolide antibiotics) and should not be prescribed (Erickson & Jones, 2000).

Nursing Management

Educate parents and children to avoid triggers that cause arrhythmia episodes, such as competitive athletics, swimming, loud noises, and hypokalemia.

Teach the parents and adolescents about prescription medications and over-the-counter medications to avoid, and to share the list with healthcare providers. The list is available at http://www.qtdrugs.org.

Supraventricular Tachycardia (SVT)

Supraventricular tachycardia is an abrupt onset of a rapid, regular heart rate, often too fast to count, due to a congenital heart defect or Wolff-Parkinson-White syndrome. Prolonged episodes of SVT (more than 24 hours) are life-threatening and can progress to CHF or cardiogenic shock if untreated.

Clinical Manifestations

A heart rate of up to 260 beats/minute in infants or between 150 and 240 beats/minute in older children. Early signs in infants include poor feeding, irritability, and pallor. Older children may have palpitations, chest discomfort, dizziness, syncope, or cardiac arrest. Recurrent attacks are common.

Diagnostic Procedures

ECG diagnoses the condition. A 24-hour Holter monitor or event monitor can be used for episodic SVT; stress testing is used if exercise triggers SVT. Electrophysiologic cardiac catheterization or transesophageal ECG recording can be used to diagnose and select appropriate treatment.

Clinical Therapy

SVT episodes in a stable infant or child are initially treated with vagal maneuvers (ice to face, rectal stimulation with a thermometer, Valsalva maneuver, gag reflex, blowing forcefully on the thumb) to slow the heart rate.

IV adenosine is indicated when the vagal maneuvers are unsuccessful. Digoxin, amiodarone, or propranolol may be used when more aggressive therapy is needed for acute episodes.

Synchronized cardioversion is used for urgent or life-threatening situations in a sedated child to convert the tachycardia to sinus rhythm.

Long-term digoxin and beta blockers may be given to reduce the frequency of episodes (Kaltman, Madan, Vetter, et al., 2006).

Radiofrequency ablation may be performed in the cardiac catheterization laboratory.

Nursing Management

Assessment

Monitor vital signs; use a cardiorespiratory monitor and pulse oximetry to identify deterioration of the child's condition. Identify changes in level of consciousness, color, weakness, irritability, and feeding pattern, indicating hypoxia and cardiopulmonary compromise.

Implementation

Assist with vagal maneuvers if ordered, and monitor for recurrence of the arrhythmia.

Administer medications as ordered and monitor for response.

Provide for rest and adequate nutrition.

Have emergency drugs and resuscitation equipment available at bedside.

Patient and Family Education
Educate about danger signs indicating a recurrence of SVT and the use of valsalva maneuver. Encourage parents to become trained in CPR and to have an emergency care plan.

Emphasize the avoidance of cardiac stimulant medications (e.g., decongestants) that could trigger another episode. Educate parents about prescribed medications for SVT management.

INJURIES OF THE CARDIOVASCULAR SYSTEM

Hypovolemic Shock

Inadequate tissue and organ perfusion results from the movement of blood or plasma out of the intravascular compartment. Inadequate intravascular volume leads to impaired delivery of oxygen and nutrients to cells and accumulation of toxic waste in the capillaries. Cellular hypoxia and acidosis develop simultaneously. Causes include hemorrhage, burns, nephrotic syndrome, sepsis, dehydration, diabetic ketoacidosis, and diabetes insipidus. The child's body attempts to compensate with adrenergic and renal mechanisms until 20% to 25% of volume loss occurs, and then life-threatening hypotension and hypoxemia occur.

Clinical Manifestations

Early shock—persistent tachycardia of more than 130 beats per minute, increased respiratory effort, capillary refill time of more than 2 seconds, weak distal pulses, pallor or mottled color, cold extremities, BP often normal for age, child irritable and anxious, decreased urine output (less than 1–2 mL/kg/hour in newborns and less than 0.5–1.0 mL/kg/hour in infants and children).

Uncompensated shock—tachycardia, tachypnea, absent distal pulses, decreasing systolic BP, capillary refill time of more than 3 seconds, cold extremities, cyanosis, confusion, lethargy, decreased level of consciousness, oliguria. Progresses to cardiopulmonary failure if untreated.

Diagnostic Procedures

No laboratory values diagnose the volume deficit rapidly. Hematocrit and hemoglobin, arterial blood gases, serum electrolytes, glucose, osmolality, blood urea nitrogen, and urinalysis are indicated.

Clinical Therapy

Establish and maintain a patent airway, give supplemental oxygen, and control bleeding.

Start an IV or intraosseous line to give large volumes of Ringer's lactate that has buffers to counteract acidosis (Ecklund & Ecklund, 2007). A fluid volume of 20 mL/kg is administered rapidly over 5 minutes and repeated in 5 minutes if the child's physiologic condition does not improve. Packed red blood cells are often administered when no response to the fluid boluses.

Inotropic medications to sustain cardiac output and increase renal perfusion are indicated for some children.

Monitor the child's circulatory status, especially when the liver or spleen is injured, for signs of continued bleeding.

Nursing Management

Assessment

Assess the severity of acute illnesses to determine if dehydration is present. If external bleeding is apparent, determine the amount of blood lost. Assess for a potential injury causing internal bleeding if no external bleeding.

Frequently assess the child's vital signs, capillary refill time, level of consciousness, color, and skin temperature. Monitor urine output and specific gravity hourly. Signs of the child's improved status include the following:

- A decrease in heart rate, respiratory rate, and capillary refill time
- An increase in systolic BP and urine output
- Improved color, level of consciousness, and skin temperature
- Regaining of lost weight

Implementation

Assist with the child's assessment and IV access. Calculate and prepare the IV fluid boluses needed for the child's weight (20 mL/kg). Ensure rapid fluid administration by IV push or pressure bag. Monitor the child's physiologic response to the fluid bolus within 5 minutes.

Keep the child warm. Use warmed IV fluids for resuscitation.

When packed red blood cells are given, verify that the correct blood has been obtained. Change the IV fluid to normal saline. Assess the child carefully for a transfusion reaction.

Support to the child and family during the acute phase of treatment. When the parent is present during the resuscitation, assign a healthcare provider to provide information and support. Explain the care being provided and how it helps the child. Listen to parent concerns and correct any misconceptions.

Distributive Shock (Septic Shock)

Distributive shock is an abnormal distribution of blood volume usually resulting from a decrease in systemic vascular resistance, allowing blood to accumulate in the extremities. Less blood returns to the heart, so preload and cardiac output fall. Common causes include sepsis, anaphylaxis, and spinal cord injury.

Clinical Manifestations

Septic shock has three phases: compensated, uncompensated, and refractory.

Compensated phase—tachycardia and tachypnea; fever (more than 38°C, or 100.4°F) or hypothermia (less than 36°C, or 96.8°F); warm, dry extremities; a bounding pulse and a brisk capillary refill time; normal urine output; diminished level of responsiveness.

Uncompensated phase—hypotension and inadequate oxygen and nutrient delivery to the tissues; fever or hypothermia; poor tissue perfusion of the vital organs; multiple organ failure begins.

Refractory phase—shock becomes irreversible, cardiac output falls.

Clinical Therapy

Treatment of sepsis, with appropriate antibiotics effective for the organisms, is indicated.

Aggressive fluid administration is used to stabilize the circulation and ensure adequate tissue perfusion.

Hemodynamic monitoring and vasopressors are used to maintain the BP. Metabolic acidosis is treated.

Nursing Management

See Hypovolemic Shock section.

17 ALTERATIONS IN IMMUNOLOGIC FUNCTION

To understand normal actions of the immune system, an overview of the types of cells and tissues in the immune system, as well as the classes of immunoglobulins, is necessary.

IMMUNODEFICIENCY DISORDERS

Immunodeficiency, a state of decreased responsiveness of the immune system, can occur to varying degrees in response to several congenital or acquired events and causes a deficiency in B cells, T cells, or both.

Congenital or **primary immunodeficiency** occurs when infants are born with a lack of humoral antibody formation (B-cell disorder), a deficient cellular immune system (T-cell disorder), or a combination of both defects.

Acquired or **secondary immunodeficiency,** as in human immunodeficiency virus (HIV) infection.

See Table 17–1.

Severe Combined Immunodeficiency Disease

Severe combined immunodeficiency disease (SCID) is a congenital condition characterized by severely impaired humoral and cellular immunity, which is manifested by lack of appropriately functioning T cells and B cells (Davies, 2005; Tezcan, et al., 2005). SCID occurs in X-linked recessive and autosomal recessive forms. The disorder is more common in males than females. Without appropriate treatment, children born with severe combined immunodeficiency disease usually do not survive more than 1 year (Cleary, Insel, & Lewis, 2005; Davies, 2005; Kobrynski, 2006).

Clinical Manifestations
Susceptibility to infection during the first few months.

Manifestations include oral candidiasis, failure to thrive, skin infections, persistent respiratory infections, and diarrhea (Box 17–1).

Diagnostic Tests
Complete blood count

Erythrocyte sedimentation rate

B- and T-cell lymphocyte counts (see Table 17–2)

Table 17–1   Laboratory Findings for Selected Congenital Immunodeficiency Disorders

Disorders	Laboratory Findings
B cell	
X-linked hypogammaglobulinemia	Reduced IgA, IgM, IgE, IgG (<100 mg/dL), absence of B cells in peripheral blood, normal T cells
Selective IgA deficiency	IgA <10 mg/dL
Common variable immuno-deficiency	IgA, IgM reduced; IgG <250 mg/dL
T cell	
DiGeorge syndrome	Lymphopenia; absent T-cell functions, decreased T cells, normal B cells
Immunodeficiency with hyper-IgM	Reduced IgG, IgA; elevated IgM; mutations in T-cell surface proteins
Combined	
Severe combined immunodefi-ciency syndrome	Complete absence of T and B cells and NK immunity
Wiskott-Aldrich syndrome	Thrombocytopenia, low platelet volume, nonfunctional B cells, normal IgG, decreased IgM, increased IgA, increased IgE; inability to respond to polysaccharide antigens

Note: IgA, immunoglobulin A; IgE, immunoglobulin E; IgG, immunoglobulin G; IgM, immuno-globulin; NK, natural killer.

Immunoglobulin levels are significantly reduced. Refer to Table 17–1 for laboratory findings in SCID.

A chest radiograph is conducted to assess thymus size.

Clinical Therapy

Intravenous immune globulin is administered to provide protection until humoral immunity is established.

Hematopoietic stem cell transplantation offers the best hope for children with SCID.

Box 17–1	Warning Signs of Primary Immune Deficiency

Persistent, frequent, and unusual types of infections

Infections that are resistant to treatment

Failure to thrive

Delayed development

Family history of primary immunodeficiency

Table 17–2 Cells Evaluated in Laboratory Studies for Immune Conditions

Test and Type of Cell Evaluated	Action	Implication of Increased or Decreased Levels
White blood cell count		
Neutrophil (polys) (54%–62%)	Phagocytic cell that defends against bacteria	Increased in bacterial infection, inflammatory processes, and some malignancies
Eosinophil (1%–3%)	Associated with antigen–antibody reaction	Increased in allergic reaction; decreased in children receiving corticosteroids
Lymphocytes (T, B, and non-B/non-T [natural killer]) (25%–33%)	Major components of immune system	Increased in many infections; decreased in children with immune deficiency
Immunoglobulins (Ig)		
IgM, IgG, IgA, IgD, IgE	Many roles in a number of immunologic reactions	Increased in presence of infection or allergic response; decreased in children with immune deficiency

T-cell function is restored with the transplantation, and new cells appear 3 to 4 months after infusion of the donor stem cell.

Prevention and prompt treatment of infection is essential. Antibiotic therapy is targeted at infectious agents. Antibiotic prophylaxis and special immunization recommendations are needed. Children with T-cell deficiencies should receive cytomegalovirus-negative irradiated blood products due to the risk of infection and graft-versus-host disease from lymphocytes in the donor blood (Kobrynski, 2006).

Nursing Management

Assessment and Diagnosis

Obtain a thorough history of infections, including age of onset, type of causal organism, frequency, and severity.

Assess family history, and determine whether the child has had any unusual reactions to vaccines, medications, or foods.

Measure the child's height and weight accurately to identify failure to thrive.

Assess the child's nutritional intake and fluid and electrolyte balance.

Assess for any evidence of infections involving the skin, subcutaneous tissues, respiratory system, or mucous membranes.

Palpate the abdomen for hepatomegaly and the lymph nodes for lymphadenopathy.

Perform a developmental assessment, and assess for delays in achievement of developmental milestones.

Assess family support systems and coping mechanisms when the child is diagnosed with the disorder.

Implementation
Prevent Systemic Infection
Frequent and thorough hand hygiene is essential.

Standard precautions are always used, and transmission-based precautions are established when indicated.

Implement sterile or aseptic technique when caring for all sites where needles, catheters, central lines, endotracheal tubes, pressure-monitoring lines, peripheral intravenous lines, or other invasive equipment enters the child's body.

Food and other items entering the hospital room may require special treatment.

Place the child in a positive pressure isolation room; contact with infectious individuals should be avoided.

Inform parents that because of the risk of infection to the child, live vaccines are avoided. Refer to current immunization guidelines for the immunocompromised child at http://www.cdc.gov.

Promote Skin Integrity
Provide thorough and frequent skin care, and closely observe all possible pressure areas for signs of breakdown or infection.

Implement measures to avoid skin trauma.

Reposition the child frequently, and encourage range-of-motion exercises.

Promote Nutritional Balance
Encourage adequate fluid and nutritional intake.

Provide foods that the child prefers and those with high nutritional value.

Offer small, frequent feedings of high-calorie, protein-rich foods.

Protein intake can be increased by adding dried milk powder to foods.

Energy intake can be increased by adding small amounts of fats and special nutritional formulas to the diet.

Only pasteurized milk products should be used to avoid potential infection.

Refer to a dietitian as needed to plan with parents for the best individualized diet for the child.

Manage Medication Therapy
Administer IVIG as prescribed.

Monitor for side effects of antibiotics, such as overgrowth of resistant organisms.

Provide Emotional Support and Referrals
SCID is a life-threatening and devastating disease.

Evaluate the family's knowledge about the disease and provide education on infection control measures and signs of infection.

Involve the parents by encouraging them to assist in and manage care for their child.

Listen closely to their concerns and encourage them to discuss their fears.

Offer referrals to an appropriate support group or counselor if needed.

Genetic counseling should be encouraged.

Wiskott-Aldrich Syndrome

A combined congenital immunodeficiency syndrome, Wiskott-Aldrich syndrome (WAS) is an X-linked recessive disorder that occurs in males and causes mutation in the WAS gene and changes in the WAS protein (Kobrynski, 2006).

Clinical Manifestations

Thrombocytopenia, which leads to bleeding, evidenced by petechiae, hematuria, bloody diarrhea, and hematemesis

Eczema and recurrent infections in infancy and childhood. Infections including otitis media, bacterial pneumonia, and skin infections are common (Ochs & Thrasher, 2006).

Diagnostic Tests
Complete blood count

Platelet count

Immunoglobulin levels

Stool for guaiac

Clinical Therapy
Antibiotic prophylaxis with platelet infusions, and intravenous immune globulin infusions

Splenectomy, if hypersplenism is present

Hematopoietic stem cell transplantation is the only cure.

Nursing Management
Nursing care is similar to that for the child with SCID.

Assessment
Assess for splenomegaly, cervical lymphadenopathy, and hepatomegaly.

Observe for excessive bleeding from any wounds or bleeding from the gastrointestinal tract.

Thorough assessments for signs of infection.

Implementation
Refer the parents for genetic counseling to help them understand the transmission of the disease and the probability of having another child with the same disorder.

Referral to family counseling may be appropriate.

Provide support during the process of transplantation.

Arrange for psychological support for those parents who may be overwhelmed with guilt from learning that the illness is inherited.

Human Immunodeficiency Virus and Acquired Immunodeficiency Syndrome
Clinical Manifestations
See Table 17–3 for HIV staging.

The neonate is asymptomatic at birth. The time period for the development of opportunistic infections varies; however, the interval from HIV infection to the onset of overt acquired immunodeficiency syndrome (AIDS) is shorter in children than in adults and shorter in children infected perinatally than in those infected through transfusion. See Table 17–4 for clinical manifestations of HIV in children.

Table 17–3 Clinical Staging of Pediatric Human Immunodeficiency Virus (HIV) Infection (Children Younger Than 13 Years of Age)

Diagnosis of HIV infection in children

    HIV infected (two or more positive tests for HIV or clinical signs and symptoms of HIV infection or an AIDS-defining illness)

    Perinatally exposed (born to a mother known to be infected with HIV)

    Seroconverter (born to a mother known to be infected with HIV, but has had two negative HIV tests)

When infected, the child with HIV is classified as

    Category N (not symptomatic)

    Category A (mildly symptomatic)

    Category B (moderately symptomatic)

    Category C (severely symptomatic)

Source: Adapted from *Red Book: 2006 Report of the Committee on Infectious Diseases* (27th ed., pp. 380–381), American Academy of Pediatrics, 2006, Elk Grove Village, IL: Author.

Table 17–4 Clinical Manifestations of Human Immunodeficiency Virus in Children

Etiology	Clinical Manifestation
Frequent, chronic, or unusual infections due to poor immune response	Chronic bilateral otitis media
	Oral candidiasis
	Pneumocystis jiroveci pneumonia (PCP)
	Skin disorders
	Fever
Poor nutritional intake owing to lack of appetite caused by disease and medications	Failure to thrive (eating disorder of childhood)
	Weight and body mass index below 10th percentile
	Chronic diarrhea
	Skin irritation
Immune system overgrowth to compensate for lack of proper immune response	Hepatosplenomegaly and lymphadenopathy

Note: Be alert for the possibility of HIV infection in infants with some combinations of the clinical manifestations, especially in infants known to be at risk.

Most children with AIDS have nonspecific findings, including:

- Lymphadenopathy
- Hepatosplenomegaly
- Nephropathy

- Oral candidiasis
- Failure to thrive and weight loss
- Delayed development
- Chronic diarrhea
- Chronic eczema and dermatitis
- Fever of unknown origin
- Specific symptoms usually appear within 2 years in children who acquire HIV infection perinatally.
- Bacterial and opportunistic infections, such as *Streptococcus, Haemophilus influenza, Salmonella,* and *Pneumocystis jiroveci* pneumonia (formerly known as *pneumocystis carini),* and malignancies, such as lymphomas, frequently occur as the disease progresses.
- Lymphoid interstitial pneumonitis
- Encephalopathy, resulting in developmental delay or a deterioration of motor skills and intellectual functioning (Plowfield, 2007; Kline, 2006)

Diagnostic Tests

Serologic tests for detection of the virus are monitored in infants born to HIV-infected mothers. These tests are performed within 48 hours of birth.

Infants with initially negative virologic tests should be retested at 1 to 2 months. Tests are repeated at 3 and 6 months, and then again between 12 and 18 months.

Because an infant born to an HIV-infected mother may have maternal antibodies up to 18 months of age, routine antibody tests are not helpful for diagnosing HIV infection in infants (Alvarez & Rathore, 2007).

Preferred tests are the HIV DNA polymerase chain reaction (PCR) or the HIV RNA assay (viral load).

Any positive result is confirmed by retesting.

CD4+ percentage or counts should be performed at least every 3 to 4 months to evaluate the child's immune status (U.S. Department of Health and Human Services, 2008a).

Clinical Therapy

Medical management begins with prevention of the spread of HIV from mother to newborn.

Early identification of infected infants is important to ensure the most effective treatment.

HIV-infected mothers should be identified during pregnancy, and their infants should undergo periodic laboratory testing, as described earlier.

All infected mothers should receive combination antiretroviral therapy after the first trimester of pregnancy. Monotherapy is no longer recommended in the United States; however, if a mother with HIV infection is in labor and has not been on an antiretroviral regimen, this type of treatment may be used (Cibulka, 2006).

Medication Therapy

All infants of infected mothers with indeterminant HIV infection status should start prophylaxis against PCP by the age of 4 to 6 weeks and continue to 1 year of age unless the diagnosis of HIV infection is excluded. Prompt therapy with anti-infectives is used for bacterial and viral opportunistic infections. The need for prophylaxis after 1 year of age is dependent on the child's degree of immunosuppression (AAP, 2006; Baker, 2007).

Treatment for the child diagnosed with HIV involves highly active antiretroviral therapy (HAART). Initial medication therapy should include a combination of several antiretroviral (AVR) drugs. At least three drugs from a minimum of two different categories should be used: the nucleoside/nucleotide reverse transcriptase inhibitors, abacavir, didanosine, emtricitabine, laminvudine, stavudine and zidovudine; protease inhibitors atazanavir, fosamprenavir, lopinavir/ritonavir, nelfinavir and ritonavir; the nonnucleoside reverse transcriptase inhibitors efavirenz and nevirapine; and the fusion inhibitor enfuvirtide are all approved for use in children (Alvarez & Rathore, 2007;U.S. Department of Health and Human Services, 2008a; U.S. Department of Health and Human Services, 2008b).

Nursing Management

Assessment and Diagnosis

For infants at risk of HIV infection, obtain the HIV test results of the mother, if available. When the mother's results are positive, the infant should be screened for HIV infection according to the Centers for Disease Control and Prevention guidelines as described in the Diagnostic Tests section.

Facilitate the screening, and explain the necessity of the screening to the family.

Physiologic Assessment

Observe and evaluate potential sites of infection.

Assess breath sounds, respiratory status, arterial blood gases, level of consciousness, and mental status.

Assess the child's height and weight frequently. Observe for signs of failure to thrive, and assess for anemia.

Assess for *Candida* infections in the mouth and the diaper area.

Note any developmental delays in motor skills or intellectual functioning.

Psychosocial Assessment

Assess family support systems and coping mechanisms, as the stressors of caring for a child with HIV infection may overwhelm parents.

Assess the family's ability to care for the child. Inquire about the extended family's ability to provide daily care as well as emotional support.

Support the family when they decide to inform a school-age child or adolescent of the diagnosis.

When assessing an adolescent with HIV infection, evaluate the teen's understanding of how HIV is transmitted and the response to the diagnosis.

Implementation

Prevent disease by evaluating test results and instituting measures to prevent perinatal transmission of HIV to the infants of infected mothers.

Testing, prophylaxis for HIV-exposed infants and opportunistic infections, and follow-up visits for evaluation of general health and development for all infants at risk of the disease are advised.

Educate sexually active adolescents on the importance of practicing safe sex and the ramifications of high-risk sexual behaviors and intravenous drug abuse.

Adolescents who are sexually active should be offered HIV testing. Many states have provisions that allow teens to be tested for HIV without parental knowledge (CDC, 2006e).

Prevent Infection

Prevent infection with HIV, and prevent infections of various types in children with HIV infection:

- Protect the neonate from HIV-infected maternal secretions.
- Bathe the newborn as soon as possible after delivery, and wash the eyes and face before administration of prophylactic eye drops or ointment.
- Avoid invasive procedures in the newborn.

- Encourage the mother to formula-feed rather than breastfeed (Luxner, 2003; NIAID, 2004).
- Properly dispose of needles and contaminated materials or equipment to reduce the transmission of HIV.
- Frequent hand hygiene and limiting exposure of the child to individuals with upper respiratory or other infections are the best interventions to protect the child with HIV from acquiring other infections.
- A modified immunization schedule is recommended (see chapter 7).

Tuberculosis is more common in children with HIV infection; therefore, annual skin tests that are performed and read by health professionals are recommended (AAP, 2006).

Promote Medication Regimen Adherence

A treatment regimen with antiretroviral therapies for the child with HIV infection may be complex, time consuming, and costly, presenting an overwhelming challenge to the child and the family.

Adherence to the prescribed antiretroviral regimen is imperative, as nonadherence will likely result in increased morbidity and mortality.

Use behavior modification techniques and positive reinforcement to promote the child's adherence.

Promote Respiratory Function

Encourage the child to cough and deep breathe every 2 to 4 hours to improve respiratory function.

Blowing cotton balls with a straw, blowing bubbles, or other games may engage the interest of a younger child.

Reposition infants frequently so that all areas of the lungs can fully expand.

Rest periods to conserve energy and lower the body's demand for oxygen should be included in the plan of care.

Promote Adequate Nutritional Intake

Because many children with HIV infection have failure to thrive, nutrition is an important part of their care.

A nutritionist should be involved in planning an appropriate diet for the child that provides necessary calories, protein, and other nutrients.

Vitamins may be especially lacking in the diets of infected children.

Antioxidants (vitamin A, vitamin E, zinc, and selenium) are known to enhance general immune system function and should be consumed at recommended levels.

Adequate nutrition is sometimes provided by hyperalimentation, nasogastric feeding, or gavage feeding.

Alternative formulas may be recommended.

Anti-diarrheal medications may be prescribed for older children.

Carefully monitor hydration status, skin turgor, and urine output. Provide careful perineal skin care to prevent infection.

The frequency of *Candida* infections leads to blisters, cracking, and discharge involving the oral mucous membranes.

Mouth care with a non-alcohol-based solution, such as normal saline, to keep the child's lips and mouth moist should be performed every 2 to 4 hours.

Precautions to guard against foodborne illness are particularly important for the HIV-infected child.

Provide Emotional Support
Spend time with the family to provide them with an opportunity to discuss their fears and feelings.

Clarify any misconceptions the older child with HIV infection may have about the transmission of the disease. Routes of transmission and the need for safe sexual practices must be clearly discussed with adolescents.

Providing support for adolescents is particularly important, as the dependence that this chronic and terminal disease brings can make it difficult to meet the developmental task of independence.

Adolescents may benefit from contact with other infected peers.

Discharge Planning and Community Care
Be honest and direct. Education is essential and begins at the time of admission or diagnosis.

Explain that there is no evidence that casual contact among family members can spread the infection.

Discuss the family's finances as well as health insurance coverage for the child's care.

Assess the family's ability to provide nutritious food, required medications, and a supportive environment.

Refer to services, as needed, to ensure provision of quality care for the child after discharge.

Support groups, home healthcare nursing services, financial assistance, and psychological counseling are usually needed at some point during the child's illness, and the family should be aware of the availability of such services.

Assist the family with coping mechanisms to deal with feelings of guilt about the child's condition.

AUTOIMMUNE DISORDERS

In an immune system damaged by pathologic changes, an immune response may occur to some of the body's own proteins, resulting in the production of autoantibodies. These pathologic conditions in which the body directs the immune response against itself—identifying *self* as *nonself*—are called *autoimmune disorders*.

Systemic Lupus Erythematosus

Systemic lupus erythematosus is a chronic inflammatory, autoimmune disease of unknown origin that involves many organ systems.

It is characterized by the presence of anti-nuclear antibodies (ANA) (Gottlieb & Ilowite, 2006).

It is primarily diagnosed in adulthood; however, 15% to 50% of cases are diagnosed in childhood, usually adolescence (Marinescu & Ilowite, 2007; Stichweh, Arce, & Pascual, 2004).

The disease is more common in African Americans, Hispanics, Native Americans, and Asians than in Caucasians. The disease is more severe in African Americans and Hispanics (Gottlieb & Ilowite, 2006).

Females are affected more than males, with a 3:1 ratio prior to puberty and a 9:1 ratio after puberty (Gottlieb & Ilowite, 2006; Marinescu & Illowite, 2007).

Systemic lupus erythematosus is characterized by periods of remission and exacerbation (flares). Flares are triggered by a variety of causes, including sun exposure, an upper respiratory infection or other infection, and stress.

Clinical Manifestations
See Table Table 17–5.

Manifestations of systemic lupus erythematosus may be acute with onset of nephritis, arthritis, or vasculitis or may be noted as a gradual onset with nonspecific symptoms.

Table 17–5 Clinical Manifestations of Childhood Onset Systemic Lupus Erythematosus

System	Clinical Manifestations
Integumentary	A butterfly rash on the face, consisting of a pink or red rash over the bridge of the nose extending to the cheeks, is a characteristic finding
	Photosensitivity
	Alopecia
	Mouth or nose ulcers
Hematologic	Fatigue
	Fever
	Easy bruising
	Bloody stools
	Nosebleeds
Musculoskeletal	Joint pain
	Swollen, inflamed joints
	Myalgias
	Muscle weakness
Neurologic	Headache
	Peripheral neuropathy
	Pychosis
	Seizures
	Mood disorder
	Cognitive disorder
	Stroke
Pulmonary	Chest pain
	Dyspnea
	Pulmonary hypertension
	Pulmonary embolism
Cardiac	Arrhythmias
	Chest pain
	Friction rub
	Raynaud's phenomenon (fingers turning white and/or blue in the cold)

Table 17–5   Clinical Manifestations of Childhood Onset Systemic Lupus Erythematosus (Continued)

System	Clinical Manifestations
Renal	Hematuria
	Hypertension
	Proteinuria
Gastrointestinal	Abdominal pain (may rotate to the shoulder)

Source: Adapted from "Systemic Lupus Erythematosus in Children and Adolescents," by B. S. Gottlieb & N. T. Ilowite, 2006, *Pediatrics in Review, 27*(9), 323–328; "Systemic Lupus Erythematosus," by R. E. Petty & R. M. Laxer, 2005, in J. T. Cassidy, R. E. Petty, R. M. Laxer, & C. B. Lindsley (Eds.), *Textbook of Pediatric Rheumatology* (5th ed., pp. 342–391), Philadelphia: Elsevier Saunders; and "Update on Pediatric Systemic Lupus Erythematosus," by D. Stichweh, E. Arce, & V. Pascual, 2004, *Current Opinion in Rheumatology, 16*, 577–587.

Symptoms vary and depend on the organ involved and the amount of tissue damage that has occurred.

Initial symptoms include fever, chills, fatigue, oral ulcers, malaise, and weight loss. The most common symptoms are rash, fever, mucositis, and arthritis. A butterfly rash on the face, consisting of a pink or red rash over the bridge of the nose extending to the cheeks, is a characteristic finding (Gottlieb & Ilowite, 2006).

Diagnostic Tests

Blood tests reveal: anemia, an elevated blood urea nitrogen (BUN), abnormal plasma proteins, abnormal erythrocyte sedimentation rate (ESR), presence of antinuclear antibodies, and a positive lupus erythematosus (LE) cell reaction, which indicates nonspecific inflammation.

Coombs test is positive.

Radiologic examinations include chest radiographs and CT scans, as well as MRI of affected joints.

A 24-hour urine collection and imaging studies, as well as renal biopsies, may be performed to evaluate lupus nephritis.

Urinalysis may reveal proteinuria.

Clinical Therapy

Medications include corticosteroids (prednisone and methylprednisolone), antimalarial preparations (hydroxychloroquine), NSAIDs (naproxen and ibuprofen) and immunosuppressants (cyclophosphamide, azathioprine, methotrexate, cyclosporine, mycophenolate mofetil; Buka & Cunningham, 2005; Gottlieb & Ilowite, 2006; Marinescu & Ilowite, 2007; O'Neill & Isenberg, 2006).

Diet may be restricted if the child has excessive weight gain or fluid retention from steroids and renal damage.

Nursing Management
Assessment and Diagnosis
Since systemic lupus erythematosus generally consists of multiorgan involvement, careful assessment of each of the systems is essential to detect any complications as early as possible.

A thorough physiologic assessment and a thorough psychosocial assessment are essential.

Assess the child's nutritional status, including baseline weight and history of recent weight loss or weight gain.

The skin is assessed for rashes, ulcer photosensitivity, ecchymosis, petechiae, cyanosis, and hair loss.

Respiratory assessment includes breath sounds and respiratory rate and assessing for pleural effusion or pleuritis.

Cardiovascular assessment includes vital signs and heart tones and assessing for symptoms of pericarditis or friction rub.

Musculoskeletal assessment includes joint pain, joint deformity or discomfort, pain, weakness, and ability to perform activities of daily living.

Neurologic assessment includes changes in affect or cognitive abilities and seizure activity.

Gastrointestinal assessment includes palpating the spleen to detect splenomegaly, abdominal pain, and anorexia.

Assess family interactions, exploring stressful situations such as divorce or trauma.

Treatment-related restrictions associated with medications and changes in appearance, such as weight gain, cushingoid appearance, and skin rashes, can lead to withdrawal, depression, and suicidal tendencies.

Perform psychological assessments periodically as the child grows and adapts to the disorder or faces new developmental challenges with a chronic disease.

Evaluate school performance.

Implementation

Prevent Infection

Infections are a leading cause of death for patients with systemic lupus erythematosus.

Prophylactic antibiotics may be required for dental work and surgical procedures.

Instruct the patient and family to inform all healthcare providers of the disease to plan for prophylactic measures.

Emphasize the importance of receiving recommended immunizations and of obtaining a yearly influenza vaccine to prevent infection.

Instruct the family on hand hygiene and infection control measures in the home.

Warn adolescents about the dangers of tattooing and body piercing because of the risk of infection.

Maintain Fluid Balance

Because most children with systemic lupus erythematosus have renal involvement, nursing care includes maintaining accurate intake and output measurements and frequent evaluation of the child's fluid and electrolyte status and weight.

Promote Adequate Nutrition

The diet may be restricted depending on renal involvement, weight gain, weight loss, or other complications.

The child is at risk for weight gain associated with treatment with steroids and a decreased activity level during exacerbations of this disease.

A well-balanced, nutritious diet with calcium and vitamin D supplements to support bone density as well as appropriate fluid intake for age should be encouraged.

Promote Skin Integrity

Presence of the ulcers on mucous membranes can cause weakening of the tissues, placing the child at increased risk for infection.

Provide instructions on oral care to maintain intact oral mucosa.

Encourage the use of good hygienic measures and a mild soap for the skin.

Recommend that adolescents limit their use of cosmetics, especially oil-based formulations.

Reinforce the importance of avoiding sunlight as much as possible and the use of sun protection factor (SPF) of 30 or higher at all times when in the sun.

Encourage the child to wear protective clothing to limit exposure to sunlight.

Encourage the adolescent to avoid the use of tanning beds.

Provide instructions on oral care to maintain intact oral mucosa.

Provide instructions on the care of the head if alopecia occurs.

Promote Rest and Comfort

Encourage frequent rest periods such as naps.

Encourage a nutritious diet to maximize energy stores.

A physical therapist can plan a therapeutic exercise program to encourage mobility and increase muscle strength.

Implement measures such as application of heat to painful areas.

Avoidance of Triggers for Disease Flares

Many children and their parents can recognize the signs of an impending exacerbation and the triggers that precede them.

Partner with the parents and child to implement measures to avoid these triggers.

Discuss preventive behaviors such as avoiding sun exposure and stressors.

Female adolescents who are sexually active should avoid birth control pills that contain the hormone estrogen because the extra estrogen may exacerbate symptoms. Alternate birth control methods should be discussed with the adolescent.

Provide Emotional Support

Adolescents may have an altered body image as a result of rash, alopecia, arthritic changes in the joints, and chronic disease.

Referral to a lupus support group, social services, or counseling may be helpful.

Juvenile Arthritis

Juvenile arthritis refers to chronic joint inflammation diagnosed prior to 16 years of age and results in decreased mobility, swelling, and pain.

Occurs twice as often in females than males; peak age of onset is between 1 and 3 years of age (Cassidy & Petty, 2005).

There are three major types of JRA: pauciarticular arthritis, systemic arthritis, and polyarticular arthritis.

- *Polyarthritis* involves five or more joints during the first 6 months after diagnosis, particularly the knee, wrist, elbow, and ankle joints. The small joints of the hands and feet may be affected as well as the neck and the temporomandibular joints. This type of arthritis affects approximately 30% of children with juvenile arthritis. This classification is further identified as RF positive or RF negative. Only 3% to 5% of these children are RF positive (Petty & Cassidy, 2005a). Approximately 5% of these children will have eye inflammation (uveitis).

- *Oligoarthritis arthritis* primarily affects the knees, ankles, and elbows, and occurs more frequently in females. Approximately 50% to 60% of children with juvenile arthritis have oligoarthritis. It generally manifests between 2 and 4 years of age. Four or fewer joints are affected in this type of juvenile arthritis. Uveitis occurs in 15% to 20% of children with oligoarthritis (Petty & Cassidy, 2005b).

- *Systemic arthritis* affects males and females equally and is characteristically manifested by high fever, polyarthritis, and rheumatoid rash. Systemic arthritis affects internal organs and joints. Approximately 10% to 15% of children with juvenile arthritis have systemic arthritis with no peak age of onset reported (Petty & Cassidy, 2005c).

Clinical Manifestations

Juvenile arthritis may be restricted to a few joints or be systemic with involvement of multiple joints.

Symptoms can include fever, rash, lymphadenopathy, splenomegaly, and hepatomegaly.

The child may develop a limp or obviously favor one extremity over the other.

Pain, stiffness, loss of motion, and swelling occur in the large joints such as the knees.

Older children may develop symmetric involvement of the small joints of the hand.

Disease is frequently chronic, extending over several years after an initial manifestation with pain and other symptoms.

Remissions and exacerbations are characteristic.

Diagnostic Tests

In some children, rheumatoid factor, human leukocyte antigen (HLA) B27, and antinuclear antibody (ANA) tests are positive.

Erythrocyte sedimentation rate (ESR) and C-reactive (CRP) tests may be helpful in determining the amount of inflammation (Cassidy & Petty, 2005).

Clinical Therapy

Goals of treatment are to relieve pain, control inflammation, manage systemic complications, preserve joint function and range of motion, and promote normal physical, psychosocial, behavioral, and vocational development (Cassidy & Petty, 2005; Emery, 2004).

Medications include NSAIDs (aspirin, ibuprofen, naproxen, tolmetin, diclofenac, meloxicam), disease-modifying antirheumatic drugs (methotrexate, sulfasalazine), corticosteroids (methylprednisolone, triamcinolone hexacetonide), and biologic response modifiers (etanercept; Cassiday & Petty, 2005; Emery, 2004; Marinescu & Ilowite, 2007).

Physical and/or occupational therapy increases strength and mobility of joints while protecting them from injury.

Exercise such as swimming is encouraged because it involves a majority of the muscles and joints with minimal impact and stress on joints. Surgery is occasionally performed to relieve pain and maintain or improve joint function in children with joint contractures.

Children less than 6 years of age with oligoarthritis or polyarthritis who have a positive ANA test should have an eye exam every 3 to 4 months. Children 7 or older or those with a negative ANA test need an exam every 6 months. Because uveitis is very rare in children with systemic arthritis, the recommended frequency for eye exams is every 12 months (Marinescu & Ilowite, 2007).

Nursing Management

Assessment

A careful history is important because it is sometimes the primary mode of diagnosis.

Assess for joint swelling and deformities, pain, decreased mobility, morning stiffness, fever, nodules under the skin, delayed growth, and enlarged lymph nodes.

Implementation

Promote Improved Mobility

Physical therapy as prescribed

Range-of-motion exercises, stretching, hydrotherapy, and swimming as indicated

Encourage the child to perform activities of daily living.

Exercise may be painful or even difficult for the child.

Emphasize the importance of establishing a regular exercise and activity routine.

Encourage periods of rest during exacerbations, as the child fatigues more easily.

Teach the child methods to reduce stress on joints, such as using wrist splints when lifting.

Encourage Adequate Nutrition

Promote general health by encouraging a well-balanced diet.

Encourage adequate hydration to reduce the risk of constipation associated with immobility.

Dietary consultation will help ensure that the child receives adequate calories and a well-balanced diet.

Monitor the child's food and liquid intake and output.

Manage Side Effects of Medication

Aspirin and corticosteroids may lead to gastric irritation. To decrease the risk of stomach irritation or pain, aspirin should be administered with food, milk, or a prescribed antacid.

Monitor for signs and symptoms of aspirin toxicity, including tinnitus, decreased hearing, nausea, vomiting, drowsiness, irritability, and rapid, shallow breathing.

Caution the family not to use products with aspirin or nonsteroidal anti-inflammatory agents; contact a health professional for treatment of childhood illnesses.

Community Care

The child will need assistance to facilitate performance in school. Walking in hallways, reaching a locker, writing, and other activities may produce pain; partner with family and school personnel to plan alternative approaches.

Assist the family to adjust to the periodic disruption of family life when the child has exacerbations. Provide support and referral to other families experienced with juvenile arthritis.

ALLERGIC REACTIONS

Allergy

Allergy is an abnormal or altered reaction to an antigen. Antigens responsible for clinical manifestations of allergy are called *allergens*.

Allergens can be ingested in food or drugs, injected, absorbed through contact with unbroken skin, and inhaled (Box 17–2). An allergic reaction is an antigen–antibody reaction and can manifest itself as:

- Anaphylaxis
- Atopic disease
- Serum sickness
- Contact dermatitis

See Table 17–6 for a list of the various clinical manifestations common in allergic reactions.

Box 17–2	Common Childhood Allergens

Common childhood allergens include

Animal dander	Medications, such as penicillin	Seafood
Cockroaches	Mites	Shellfish
Cow's milk	Mold	Soy
Dust	Plant pollens	Tree nuts
Egg whites	Peanuts	Wheat

Table 17–6 Clinical Manifestations of Allergic Reactions in Children

System	Clinical Manifestations
Respiratory system	Wheezing
	Rhinitis (seasonal and perennial)
	Cough
	Adventitious breath sounds
	Inspiratory stridor
	Edema of glottis
	Nasal congestion or discharge
Gastrointestinal system	Abdominal pain and colic
	Mouth sores
	Constipation
	Diarrhea
	Bloody stools
	Geographic tongue
	Vomiting

Table 17–6 Clinical Manifestations of Allergic Reactions in Children (Continued)

System	Clinical Manifestations
Skin	Angioedema
	Urticaria
	Eczema
	Atopic dermatitis
	Erythema multiforme
	Purpura
	Drug and food rashes
	Contact dermatitis
Nervous system	Headache
	Tension
	Fatigue
	Seizures
	Ménière syndrome
	Tremors
	Irritability
	Sleep disorders
	Decreased concentration
Eyes	Conjunctivitis
	Cataract
	Ciliary spasm
	Iritis
	Itching eyes
	Tearing
Hematologic	Thrombocytopenic purpura
	Hemolytic anemia
	Leukopenia
	Agranulocytosis
Musculoskeletal system	Arthralgia
	Myalgia
	Torticollis
Genitourinary system	Dysuria
	Vulvovaginitis
	Enuresis
Miscellaneous	Anaphylactic shock
	Serum sickness

The **hypersensitivity response,** an overreaction of the immune system, is responsible for allergic reactions. Hypersensitivity reactions have been classified into four types:

Type I hypersensitivity reactions, the most common allergic reactions, are immediate reactions that occur within seconds or minutes of exposure to the antigen and may progress to anaphylaxis. The release of chemical substances such as histamine is responsible for the signs and symptoms exhibited. The first time a child is exposed to the allergen, there is no reaction. With every exposure thereafter, however, the allergic child may have a reaction to the allergen.

Type II hypersensitivity reaction is immediate, within 15 to 30 minutes after exposure to the antigen.

Type II sensitivity reaction is immediate, within 15 to 30 minutes after exposure to the antigen. Type III hypersensitivity reaction may be difficult to distinguish from type II reaction. Hypersensitivity reactions generally peak within 6 hours.

Type IV reactions are delayed responses that do not appear until several hours after exposure and require 24 to 72 hours to fully develop. A type IV reaction, which is not confined to any specific tissue, is elicited by relatively complex antigens such as those of bacteria and viruses and by simple antigens such as drugs and metals.

Nursing Management
Implementation
Educating the child and family on methods to minimize or avoid exposure to allergens is important.

Parents of children who have had severe reactions to bee or wasp stings should be taught how to take precautions (avoid bright-colored clothing and avoid perfumed soaps and lotions) and how to provide emergency treatment if the child is stung.

An EpiPen may be prescribed, and the parents and child will require instructions on its proper use.

Partner with the family to determine effective measures to allergy-proof their home. Pets, dust, carpets, fabrics, feather pillows and bedding, and cigarette smoke can all cause allergic reactions.

When the child has type I reactions to an environmental substance, avoidance of the allergen is most critical.

In addition, care providers, families, and school personnel must be able to treat anaphylaxis if exposure to the allergen occurs.

School nurses keep records regarding children's allergies and inform school personnel about the allergies and cautions that should be followed.

Be sure to label the child's chart and bed and apply a red armband to the child to alert others to allergies when the child is hospitalized.

Nurses must be aware of the resuscitation procedures and equipment in all facilities, such as hospital units, offices, childcare centers, and schools.

Anaphylaxis

Anaphylaxis is a potentially life-threatening systemic reaction to an allergen. Symptoms can occur within minutes or up to 2 hours after exposure to an allergy-causing substance.

Clinical Manifestations

See Table 17–7 for clinical manifestations of anaphylaxis.

Clinical Therapy

Essential to preservation of life is the immediate recognition and treatment of anaphylactic reaction.

Establish a stable airway.

Epinephrine is the medication of choice for treating an anaphylactic reaction (Sampson & Leung, 2007).

Epinephrine may be administered subcutaneously, intramuscularly, or via an endotracheal tube. Epinephrine reverses the symptoms of an anaphylactic reaction by causing vasoconstriction and reversing airway constriction.

Antihistamines, such as diphenhydramine (Benadryl), and steroids are often administered to the child experiencing an anaphylactic reaction.

Place the child in a supine position, and elevate the legs to increase venous return.

Obtain intravenous access for fluid resuscitation. Large volumes of fluids may be required to treat hypotension caused by increased vascular permeability and vasodilation.

Administer oxygen.

The child may require endotracheal intubation and mechanical ventilation.

Monitor the child for an observation period of at least 4 hours following a prolonged episode (Sheffer, Feldweg, & Castells, 2006).

Table 17–7 Clinical Manifestations of Anaphylactic Shock

System	Clinical Manifestations	
Respiratory	Wheezing	
	Stridor	
	Dyspnea	
	Laryngospasm	
	Bronchospasm	
	Pulmonary edema	
	Cyanosis	
Cardiovascular	Profound hypotension	
	Tachycardia	
	Dysrhythmias	
	Decreased central venous pressure	
Neurologic	Anxiety	
	Restlessness	
	Lethargy	
	Progression to coma	
Gastrointestinal	Vomiting	
	Diarrhea	
	Abdominal pain	
Integumentary	Edematous face, lips, tongue, hands, feet	Assess for edema and rashes.
	Skin warm	Assess skin temperature.
Renal	Oliguria progressing to anuria	Assess urine output hourly.
		Monitor intake hourly.
		Monitor serum blood urea nitrogen and creatinine.

Patient and Family Education

Prevention of reexposure to the allergen is essential.

Determining the cause of anaphylaxis, if uncertain, may require numerous diagnostic studies. Previous tolerance of a substance does not rule it out as the trigger. Direct skin testing and radioallergosorbent testing are available for some antigens.

Nursing Management

Assessment

Assess the child for respiratory distress, hypotension, tachycardia, and edema.

Assess breath sounds for wheezing.

Assess all vital signs, including peripheral pulses.

Monitor urine output hourly.

Monitor oxygen saturation.

Assess skin temperature, color, and moisture.

Implementation

Emergency management of anaphylaxis is the administration of epinephrine, oxygen, and fluids.

Maintain the child on bed rest immediately after anaphylaxis until the observation period has concluded.

Provide the child and family the opportunity to express anxiety and concerns.

For home care, partner with the family to assure that the child and family members can properly administer epinephrine.

Emphasize to the family that the child should always wear a medical identification tag and should always have an EpiPen immediately available for emergencies.

Ensure that the childcare providers or school officials can recognize the signs and symptoms of anaphylaxis and can appropriately administer epinephrine.

Instruct the child and family to activate the emergency medical system (911) as soon as epinephrine is administered.

Food Allergy

Food allergy is an IgE-mediated reaction that is potentially systemic, characteristically rapid in onset, and may be manifested as swelling of the lips, mouth, uvula, or glottis, generalized urticaria, atopic dermatitis, and, in severe reactions, anaphylaxis. An estimated 6% of all children have some type of food allergy (Chehade, 2007).

Food allergy is the most common cause of anaphylaxis, and is most prevalent in children with a family history of allergic reactions to various substances and foods (atopy).

The most common food allergens are fish, shellfish, peanuts, tree nuts, eggs, soy, wheat, corn, strawberries, and cow milk products.

About 1% of children have an allergy to peanuts, and the incidence is increasing. A majority of the 150 deaths from food allergies that occur annually in the United States are due to peanut allergy (Palmer & Burks, 2006).

Nursing Management

Instruct parents of infants to introduce new foods at a rate of not more than one new food every 3 to 5 days. Discuss any changes in diet or preparation of formula.

Reassure parents that the child's symptoms will disappear when the offending foods are removed from the diet.

Be alert for skin, respiratory, and other characteristic manifestations of allergy. Refer such cases to an allergist immediately for diagnosis.

Assist in testing and instruction. If an allergy is identified, help the family to identify and eliminate the offending foods.

Emphasize the importance of reading food labels for hidden foods that can trigger an allergic reaction (Simons, Weiss, Furlong, et al., 2005).

An EpiPen® should be available and accessible at home and school.

The child with a food allergy should wear medical alert identification.

Be sure that school personnel are informed about the allergy and that a food allergy plan is in place.

Latex Allergy

Latex allergy is caused by an immunoglobulin E–mediated response that develops after repeated exposure to latex. A reaction to latex products can be manifested as an irritant reaction of the skin with redness, inflammation, and blisters (type IV delayed hypersensitivity) or type I hypersensitivity, which is immediate and often has systemic manifestations (e.g., itchy eyes, asthma, or anaphylaxis).

An estimated 10% to 17% of healthcare workers are thought to be sensitive to latex. In addition, 40% to 65% of children with spina bifida and congenital genitourinary defects and approximately one-third of children with three or more surgeries are sensitive to latex (Paskawicz, 2005). Healthcare personnel are also at risk for latex allergy because of exposure in the workplace (Box 17–3).

Nursing Management

Assessment

Children and adolescents at high risk should receive allergy testing for latex.

The radioallergosorbent test (RAST) is most often used.

| Box 17-3 | Measures to Protect Against Latex Allergy |

Healthcare personnel are at high risk of developing latex allergy because of intense exposure to products containing latex. Nurses can protect themselves by using the following measures:

- Decrease exposure by choosing alternative products when available (use synthetic rubber, polyethylene, nitrile, neoprene, and vinyl gloves).
- Use powder-free gloves if using latex gloves (the powder has high amounts of latex that can be inhaled).
- Avoid use of oil-based hand creams and lotions before putting on latex gloves, as these preparations break down the latex.
- When symptoms of sensitivity to latex occur on exposure (rash, hives, nasal congestion, conjunctivitis, cough, or wheeze), contact the employee health department of your facility.
- If diagnosed as latex allergic, avoid all contact and wear a medical alert bracelet.

Implementation

When a positive skin test has occurred or when the child has had a reaction to latex, all latex products must be removed from the allergic individual's environment.

Alternative products, such as nonlatex gloves and catheters, must be used when providing health care.

Emphasize to the family that the child with latex allergy should also wear a medical alert identification bracelet at all times.

Educate families about the need to have an epinephrine kit readily available at home and school.

Be alert for any signs of hypersensitivity when the child is receiving health care, and be prepared with drugs and equipment to treat anaphylaxis.

Emphasize to parents and children that many everyday products contain latex, including latex balloons, condoms, and many toys.

18 ALTERATIONS IN HEMATOLOGIC FUNCTION

An understanding and application of the normal blood values in children are needed when caring for children with alterations in hematologic function (see chapter 5).

ANEMIA

Iron Deficiency Anemia

Iron deficiency anemia is the most common type of anemia and nutritional deficiency among children (Carley, 2003). This can result from a variety of causes, including the following:

- Anemia secondary to blood loss
- Malabsorption
- Poor nutritional intake
- Increased metabolic demands—for example, growth spurts
- Lead poisoning

Clinical Manifestations (Acute)

Pallor

Fatigue

Irritability

Clinical Manifestations (Chronic)

Nail deformities

Growth retardation

Developmental delay

Tachycardia

Systolic murmur

Diagnostic Tests

Clinical presentation

Laboratory studies that assist in diagnosis: hemoglobin, hematocrit, red blood cell count, mean corpuscular value, and reticulocyte count are evaluated.

Serum ferritin concentration measures iron storage (Coyer, 2005).

Red blood cells are microcytic and hypochromic (Carley, 2003).

See chapter 5 for normal blood values.

Clinical Therapy

Oral elemental iron preparations

Diet high in foods with iron

Nursing Management

Assessment

Screening is recommended at 9 to 12 months of age and 15 to 18 months of age.

Review laboratory findings.

Make height and weight comparisons for the child across time.

Perform developmental screening tests for developmental delay.

Obtain diet history.

Implementation

Family-centered care focusing on prevention, dietary management, medication therapy, and follow-up.

Intervention

Dietary Management

Long-term treatment focusing on the following is preferred for iron deficiency anemia:

- Plan a diet with foods rich in iron (Table 18–1).
- Infant over 6 months of age should have breast milk or iron-fortified formulas.
- Avoid cow's milk feeding during infancy to prevent bleeding from the gastrointestinal tract.
- Finger foods rich in iron for toddlers depending on age, such as thinly sliced meats should be provided.

Table 18–1   Food Sources of Iron and Vitamin C

Iron-Rich Foods	Food Sources of Vitamin C
Meats, fish, poultry	Orange juice
Vegetables	Citrus fruits
Dried fruits	Strawberries
Legumes	Tomatoes
Enriched grain products	Broccoli and other green leafy vegetables
Whole-grain cereals	Potatoes
Iron-fortified dry cereals	Some dry cereals

- Encourage adolescents to eat foods with high iron content and vitamin C, such as hamburgers and dried fruit.

Medication Therapy

Oral iron preparations are administered to correct the anemia. Ferrous sulfate should be administered using the following guidelines:

- On an empty stomach if possible
- With vitamin C
- With a straw or placed on the back of the tongue to avoid staining teeth
- Without dairy foods that decrease the absorption of iron
- With small amounts of appropriate food choices if necessary

Side effects of iron sulfate exist and must be communicated by parents to healthcare providers:

- Black stools
- Constipation
- Gastrointestinal discomfort

Monitor for signs and symptoms of iron overload, including the following:

- Abdominal pain
- Vomiting
- Bloody diarrhea
- Shortness of breath

Severe overdose may be fatal: Keep iron preparations securely locked away from children.

Patient and Family Education

Medication administration and secure storage

Dietary management

Normocytic Anemia

Normocytic anemia is anemia in which cells are of normal shape and size but are decreased in number secondary to an increase in the destruction of red blood cells or decreased production of red blood cells.

This condition is treated by correcting the cause, which can be any of the following:

- Chronic hemolytic anemia
- Pancytopenia
- Disseminated intravascular coagulation
- Glucose-6-phosphate dehydrogenase deficiency
- Hemolytic uremic syndrome
- Juvenile arthritis
- Chronic liver disease

Sickle Cell Disease

Sickle cell disease is a hereditary hemoglobinopathy characterized by the partial or complete replacement of normal hemoglobin with abnormal hemoglobin S (HgbS) in red blood cells. This causes occlusion of small blood vessels, ischemia, and damage to affected organs. Sickle cell trait (carrying one gene for the disease) affects 1 in 12 African Americans and 1 in 16 Hispanic Americans (The American Sickle Cell Anemia Association, 2005). Sickle cell anemia (HgbSS disease), an autosomal recessive disorder, is the most common type of sickle cell disease and will be the focus of this discussion.

In sickle cell anemia, the hemoglobin in the red blood cell acquires an elongated crescent or sickle shape. Sickling may be triggered by fever, hypoxia, emotional stress, or physical stress. Precipitating factors for sickle cell crisis include increased blood viscosity (such as from a low fluid intake or fever) and hypoxia or low oxygen tension. Potential causes of hypoxia or low oxygen tension include high altitudes, poorly pressurized airplanes, hypoventilation, vasoconstriction when cold, or an emotionally stressful event. Any condition that increases the body's need for oxygen or alters the transport of oxygen (such as infection, trauma, or dehydration) may result in sickle cell crisis. The sickled cells are rigid and obstruct capillary blood flow. Microscopic obstructions lead to engorgement and tissue ischemia. This local tissue hypoxia causes further sickling and ultimately large infarctions.

Clinical Manifestations

Pain

Sickle cell crisis, including vaso-occlusive crisis, splenic sequestration, or aplastic crisis

See Box 18–1 for the precipitating factors contributing to sickle cell crisis.

Box 18–1	Precipitating Factors Contributing to Sickle Cell Crisis
Fever	Alcohol consumption
Dehydration	Pregnancy
Altitude	Elevated hemoglobin levels
Extremes in temperature	Elevated reticulocyte counts
Vomiting	Excessive exercise or physical activity
Emotional distress	Acidosis
Fatigue	

Diagnostic Tests

Initial diagnosis made from cord blood using hemoglobin electrophoresis.

Sickledex is used for quick screening for those older than age 6 months.

Hemoglobin electrophoresis is performed to verify positive Sickledex test results.

Complete blood count reveals degree of anemia.

Reticulocyte count is elevated in sickle cell anemia.

Clinical Therapy

Management focuses on pain control, hydration, oxygenation, prevention/treatment of infection, and prevention of associated complications.

Pain control with parenteral analgesics such as dilaudid and morphine; parenteral ketoralac or oral ibuprofen may be administered as adjunctive therapy.

Oral and intravenous fluid replacement promotes pain relief as dehydration is often a cause of crisis, reduces viscosity of blood.

Oxygen administration provides comfort; decreases incidence of pulmonary complications.

Prevention and treatment of infection: it is essential that child receives recommended immunizations; should receive 23-valent pneumococcal vaccine (Pneumovax) at 2 and 5 years of age (Quinn, Rogers & Buchanan, 2004); children 6 months of age and older should receive an annual influenzae vaccine; children 2 years of age and older should receive the meningococcal vaccine (Mehta, Afenyi-Annan, Byrns, et al., 2006).

Daily penicillin prophylaxis for children ages 2 months to 5 years to prevent life-threatening infection with *Streptococcus pneumonia.* Continued past age 5 if child has had spleenectomy or is considered at high risk for the infection (Saunthararajah, Vichinsky, & Embury, 2005).

Transfusion of normal red blood cells for children who have splenic sequestration, stroke, acute chest syndrome, severe anemia, and surgery. Blood transfusions improve tissue oxygenation, reduce sickling, and temporarily reduce the percentage of Hb S. Chronic transfusions may be indicated in the child with sickle cell anemia who has had a stroke (Lindsey et al., 2005; Platt & Eckman, 2006).

A chelating agent is administered if the child develops iron overload from chronic transfusions.

Other therapies: hydroxyurea may be used to improve fetal hemoglobin levels; FDA labeling related to indications for the use of this drug refers only to adults, necessitating off-label usage in the pediatric population (Heeney & Ware, 2008). Hematopoietic stem cell transplantation (HSCT) is the only known cure for sickle cell anemia and has been used in children younger than 16 years with complications related to the disease. The treatment, however, is limited to children who have a family donor who is genotypically identical. The survival rate for children who have been able to receive an HLA-identical sibling donor stem cell transplant is 93% (Platt & Eckman, 2006).

Nursing Management

The focus of nursing management is identification of children at risk, early recognition and prevention of crisis, promotion of growth and development, prevention of complications, and family support.

Assessment

Physical assessment with detailed history and assessment of developmental milestones

Pain assessment

Psychosocial assessment, including self-concept and self-esteem, body image, and social interactions

Assessment of family resources

Assessment for signs of complications associated with sickle cell anemia

Implementation

Promote increased tissue perfusion with transfusions and activity monitoring.

Promote hydration orally and intravenously.

Manage pain with appropriate analgesics and other measures.

Prevent infection with antibiotic prophylaxis, immunizations, and prompt recognition of infection.

Ensure adequate nutrition with a high-protein and high-calorie diet. Emphasize the importance of folic acid and vitamin C supplements as prescribed.

Prevent complications of crisis, observing for worsening anemia/shock.

Provide emotional support for client and family.

Provide assistance with discharge planning and home care needs.

Patient and Family Education
Provide information on the disease and treatments.

Assess knowledge on potential crisis situations and when to seek medical attention.

Partner with family to explore resources.

Discuss signs of dehydration.

Provide information on red blood cell transfusion therapy and use of chelating agents for iron overload.

Assist the family with information for care of the child at school.

Refer family for genetic counseling as needed.

Assist with resources for financial and emotional support for this chronic disease.

**Expected Outcomes for the Child and Family
with Sickle Cell Disease**
Management of pain

Maintenance of adequate hydration

Prevention of infection

Prompt identification of complications

Maintenance of normal growth and development

Support for the family to deal with the chronic nature of the disease and care

Thalassemias

Thalassemias most often occur in people of Mediterranean descent and are a group of inherited blood disorders of hemoglobin synthesis. These blood disorders cause mild to severe anemia and are classified in types of β-thalassemias and α-thalassemias. The most common type is β-thalassemia major, also known as *Cooley's anemia*.

β-Thalassemia stems from a defective hemoglobin chain resulting in impaired production of the beta chain of hemoglobin A. In α-thalassemia, the defect occurs on the alpha chain of the adult hemoglobin. The severity of both disorders depends on the number of defective genes. The three types of β-thalassemia are (Richardson, 2007):

- β Thalassemia minor, or thalassemia trait (produces mild anemia)
- β Thalassemia intermedia (produces moderate anemia, may require transfusions)
- β Thalassemia major (produces anemia requiring transfusion)

The four types of α-thalassemia are (DeBaun & Vichinsky, 2007; Richardson, 2007):

- α-thalassemia silent carrier—defect in a single alpha chain–forming gene
- α-thalassemia trait—defect in two genes
- Hemoglobin H disease—defect in three genes
- α-thalassemia major—defect in all four alpha-forming genes

Clinical Manifestations of β-Thalassemia

Clinical manifestations of β-thalassemia are caused by the defective synthesis of hemoglobin, structurally impaired red blood cells, and the shortened life span of the RBCs. The infant with β-thalassemia major manifests pallor, failure to thrive, hepatosplenomegaly, and severe anemia that leads to chronic hypoxemia (Richardson, 2007).

See Table 18–2 for clinical manifestations of β-thalassemia.

Clinical Manifestations of α-Thalassemia

The child with a one-gene defect (alpha thalassemia silent carrier) is generally symptom free, while the child with a two-gene defect (alpha thalassemia trait) may have mild anemia. Manifestations of hemoglobin H disease include anemia and splenomegaly. Alpha-thalassemia major results in hydrops fetalis, intrauterine congestive heart failure cardiomegaly, hepatomegaly, and death. Bone marrow transplant is the only cure (DeBaun & Vichinsky, 2007; Richardson, 2007).

Diagnostic Tests

Prenatal testing is performed using chorionic villus sampling or amniocentesis.

Hemoglobin electrophoresis reveals a decreased production of one of the globin chains in hemoglobin and an elevated F and A hemoglobin.

A complete blood count (CBC) reveals a decreased hemoglobin, hematocrit, and reticulocyte count (DeBaun & Vichinsky, 2007).

Table 18–2   Clinical Manifestations of β-Thalassemia

Body Organs	Clinical Manifestations
Red blood cells (anemia)	Pallor
	Fatigue
	Folic acid deficiency
Skeletal changes	Osteoporosis
	Delayed growth
	Susceptibility to pathologic fractures
	Facial deformities: enlarged head, prominent forehead and parietal bossing, prominent cheek bones, broadened and depressed bridge of nose, enlarged maxilla with protruding front teeth, eyes with mongolian slant and epicanthal fold
Heart	Chronic congestive heart failure
	Murmurs
Liver/gallbladder	Hepatomegaly
Spleen	Splenomegaly
Endocrine system	Delayed sexual maturation
	Symptoms of diabetes (see chapter 22)
Skin	Darkening of skin

Source: Data from "Hemoglobinopathies," by M. R. DeBaun & E. Vichinsky, 2007, in R. M. Kliegman, R. E. Behrman, H. B. Jenson, & B. F. Stanton (Eds.), *Nelson Textbook of Pediatrics* (18th ed., pp. 2025–2038). Philadelphia: Saunders Elsevier; and "Microcytic Anemia," by M. Richardson, 2007, *Pediatrics in Review, 28*(1), 5–14.

Clinical Therapy

Supportive, involving transfusions of normal cells every 2 to 4 weeks for those with severe disease

Treatment of iron overload with chelating agents

Potential splenectomy

Hematopoietic stem cell transplantation (HSCT) in newly diagnosed cases

Nursing Management

Nursing care focuses on observing for complications of transfusion therapy, supporting the child and family in dealing with a chronic life-threatening illness, and referring the family for genetic counseling.

Assessment
Assess for classic manifestations listed previously.

Assess heart sounds, breath sounds, and respiratory effort.

Assess for signs of infection.

Assess for signs of iron overload: abdominal pain, vomiting, and bloody diarrhea.

Implementation
Monitor the child receiving blood transfusions.

Teach parents how to administer chelating agents for iron overload.

Provide parents with necessary information for treatment, complications, and follow-up treatment for the child.

Teach parents that diet should include folic acid and ascorbic acid (vitamin C); iron should not be administered and foods rich in iron should be avoided.

Age-appropriate care in school and at home is a lifelong commitment for the nurse and the family.

Evaluation
Expected outcomes for the child with thalassemia include the following:
- no signs of infection
- demonstrates effective tissue perfusion throughout the body
- participation in age-appropriate, safe activities
- demonstrates positive body image
- demonstrates effective tissue perfusion throughout the body
- family understanding of treatment regimen and signs of potential complications

Hereditary Spherocytosis
Hereditary spherocytosis (HS) is an autosomal dominant hemolytic disorder in which the red blood cell membrane is fragile due to a defect in the protein spectrin and assumes a spherical doughnut shape. The blood cells are sequestered and hemolyzed in the spleen, leading to anemia in the child (Gallagher, 2007; Linker, 2008).

Clinical manifestations appear in the neonatal period or during early infancy and include anemia with varying severity and mild jaundice.

Aplastic crisis and gallstones are complications that may be associated with hereditary spherocytosis.

Complete blood count reveals anemia and microscopic examination reveals the abnormally shaped cells.

Hyperbilirubinemia in the newborn may require phototherapy or exchange transfusions. Surgical removal of the spleen, generally around the age of 5 years, produces a clinical cure by eliminating hemolysis; however, it does not correct the red blood cell defect. Removal of the spleen increases the risk of infection and sepsis.

Nursing care for the child with hereditary spherocytosis is the same as care for the child with anemia.

Aplastic Anemia

Aplastic anemia is a congenital or acquired condition that results from failure of the bone marrow to produce adequate numbers of circulating blood cells. Most aplastic anemia is immune-mediated and results from a combination of environmental exposure and an individual's genetically determined response to the causative environmental agent (Corbeel, 2005; Young, Calado, & Scheinberg, 2006).

Clinical Manifestations

Manifestations vary depending on the degree of thrombocytopenia, anemia, and neutropenia and include:

Bleeding

Purpura and petechiae

Bloody stools

Epistaxis

Retinal bleeding

Weakness, pallor, and fatigue

Tachycardia

Death may occur secondary to hemorrhage, sepsis, and malignancy.

Diagnostic Tests

Complete blood count reveals anemia, leukopenia with marked neutropenia, thrombocytopenia, and pancytopenia.

Serum iron is elevated.

Bone marrow aspiration reveals yellow, fatty bone marrow instead of red bone marrow.

Clinical Therapy

Determine risk factors.

Supportive treatment of transfusions, including packed cells and platelets.

Immunosuppressive therapy

Antibiotics are indicated if confirmed infection.

HSCT if indicated.

Nursing Management
Prevent bleeding.

Administer and monitor blood transfusions.

Prevent infection.

Encourage mobility as tolerated.

Educate parents and child about disorder.

Provide emotional support.

Conserve patient energy.

Observe for complications associated with transfusions.

Assist family with resources related to life-threatening disease.

BLEEDING DISORDERS
Bleeding disorders include both hereditary and acquired disorders resulting in various bleeding tendencies. Hereditary disorders include hemophilia and von Willebrand disease. Acquired disorders include disseminated intravascular coagulation, Henoch-Schönlein purpura, idiopathic thrombocytopenic purpura, and meningococcemia.

Hemophilia
Hemophilia is defined as a group of hereditary bleeding disorders resulting from specific clotting factor deficiencies. Types of hemophilia include hemophilia A (factor VIII deficiency), hemophilia B (factor IX deficiency), also known as *Christmas disease,* and hemophilia C (factor XI deficiency; (Curry, 2004).

Clinical Manifestations
Hemophilia is manifested in different children by bleeding tendencies that range from mild to moderate or severe.

Spontaneous bleeding

Hemarthrosis (bleeding into a joint space)

Deep tissue hemorrhage

Limited motion

Pain

Tenderness and joint swelling

Bone changes

Contractures

Disabling joint deformities

Easy bruising

Nosebleeds

Hematuria

Bleeding after tooth extractions, minor trauma, or minor surgical procedures

Diagnostic Tests

Chorionic villa sampling

Amniocentesis

History and physical examination

Factor VIII or IX levels are decreased.

Prolonged activated partial prothrombin time

Prothrombin time, thrombin time, fibrinogen, and platelet count are normal.

See chapter 5 for diagnostic tests for clotting disorders.

Clinical Therapy

Factor replacement therapy with factor concentrate

Prompt and adequate treatment to prevent serious bleeding episodes

For mild hemophilia, desmopressin acetate to increase factor VIII activity (Curry, 2004; Manno & Larson, 2005)

Nursing Management

Important nursing care focuses on identifying the child with hemophilia and implementing measures to prevent serious bleeding events through collaboration with the child and family.

Assessment

Perform history and physical assessment.

Assess for evidence of bleeding, ecchymosis, petechia, hematuria.

Assess for any joint pain, swelling, or permanent deformity.

Perform pain assessment.

Perform neurological assessment due to risk of intracranial hemorrhage.

Evaluate achievement of expected growth and development stages.

Assess older children's and parents' understanding of the disease, limitations, and their adaptation to the disease.

Assess child and family's coping strategies and support systems.

Determine ability of family resources to manage procedures and treatment.

Implementation
The goals of nursing care include the prevention and control of bleeding episodes, limiting joint involvement, managing pain, and providing support to the child and family. Short- and long-term interventions are necessary.

Patient and Family Education
Safe and age-appropriate toys

Adapted home environment

Bleeding episode education

Seeking medical attention

Medical identification tag

Preparation and administration of factor concentrate

Individual school health plan

Physical rehabilitation as needed for joint deformities

Evaluation
Expected outcomes for the child include the following:
- Free from injury
- Normal joint mobility
- Pain successfully managed
- Normal growth and development demonstrated
- Adequate knowledge of disease management and treatment demonstrated
- Adequate support provided to family to manage disease

Von Willebrand Disease

Von Willebrand disease is the most common hereditary bleeding disorder and occurs in up to 3% of the world's population. There are a variety of subtypes of this disorder that are classified based on the amount and functionality of the von Willebrand factor (vWF), a plasma protein and the carrier for clotting factor VIII. The most common form of the disorder is transmitted as an autosomal dominant trait, and can occur in both males and females. The gene for the disease is located on chromosome 12 (Curry, 2004).

Clinical Manifestations

Easy bruising

Epistaxis

Gingival bleeding

Ecchymosis

Increased bleeding with lacerations, during surgery, and during dental extractions

Menorrhagia in teenage girls

Gastrointestinal bleeding may occur

Diagnostic Tests

Decreased von Willebrand factor levels, von Willebrand factor antigen levels, and factor VIII activity

Reduced platelet agglutination

Prolonged bleeding time

Prolonged or normal activated partial thromboplastin time (APPT)

Clinical Therapy

Infusion of von Willebrand protein concentrate as indicated

Desmopressin (DDAVP) is administered to promote release of stored vWF and to prevent bleeding associated with dental or surgical procedures.

Nursing management is the same as for a child with hemophilia.

Henoch-Schönlein Purpura

Henoch-Schönlein purpura (HSP) is described as an inflammation of the small blood vessels. The cause of HSP is unknown; however, IgA is known to play a role in the development of the illness, which generally follows an upper respiratory infection (Roberts, et al., 2007; Saulsbury, 2007).

Child typically presents with slightly raised purpuric lesions (palpable purpura), joint pain (arthritis), colicky abdominal pain, gastrointestinal bleeding represented by blood in the stool, and hematuria (Chen, Change, Chu, et al., 2007; Saulsbury, 2007).

Generally, this is a self-limiting disease.

Severity of the renal involvement (nephritis) is the primary prognostic factor, with 30% to 50% having long-term problems (Saulsbury, 2007).

Clinical Therapy

Management focuses on supportive care directed at the systems involved.

Child should be monitored for rare but serious complications, including hemorrhage in any body system (Roberts, Waller, Brinker, et al., 2007).

While the IgA concentration is elevated in approximately 50% of patients with HSP, there is no defining laboratory test that confirms the diagnosis.

Tests may be performed to rule out other illnesses (Roberts et al., 2007; Saulsbury, 2007).

Supportive care focuses on controlling gastrointestinal symptoms, joint pain, and renal involvement. Steroids may be used.

Nursing Mangement

Care is centered on management of the presenting symptoms.

Assess the child's skin for changes in the purpuric lesions.

Perform careful abdominal assessment and joint assessment.

Stools should be evaluated for occult blood.

Monitor urine output and test urine for the presence of blood.

Perform daily weights and careful assessment for the development of edema.

A full multisystem assessment aids in detection of complications related to hemorrhage in body systems.

Any abnormalities should be reported to the physician.

Teaching related to corticosteroid therapy is essential.

HSP generally is self-limiting, but the nurse should be diligent not only in monitoring the child for progression of the disease but in supporting the family during the illness.

Idiopathic Thrombocytopenic Purpura

Idiopathic thrombocytopenic purpura, also known as immune thrombocytopenic purpura, is the most common bleeding disorder in children and is characterized by an increased destruction of platelets in the spleen. The cause of ITP is unknown; however, the child has typically been well, has a history of recent viral illness, and then develops onset of bruising and bleeding that concerns parents (Buchanan, 2005; Panepinto & Brousseau, 2005).

Clinical Manifestations

Bleeding from gums, nosebleeds, and in urine and stools

Multiple ecchymoses, petechiae, and purpura

Diagnostic Tests

Platelet count is decreased (less than 20,000 µL/dL).

Hemoglobin and white blood cell count is normal.

For atypical presentation, bone marrow aspiration is used to rule out other diagnoses (Buchanan, 2005).

Clinical Therapy

Clinical therapy is dependent on platelet count and varies among healthcare providers.

Treatment may include corticosteroids, intravenous immune globulin (IVIG), and anti-Rh (d) immune globulin (Wang, Wiley, Luddy, et al., 2005).

Platelet administration is indicated only if intracranial hemorrhaging occurs. Administered platelets will be destroyed.

Sixty to 80% of patients with ITP will recover completely; however, others will develop chronic disease (Wang et al., 2005).

Splenectomy may be the treatment of choice for those with chronic disease who do not respond to treatment.

Nursing Management

Nursing care focuses on controlling and preventing the number of bleeding episodes.

Assess for evidence of bleeding, including ecchymosis, petechiae, and purpura.

Assess for hepatosplenomegaly.

Monitor for nosebleeds, oozing at intravenous sites, gastrointestinal bleeding, and indications of intracranial bleeding such as vomiting and seizures.

Preventive measures include teaching parents to use acetaminophen instead of aspirin, to avoid activities that may increase injury, and to recognize signs and symptoms of bleeding.

Disseminated Intravascular Coagulation

Disseminated intravascular coagulation (DIC) is a life-threatening clotting disorder occurring as a complication of other serious illnesses in children.

Clinical Manifestations

Clinical manifestations of DIC result from bleeding and clotting disorders. Bleeding ranges from minor oozing to hemorrhage. Clinical manifestations include:

Petechiae, purpura, ecchymosis, and bleeding or oozing from wounds, intravenous access site, or body orifices

Pallor, cool extremities, cyanosis of extremities

Tachycardia, hypotension, tachypnea, decreased breath sounds

Weakness, malaise

Confusion, coma, seizures

Oliguria, anuria, hematuria

Occult blood in stool or emesis, abdominal distention, bleeding from mucous membranes

Diagnostic Tests

Prothrombin time and partial thromboplastin time are prolonged.

Platelet count and fibrinogen levels are decreased.

Levels of fibrin-fibrinogen split products are high.

Clinical Therapy

Management is supportive and includes:

Identification and treatment of underlying disorder

Replacement of depleted coagulation factors, fibrinogen, and platelets

Heparin

Nursing Management

Critical nursing care focuses on the assessment of bleeding, preventing further injury, and administration of prescribed therapies while treating the underlying disorder.

Assessment

Careful assessment of all systems on a continual basis is essential.

Assess extremities for capillary refill, warmth, and pulses.

Frequently assess vital signs and level of consciousness.

Monitor oxygen saturation and arterial blood gases.

Observe for petechiae, ecchymoses, and all body orifices and skin breaks for oozing blood every 1 to 2 hours.

Examine stool for the presence of blood, and measure blood loss as accurately as possible.

Assess intake and output.

Monitor urine for presence of blood.

Monitor for signs of hypovolemic shock.

Monitor BUN and creatinine to assess renal function.

Implementation

Institute bleeding control precautions.

Administer replacement blood products.

Maintain patency of airway and implement safety measures to preserve endotracheal tube position.

Report any signs of complications.

Implement measures to maintain skin integrity, such as gentle and frequent repositioning.

Identify the family's coping strategies and support system to facilitate their ability to manage this life-threatening crisis.

Meningococcemia

Meningococcemia is a virulent disease process that develops in some individuals infected with *Neisseria meningitidis*. Meningococcemia occurs primarily in young children and has a mortality rate of approximately 10%, with another 10% to 20% suffering sequalae such as limb amputation and hearing loss. Endotoxins from the bacteria are thought to impair protein C, which causes thrombosis formation. The virulence of meningococcal disease is 50 to 100 times that of other gram-negative infections (Milonovich, 2007).

Clinical Manifestations

Onset is sudden.

Often, respiratory infection is followed by fever, myalgias, weakness, headache, diarrhea, and vomiting.

The petechial rash characteristic of this disease may develop before other serious symptoms and progresses rapidly (Milonovich, 2007; Woods, 2007).

Symptoms can progress to a critical level within 12 to 48 hours of onset.

The child's condition may deteriorate rapidly within a period of a few hours.

The clotting cascade is initiated, resulting in bleeding and thrombosis in the tissues (Milonovich, 2007).

The child is critically ill and demonstrates multisystem disease. Frequently, the skin is pink and then black as the tissues are damaged from reduced oxygen delivery.

Diagnostic Tests

Blood cultures reveal *N. meningitidis*.

Organisms may be found in cerebrospinal fluid and synovial fluid (Woods, 2007).

Clinical Therapy

Isolation to prevent spread of infection

Antibiotics—penicillin or third-generation cephalosporin

Removal from sources of infection and multisystem shock management (Milonovich, 2007; Singh & Arrieta, 2004)

Prompt recognition and treatment with antibiotics

Fluid volume replacement to support blood pressure and correct hypovolemic shock

Treatment of septic shock with constant critical monitoring

Treatment of disseminated intravascular coagulation

Nursing Management

Assessment

Perform thorough assessment of all body systems.

Monitor level of consciousness for changes.

Monitor urinary output to evaluate renal function.

Assess for alterations in tissue perfusion by noting cold extremities and circumoral cyanosis.

Assess oxygen saturation levels and blood gas values.

Assess for indications of seizure activity.

Implementation
Manage fluids.

Maintain respiratory support.

Administer intravenous fluids for replacement, treatment of hypovolemia, and maintenance of blood pressure.

Administer antibiotics and vasopressive agents as indicated.

Maintain meticulous skin care for integrity.

Provide nutritional support.

Prevent further infections.

Maintain ventilator support and arterial lines if present.

Implement seizure precautions.

Assist with wound debridement as required. Maintain sterile technique.

Support child and family with information, resource allocation, and follow-up care.

HEMATOPOIETIC STEM CELL TRANSPLANTATION (HSCT)

Hematopoietic stem cell transplantation is a treatment used for diseases such as severe combined immunodeficiency disease, severe and unresponsive aplastic anemia, and leukemia. Hematopoietic stem cells exist primarily in the bone marrow but also circulate in the peripheral blood. These cells can grow into new body cells, and have become useful in treatment of immune and hematologic diseases when restoration of normal cells is needed. Stem cells can be obtained from bone marrow, cord blood, or peripheral blood and frozen for later use (Trigg, 2004).

Hematopoietic stem cell transplants are either autologous or allogenic. In autologous transplantation, the child's own marrow is taken, treated, stored, and reinfused after the child has received chemotherapy. Allogeneic transplantation may be syngeneic (from an identical twin), related, or unrelated. In allogeneic transplantation, the donor, often a sibling (related), has a compatible human leukocyte antigen (HLA). Human leukocyte antigens are proteins found on the surface of nearly all nucleated cells within the body, and they are responsible for regulating the immune response.

Clinical Therapy

Pretransplant phase:

- Evaluation of child, human leukocyte antigen typing, evaluation of organ function, and laboratory studies
- High doses of chemotherapy and possibly total body radiation to destroy circulating blood cells and the diseased bone marrow
- The chemotherapy program for destruction of bone marrow ranges from 7 to 10 days (Moore, 2005). During this time, the child is cared for in strict isolation in a special unit that provides a positive-pressure environment.

Transplant phase:

- Intravenous infusion with donor stem cells
- If successful, cells will migrate to bone marrow and transplant marrow will start producing hematopoietic blood cells in approximately 2 to 4 weeks.

Post-transplant phase:

- Pancytopenia lasts for several weeks after transplant.
- Major risks are infection, anemia, bleeding, and mouth sores.
- Transfusions of red blood cells and platelets may be required.
- Total parenteral nutrition may be required for some children.
- Those not receiving syngeneic transplants require immunosuppressive agents to prevent graft-versus-host disease.

Nursing Management

Assessment

Monitor for this multisystem disorder by assessing skin, mucous membranes, gastrointestinal function, respiratory function, cardiac function, and hydration status.

Conduct frequent assessment, including signs of graft-versus-host disease.

Implementation

Support the child and family with assessment of resources and use of support groups.

Ensure that the family is prepared to administer medications, recognize signs of graft-versus-host disease, provide adequate nutrition for the child, and perform other necessary care.

Provide information related to follow-up appointments and when to seek medical treatment.

Facilitate re-entry into school.

19 ALTERATIONS IN CELLULAR GROWTH

CHILDHOOD CANCER

Clinical Manifestations

Each type of childhood cancer signals its presence differently. Because many of the presenting signs and symptoms of cancer are typical of common childhood illnesses, a delay in diagnosis can occur. In some cases, no symptoms are noted until the cancer is advanced. Children more commonly present with **metastases** (spread of the cancer to a site other than its origin) at time of diagnosis than do adults due to this difficulty in recognition of the disease. Some of the common presenting symptoms of cancer are the following:

Pain may be the result of a neoplasm either directly or indirectly affecting nerve receptors through obstruction, inflammation, tissue damage, stretching of visceral tissue, or invasion of susceptible tissue.

Cachexia is a syndrome characterized by anorexia, weight loss, anemia, asthenia (weakness), and early satiety (feeling of being full).

Anemia may be experienced during times of chronic bleeding or iron deficiency. In chronic illness, the body uses iron poorly. Anemia is also present in cancers of the bone marrow when the number of red blood cells (RBCs) is reduced, in part because of the presence of large numbers of other bone marrow products. Treatment of cancer often promotes further anemia.

Infection is usually a result of an altered or immature immune system. In addition, infection occurs when bone marrow cancers inhibit maturation of normal immune system cells. Infection may also occur in children who are treated with corticosteroids. Because their immune response is altered, the normal signs of infection may not appear.

Bruising can occur if the bone marrow cannot produce enough platelets; bleeding after even minor trauma can then lead to ecchymosis.

Neurologic symptoms may result from impingement on the brain or nervous system. Signs of increased intracranial pressure, decreased or altered consciousness, eye abnormalities, or other neurologic or behavioral changes may be evident.

Palpable mass may be present for certain cancers. This is most commonly abdominal but may be mediastinal or in the neck or other sites.

A variety of other symptoms can occur depending on the location of the cancer. Subcutaneous nodules may appear if leukocytosis is present, superior vena cava syndrome or respiratory difficulty can occur with mediastinal tumors (e.g., neuroblastoma), and enlarged lymph nodes are common with lymphomas (Hon, Leung, Chik, et al., 2005).

During treatment for cancer, a number of complications and oncologic emergencies can occur.

Metabolic emergencies result from the lysis (dissolving or decomposing) of tumor cells, a process called *tumor lysis syndrome*. This cell destruction releases high levels of uric acid, potassium, calcium, and phosphates into the blood. Low levels of sodium occur, potentially leading to metabolic acidosis, cardiac arryhthmias, and/or renal failure (Alavi, Arzanian, Abbasian et al., 2006; Rheingold & Lange, 2006). A second type of metabolic emergency is septic shock. During periods of immune suppression, the child is vulnerable to overwhelming infection, resulting in circulatory failure, hypothermia or hyperthermia, tachypnea, mental changes, inadequate tissue perfusion, and hypotension. A third type of metabolic emergency occurs when large amounts of bone are destroyed by treatment, resulting in hypercalcemia (elevated serum calcium) (Spinazze & Schrijvers, 2006). Some children develop the syndrome of inappropriate antidiuretic hormone and have excessive release of antidiuretic hormone. The resulting decreased urinary output leads to water intoxication.

Hematologic emergencies result from bone marrow suppression or infiltration of brain and respiratory tissue with high numbers of leukemic blast cells (hyperleukocytosis). Bone marrow suppression results in anemia and thrombocytopenia (decreased platelets) with resultant coagulation disturbance and hemorrhage. Disseminated intravascular coagulation occurs in some children and is a life-threatening complication. Gastrointestinal and central nervous system bleeding (strokes) is common. Disruption of normal white blood cell (WBC) production and resulting hyperleukocytosis can lead to obstruction of small blood vessels throughout the body.

Space-occupying lesions can present with a variety of clinical manifestations. Extensive tumor growth may result in spinal cord compression, increased intracranial pressure, brain herniation, seizures, massive hepatomegaly, cardiac and respiratory complications, and superior vena cava syndrome (obstruction of the superior vena cava by tumor).

Secondary cancers are those that occur subsequent to the primary cancer but are of a different histologic type. *Other chronic conditions*, such as heart failure, cognitive dysfunction, mental health disruptions, and reproductive problems can occur, either due to the cancer itself or the side effects of treatment (Schultz, Ness, Whitton, et al., 2007; Twombly, 2007).

Diagnostic Tests

Complete blood count to include the following:

- RBC, WBC, platelets, complete blood count (CBC) with differential
- Hemoglobin and hematocrit
- RBC indices such as mean corpuscular volume, mean corpuscular hemoglobin concentration, and mean corpuscular hemoglobin
- WBC indices include the percent of all five types of WBCs (basophils, eosinophils, monocytes, lymphocytes, neutrophils).
- Absolute neutrophil count uses both the segmented (mature) and bands (immature) as a measure of the body's infection fighting capability; calculated by adding percentage of segmented neutrophils to percentage of bands and then multiplying this percentage by the WBC count.
- Serum chemistry, which includes electrolytes, including sodium, potassium, chloride, calcium, magnesium, phosphorus, and carbon dioxide
- Other studies may include renal function studies such as blood urea nitrogen, uric acid, and creatinine; and liver studies such as total bilirubin, alanine aminotransferase, aspirate aminotransferase, lactic dehydrogenase, alkaline phosphatase, and blood urea nitrogen.
- Certain substances, or markers, are elevated with some specific tumors—for example, alpha-fetoprotein level may be elevated in liver tumors; vanillylmandelic acid and homovanillic acid levels may be elevated in adrenal tumors; and elevated catecholamines are found in neuroblastoma.
- Bone marrow aspiration
- Bone marrow biopsy
- Lumbar puncture
- Radiographic examination
- Magnetic resonance imaging (MRI)
- Computed tomography (CT)
- Ultrasound
- Histologic or laboratory analysis of tumor cells after biopsy of tumor
- Additional studies for certain cancers such as pulmonary function tests; echocardiograms; nuclear medicine scans with radioactive

isotopes, such as gallium or iodine; bone scan with technetium 99m; or positron emission tomography and single-photon emission CT, which combine nuclear medicine with CT

■ Urinalysis

Clinical Therapy

A specialist in pediatric oncology is needed to manage the complex care required in cancer treatment.

A *protocol* is a plan of action for treatment that is based on the results of staging: type of cancer, its location, the particular cell type, and its degree of spread.

Surgery is used to remove or debulk (reduce the size of) a solid tumor; it is also used to determine the stage and type of cancer.

Chemotherapy is the administration of specific drugs that kill both normal and cancerous cells (Table 19–1).

Table 19–1   Medications Used for Cancer Chemotherapy

Medication	Action and Use	Nursing Implications
Cell cycle-specific agents Antimetabolites: 5-azacytidine, 5-fluorouracil, 6-mercaptopurine, 6-thioguanine, cytosine arabinoside (cytarabine), hydroxyurea, methotrexate	Work at synthesis phase of cell division; interfere with function of nucleic acid; inhibit DNA or RNA synthesis.	Most common side effects are nausea and vomiting, myelosuppression, stomatitis. Specific agents such as methotrexate and cytarabine can cause neurologic toxicity with high doses. Consult drug books and package inserts for detailed list of side effects.
		Obtain baseline CBC, liver function, renal function.
		Monitor I&O and body weight. Ensure hydration and output levels ordered by oncologist.
		Monitor VS and cardiovascular and respiratory function.
		Watch for bleeding and signs of infection.
		Monitor carefully during administration for signs of anaphylaxis.

Table 19–1   Medications Used for Cancer Chemotherapy (Continued)

Medication	Action and Use	Nursing Implications
Vinca alkaloids: etoposide, teniposide, irinotecan, paclitaxel, vinblastine, vincristine	Act during mitosis; bind with cell proteins to inhibit nucleic acid and protein synthesis.	Common side effects include nausea and vomiting, abdominal cramping and diarrhea, constipation, paralytic ileus, hair loss, hypotension or hypertension, peripheral neuropathy, and neurologic toxicity (latter especially with vinblastine and vincristine). Obtain baseline blood work. Consult specific drug information for period of maximum myelosuppressive effect. Be alert for bruising, infection, and other signs of myelosuppression. Monitor carefully during administration for signs of anaphylaxis.
Miscellaneous—G_1 phase activity: L-asparaginase	Causes depletion of asparagine, which is needed by cancer cells; makes cell in G phase vulnerable to other agents; interferes with prosynthesis. Used in combination with other agents in leukemia and other cancers.	Administered intravenously or intramuscularly. Major side effects are severe nausea and vomiting, hypersensitivity, renal failure, myelosuppression, and acid–base imbalance. Because of the risk of life-threatening hypersensitivity reactions, emergency medications and care must be immediately available.

Table 19–1   Medications Used for Cancer Chemotherapy (Continued)

Medication	Action and Use	Nursing Implications
		CBC, serum amylase, glucose, coagulation factors, bone marrow function, and liver function tests performed before therapy and twice weekly.
		Monitor I&O, neurologic status, gastrointestinal symptoms, and abdominal pain.
Miscellaneous—G_2 phase activity: etoposide	Works at G_2 phase; binds cellular proteins to cause metaphase arrest; also acts on S phase of DNA synthesis. Used with other agents, particularly in recurrent disease.	Administered orally and intravenously.
		Common side effects are nausea and vomiting, myelosuppression, hair loss, and diarrhea. Can cause anaphylaxis; hypotension and intravenous site pain with rapid infusion.
		Perform baseline CBC, liver, and renal function tests.
		Check intravenous site frequently because extravasation can cause necrosis.
		Monitor VS during infusion, and stop drug if hypotension occurs. Keep emergency drugs and equipment readily available.
Cell cycle-nonspecific agents		
Alkylating agents: cyclophosphamide, carboplatin, cisplatin, busulfan, chlorambucil, ifosfamide, thiotepa, mechlorethamine, melphalan, procarbazine, dacarbazine	Substitute an alkyl group for a hydrogen atom, leading to blockage of DNA replication. Used for treatment of many cancers, either alone or in conjunction with other agents.	Most are administered orally and/or intravenously. Array of side effects depending on specific drug. Some common side effects are nausea and vomiting, diarrhea, myelosuppression, hair loss, neuropathies, pulmonary toxicity, renal damage; secondary tumors later in life associated with some agents.

Table 19–1 Medications Used for Cancer Chemotherapy (Continued)

Medication	Action and Use	Nursing Implications
		Obtain CBC and full blood work before and during treatment. Monitor for side effects of the specific agents administered. Ensure generous hydration and monitor I&O. Teach family the importance of long-term monitoring for secondary tumors.
Antibiotics: doxorubicin, mitomycin C, dactinomycin, bleomycin, daunorubicin, idarubicin, mitoxantrone	Interfere with nucleic acid, inhibiting DNA or RNA synthesis. Used in combination with other agents to treat leukemia and other childhood cancers.	Most are administered intravenously. Common side effects include nausea and vomiting, myelosuppression, oral ulcers, and skin and pulmonary toxicity. Several have cumulative dose toxicity, such as cardiac abnormalities (doxorubicin) and skin/pulmonary complications (bleomycin); total dose the child has received must be monitored. Obtain baseline CBC and other blood studies and monitor throughout therapy. Monitor VS, lung function, cardiac function, and neurologic status throughout and after therapy. Be alert for signs of myelosuppression and mucosal ulcers.
Nitrosoureas: carmustine, lomustine	Cross breakage in DNA strands so that DNA and RNA replication cannot occur. Used in lymphomas and other childhood cancers. Can cross blood–brain barrier.	Administered orally (lomustine) or intravenously (carmustine). Major side effect is myelosuppression. Others include pulmonary fibrosis, eye infarction, skin changes, hair loss, nausea, and vomiting.

Table 19–1   Medications Used for Cancer Chemotherapy (Continued)

Medication	Action and Use	Nursing Implications
		Obtain baseline and periodic CBC and other studies. Monitor pulmonary function, skin, and signs of infection or bleeding.
Hormones: prednisone, prednisolone, dexamethasone	Analogue of hydrocortisone; anti-inflammatory; delayed and depressed immune response. Used in conjunction with other agents for many types of childhood cancer.	Often administered orally. Numerous side effects, including edema, moon face, mood lability, increased appetite, disturbed sleep, immunosuppression, disturbed glucose control, and osteoporosis. Teach child and family the effects of the drug. Minimize exposure to persons with infection. Monitor for infections in all systems. Monitor weight regularly. Take VS. Teach to take as directed. Drug must be tapered slowly at end of therapy.
Topoisomerase I inhibitors: irinotecan, mitoxantrone, topotecan	Inhibit the enzyme topoisomerase I in the cell nucleus, relaxing DNA and preventing its duplication. Used in conjunction with other agents to treat acute lymphocytic leukemia and other childhood cancers	Administered intravenously. Topotecan can be given intrathecally. Common side effects include nausea and vomiting, diarrhea, fever, dehydration, and myelosuppression. Can alter liver function and cause skin changes. Obtain baseline and periodic CBC and other studies, including liver function. Monitor for signs of myelosuppression, gastrointestinal distress, and change in liver function.

Note: CBC, complete blood count; I&O, input and output; VS, vital signs.

Other drugs used in the treatment of children with cancer include colony-stimulating factors, antiemetics, and nutritional supplements (Table 19–2).

Table 19–2   Colony-Stimulating Factors

Medication	Action and Use	Nursing Implications
Epoetin alfa (human recombinant erythropoietin)	This glycoprotein stimulates the bone marrow in red blood cell formation; useful when numbers of red blood cells are low due to chemotherapy effects.	Give subcutaneously or intravenously. Do not shake, and do not use if discolored or particles are present. Single-dose vials only, so discard any solution that is not used.
		Obtain blood tests before therapy and periodically after; improvement in hematocrit should be seen in 7–14 days.
		Monitor blood pressure before and during therapy, as hypertension can result.
		Monitor for change in neurologic response and headache; both seizures and strokes are possible side effects.
Filgrastim (Neupogen) and pegfilgrastim (Neulasta)	This human granulocyte colony-stimulating factor increases production of neutrophils by the bone marrow.	Administered subcutaneously and intravenously; prepare as directed for intravenous infusion to prevent its absorption by intravenous tubing.
		Single-dose vials only, so discard any solution that is not used.
		Incompatible with many medications; check package insert; do not give within 24 hours before or after chemotherapy drugs or their effect may be decreased.

Table 19–2   Colony-Stimulating Factors (Continued)

Medication	Action and Use	Nursing Implications
		Obtain baseline and twice-weekly complete blood count.
		Monitor for side effects such as bone pain and heart arrhythmias; report fevers, and be alert for other signs of infection when neutrophil count is low.
Oprelvekin (Neumega)	A hematopoietic growth factor, interleukin-11, that increases platelet count; useful in low platelet count due to chemotherapy effects on bone marrow.	Administered subcutaneously.
		Single-dose vials only, so discard any solution that is not used.
		Obtain baseline complete blood count and platelet count; monitor platelets throughout treatment.
		Monitor for side effects such as edema, fever, central nervous system changes, tachycardia, respiratory problems, and skin rash. Take daily weights and monitor for fluid retention.

Radiation therapy involves the use of unstable isotopes that release varying levels of energy to cause breaks in the DNA molecule and thereby destroy cells.

Biotherapy is the use of biologic retooling and molecular intervention to produce targeted cancer therapy; examples include biologic retooling such as development of antibodies that are tumor-specific to certain cancers, use of drugs that stimulate the body's own immune response, cancer vaccines, gene therapy, and molecular targeting (Butowski, Sneed, & Chang, 2006; Henderson, Mossman, Nairn, et al., 2005).

Bone marrow and hematopoietic stem cell transplantation (HSCT).

Complementary therapies such as nutritional supplements, oral herbal supplements, touch therapy, and mind/body interventions.

In cases that cannot be successfully treated, the focus of health care is end-of-life care, providing comfort and emotional support for the terminally ill child and family.

Nursing Management

Assessment

History to identify cancer contains several components:

- Complete a genogram to identify any family history of cancer.
- Ask about history of exposure to known carcinogens, such as whether a parent works in an industry with substances such as chemicals or asbestos that might remain on clothing worn home, whether the child has been treated with radiation or chemotherapy for a previous cancer, and if the child has an identified condition such as Down syndrome or has any recognized congenital anomalies.

Physiologic assessment must be thorough when cancer or potential cancer is diagnosed:

- When the child has some symptoms of cancer, evaluation for anemia, frequent infections, bleeding disorders, loss of weight, fatigue, pain, and changes in mental health and neurologic status should be performed.
- Height and weight should be carefully measured and compared with prior findings for the child; nutrition intake history may be pertinent.
- Assess hydration status and the tumor site if it is visible.
- Evaluate pain, fatigue, infections, bruising, shortness of breath, and elimination problems.
- Observe immunization status, developmental milestones, gait, and coordination, as well as any changes in mental status.
- All body systems need thorough assessment; neurologic, respiratory, cardiac, and gastrointestinal systems require particular attention.
- Extensive laboratory and radiologic/imaging studies are performed.

Cancer creates many emotional challenges, so thorough psychosocial assessment is needed:

- Gather information about the crisis from the perspective of the family (Kazak, Rourke, Alderfer, et al., 2007).
- Assess the family members (and child if old enough) for their understanding and acceptance of the diagnosis.
- Evaluate if the family has told the child about the diagnosis and whether the family needs assistance in deciding how to do this (Packman, Greenhalgh, Chesterman, et al., 2005).

- Ask what they have told siblings and if they need suggestions, help, and support to decide how much and when to share information with the child's siblings.
- Assess the level of anxiety during healthcare visits and scheduled treatments.
- Evaluate the family's resilience and methods of coping, such as the ability to integrate relaxing and meaningful activities into family life, the use of support systems in the extended family and community, and the ability to alter expectations to take into account the child's health status.
- Evaluate the family for stressors such as illness or death of another family member, occupational changes, financial problems, relocation, and change in vacation plans.
- Evaluate the family's knowledge of the U.S. Family and Medical Leave Act benefits, which provide for parental use of sick time, vacation, and leave without pay to treat an ill family member while safeguarding employment.

Inquire if the family's insurance carrier provides for a case manager in complex health needs such as cancer.
- Assess whether faith-based affiliations and healers are meaningful for the family.
- Ask parents about complementary therapy and medications they are obtaining from other sources and using at home.
- Evaluate the child's and family's knowledge and information sources, providing them with opportunities to ask questions.
- Assess the learning style of the child and family to adapt approaches to meet their needs.
- When the treated child is returning to school, evaluate the ability of the school to accept a medically vulnerable child into the classroom.
- Drawings, colored pictures cut out by the child to form a collage, discussion, and observation are used to assess for body image changes that occur as a result of cancer and its treatment.

Developmental assessment of children should be performed regularly during treatment for cancer, at times when the child feels well, so that results are accurate.

For the child who survives cancer, ongoing assessments are essential. Evaluate the child regularly with thorough physical, psychosocial, developmental, and cognitive assessments; carefully monitor all body systems (e.g., cardiovascular; respiratory; musculoskeletal; eye, ear, nose, and throat; genitourinary); record height and weight and general growth patterns; ask about the child's interactions with peers and performance at school; be alert for signs and symptoms that could indicate a secondary tumor or side effects of treatment.

Intervention

Ensure optimal nutritional intake because the catabolic effect of therapy and cancer lead to a malnourished state; offer frequent, small meals; arrange a nutritional consult.

Special nutritional products may be given orally, nasogastric or nasoduodenal tube feedings may be given, or total parenteral nutrition may be necessary.

Administer antiemetic drugs to lessen nausea from chemotherapy and radiation.

Chemotherapy drugs are prepared with special techniques under laminar flow devices to minimize potential toxic effects on healthcare providers using gloves and other hazardous drug protocols; follow the online guidelines of the Occupational Safety and Health Administration in "Controlling Occupational Exposure to Hazardous Drugs."

Avoid extravasation of intravenous drugs (leakage into the soft tissue around the infusion site), as permanent tissue damage can result.

Administer fluids to ensure adequate hydration during treatments.

Administer other supportive medications as ordered, such as antiemetics to control nausea, vitamin supplements, and antibiotics.

Monitor for side effects such as myelosuppression and neutropenia; treatments may include antibiotics, granulocyte colony-stimulating factors, and colony-stimulating factors (see Table 19–2).

Monitor for thrombocytopenia; protect the child from bruises, and be alert for signs of bleeding such as petechiae, nosebleeds, and dark-colored or bloody stools, and presence of blood in vomit and urine; minimize needle sticks and other intrusive procedures during periods of thrombocytopenia; platelet infusions may be needed.

Monitor for anemia; encourage high iron intake; administer infusions as needed.

Provide good oral hygiene with a soft toothbrush, foam wand, or water irrigation device and report oral breakdown promptly.

Partner with the oncologist, dentist, and nutritionist to plan treatment strategies to protect the oral health and erupting teeth of children.

Know all side effects of specific drugs administered and monitor for them; realize that some side effects are late and may be seen after therapy is completed.

Emphasize importance of all follow-up visits scheduled in the future for monitoring of late effects.

During radiation therapy, examine the skin daily during hospitalization or weekly when making home visits; leave the marks on the skin that outline the radiation target area; avoid use of lotions, powders, and soaps on the target skin area.

Management of infections is critical; children may be hospitalized and central lines inserted for antibiotic administration; blood cultures and cultures of infected body parts help to establish the causative organisms; administer medication treatment on time and as ordered; ensure that standard precautions and transmission-based precautions are followed; monitor temperature, vital signs, and assessment of all body systems at least every 4 hours.

Use pain management techniques to keep the child comfortable during diagnostic procedures and treatments; conscious sedation and local anesthetics are commonly used.

Facilitate contact with extended family members who might be of help, religious or spiritual connections, social service agencies, and other resources such as Internet and parent-support groups.

Assist parents who are concerned about job obligations and financial concerns.

Patient and Family Education
Basic information about the disease and the purpose of the tests that will be performed is needed as soon as the diagnosis is made.

Instructions often need to be repeated, as parents may not process information the first time it is presented due to their increased stress levels.

Assist the parents to plan how and when to tell the child the diagnosis.

Help the family to identify support systems, and intervene as needed to enhance these systems.

A variety of information and teaching approaches are needed, with specifics dependent on the child's particular treatment (Box 19–1).

The child undergoing treatment for cancer needs support appropriate to his or her developmental stage and cognitive level.

Box 19-1   The Family and Cancer Treatment

Most parents are not aware of the effects of cancer treatment and how they can help children through this experience. Depending on the stage and type of treatment, there are several suggestions to make to parents:

- Children in radiation and chemotherapy are fatigued. Provide extra rest periods with shorter activity periods between them.
- Have an overnight bag ready in case the child develops a complication and needs to be taken to stay in the hospital for a few days. Several hospital stays of a few days are normal during treatment.
- When concerned about a symptom in the child, ask the care provider. Parents are often key in identifying problems early.
- Parents are usually concerned about central line care but feel more comfortable after a few days of caring for the line.
- Children have poor appetites at times, and so nutritional intake is needed when they are hungry.
- Remember that the children are still at the normal developmental age. Treat them as a reflection of their ages, not as if they are older or younger.
- Try to maintain contact with the child's peer group and family members.
- Seek information from other parents and resources on cancer care.
- Remind parents to get time away and relax so that parental energy remains high and they are better able to deal with the child's therapy.

Talk with the child's teachers before the return to school after treatment to explain the child's condition and assist with plans to prepare the other children; role-play with the child how to tell friends about any changes in appearance.

Explore the option of summer camp for children with cancer.

The Make-a-Wish Foundation strives to make dreams come true for ill children by sponsoring them for a desired activity or outing; refer the child to this foundation if appropriate.

Ask how care has changed for the child's siblings and what they have been told about the disease; assist the family to talk with them and inform their teachers about the family stress.

Teach the parents how to ensure adequate nutritional intake, to be alert for signs of infection, to protect the child from exposure to communicable diseases during times of neutropenia, to administer medications at home, and how to handle vomiting and pain.

Teach the parents and family about symptoms that need to be treated immediately (Box 19-2).

Box 19–2 Reportable Events for Children Receiving Chemotherapy

Parents require verbal and written instructions about signs and symptoms to report to the child's oncologist while the child is receiving chemotherapy.

Have parents report the following events to your child's oncologist if they occur while the child is receiving chemotherapy:
• Temperature above 38°C (101°F)
• Any bleeding, such as nosebleeds, blood in stool or urine, petechiae, bruising
• Pain or discomfort with urination or defecation
• Sores in the mouth
• Vomiting or diarrhea
• Persistent pain anywhere, including headache
• Signs of infection, such as cough, fever, runny nose, tugging at ears
• Signs of infection in central lines, such as redness, drainage, or tenderness
• Exposure to communicable diseases, especially varicella (chickenpox)

Inform dentists and other healthcare providers that the child is receiving chemotherapy before procedures. Prophylactic antibiotics should be given before and after dental care.

Source: Adapted from *Pediatric Drug Guide*, by R. M. Bindler & L. B. Howry, 2005, Upper Saddle River, NJ: Prentice Hall Health.

Assist the parents and child to deal with any obstacles to normal development and functioning.

Teach home management of a vascular access device or central line, such as a Broviac catheter; details about cleaning the site, instilling heparin in the line or reservoir, and other needed care should be demonstrated and reviewed before discharge to home.

Emphasize the need for the child and family to have fun and be as normal as possible; play or recreation is needed for all family members.

Help parents to view the child as a "normal" child who is ill for a period of time but still needs to have limits set on behavior, develop healthy lifestyles, and have environmental stimulation to learn to talk, read, or perform motor and cognitive tasks.

BRAIN TUMORS

Clinical Manifestations

Central nervous system or brain tumors are the most commonly occurring solid tumors in children and the second most common malignancy after leukemia.

Brain tumors in children usually occur below the roof of the cerebellum and involve the cerebellum, midbrain, and brainstem.

The most common brain tumors in children are medulloblastoma, cerebral and cerebellar astrocytoma, ependymoma (from ependymal cells lining the brain ventricles and spinal cord canal), and gliomas of the cerebrum or brainstem; less common are supratentorial embryonal tumors and craniopharyngioma.

Children with brain tumors can manifest behavioral and neurologic changes; these may occur rapidly or slowly and subtly.

Some common symptoms include headache, nausea, vomiting, dizziness, abnormal gait and coordination, change in vision or hearing, fatigue, and mental status changes (Wilne, Collier, Kennedy, et al., 2007; Wilne, Ferris, Nathwani, et al., 2006).

Presenting signs can be categorized as follows:
- Nonspecific signs related to increasing intracranial pressure
- Secondary signs related to displacement of intracranial structures
- Focal signs suggesting direct involvement of the brain and cranial nerves

Brainstem tumors can present with weight deficits and may be mistakenly diagnosed as an eating disorder of infancy and childhood (failure to thrive).

Medulloblastomas are brain tumors in the external layer of the cerebellum, accounting for 10% to 20% of childhood brain tumors, and commonly occur in children 5 to 6 years of age. They are fast-growing and present with symptoms such as increased intracranial pressure, manifested by increased head circumference in infants, vomiting, headache, ataxia, and vision changes.

Astrocytomas arise from glial cells and can be either above or below the area between the cerebrum and cerebellum and comprise 40% to 60% of childhood brain tumors. The presenting symptoms vary and include endocrine, vision, and behavioral changes, and increased intracranial pressure and seizures.

Ependymomas commonly occur in the fourth ventricle of the posterior fossa and comprise 5% to 10% of childhood brain tumors. Impaired growth, hydrocephalus, seizures, and cranial nerve impairments are the most common manifestations.

Brainstem gliomas account for 10% to 20% of childhood brain tumors and are located in the pons and typically spread into the surrounding tissue. Cranial nerve impairments, mental status changes, and motor symptoms occur.

Diagnostic Tests

Health history and physical examination

CT

MRI

Positron emission tomography

Single-photon emission CT

Myelography

Angiography

Neurophysiologic tests (electroencephalography and brainstem evoked potentials) assess sensory pathway integrity and disease- or drug-related sensory dysfunction.

Examination for serum tumor markers such as alpha-fetoprotein and human chorionic gonadotropin are sometimes helpful.

Lumbar puncture may be used to identify abnormal cells in the cerebrospinal fluid.

Bone marrow aspiration and bone scans identify any extracranial primary neoplastic growth, as cancers in other sites can metastasize to or from the brain.

Clinical Therapy

Surgery is a common treatment and may be performed to obtain a biopsy specimen, to debulk (reduce the tumor size by partial removal) or excise the tumor, or to treat any hydrocephalus that may be present.

Radiation is commonly used.

Chemotherapy can shrink and help manage some tumors; intrathecal administration of chemotherapy is useful in some cases.

HSCT is an increasingly used treatment option.

Treatment of associated symptoms such as seizures and endocrine disturbance may be needed.

Nursing Management
Assessment

Thorough neurologic examination, including measurement of head circumference and assessment of the anterior fontanel, is necessary in children younger than age 18 months.

Perform developmental screening.

Ask about the child's social interactions, school performance, and any behavior changes that have occurred.

Intervention

Close monitoring of neurologic status is needed postoperatively and during all treatments.

Administer drugs such as chemotherapy, antibiotics, steroids, and anticonvulsants as ordered.

Explain procedures and treatments, the purpose of lines, and the use of sedation to keep the child restful, and answer any questions of the family.

Ask parents about resources such as other family members, available sick leave from work, and places to stay if they live far from the hospital.

Ensure that parents can recognize signs of infection and changes in the child's neurologic status at home.

Chemotherapy or radiation often occurs on an outpatient basis; inform parents of the desired outcome and potential side effects of these treatments.

Assist the family in obtaining any special equipment they may need to care for the child at home, such as a wheelchair, bed rails, or dressings.

Once treatment is completed, encourage regular healthcare visits to monitor for sequelae of treatment or recurrence of cancer.

NEUROBLASTOMA

Clinical Manifestations

Neuroblastoma is commonly a smooth, hard, nontender mass that can occur anywhere along the sympathetic nervous system chain; a frequent location is the abdomen, although other sites are the adrenal, thoracic, and cervical areas.

Neuroblastoma is usually diagnosed in children younger than age 5 years, with the median age at diagnosis being 2 years of age (Ater, 2007).

Characteristic signs are weight loss, abdominal distention, enlarged liver, irritability, fatigue, and fever.

Altered bowel and bladder function occur when the mass is retroperitoneal.

Dyspnea or infection may occur when the tumor is mediastinal.

Neck and facial edema may result from vena cava syndrome if the tumor is mediastinal and large.

Intracranial lesions may be present with periorbital ecchymosis.

Malaise, fever, and a limp can occur if there has been metastasis to the bone.

Bone marrow disease can manifest as *pancytopenia* (abnormal depression of all cellular blood components) with neutropenia (causing infections) and anemia (causing fatigue).

Metastatic spread can result in an array of symptoms affecting multiple organs.

Diagnostic Tests

Routine blood cell counts are needed, including CBC with differential.

Tumor markers include vanillylmandelic acid, homovanillic acid, dopamine, ferritin, neuron-specific enolase, lactic dehydrogenase, and a ganglioside, GD2.

Tests for initial tumor include the following:
- Tumor tissue diagnosis by light microscopy
- Biopsy of tumor cells plus laboratory evaluation showing increased urine or serum catecholamines (two separate measures, each more than 3 standard deviations above the norm for age)

Tests for metastases include the following:
- Bone marrow aspirate and biopsy
- Radiolabeled scanning with metaiodobenzylguanidine
- Bone scan
- Skeletal radiograph
- CT or MRI of abdomen, liver, brain, and eye orbits
- MRI of spine
- Chest radiograph with added CT or MRI if radiograph shows lesions

Clinical Therapy

Surgical excision of the mass is performed and may be the only treatment in low-risk stages.

With higher risk stages, surgery is followed by chemotherapy with a combination of drugs such as the following:
- Cyclophosphamide
- Ifosfamide

- Doxorubicin
- Cisplatin
- Carboplatin
- Teniposide
- Etoposide

Radiation is often used, especially in disseminated disease.

HSCT may be performed for advanced disease, sometimes followed by the biologic modifier *cis*-retinoic acid and fenretinide (to promote apoptosis; Ater, 2007).

Nursing Management

The presenting site of the tumor, such as the neck or abdomen, is assessed by observation and inspection; palpation is contraindicated.

Document related functioning, such as bowel and bladder function.

Take vital signs to watch for elevated temperature and vital sign changes caused by a thoracic mass.

Observe gait and coordination.

Take weight and height (or length for infant) and compare with earlier percentiles for the child.

Psychosocial assessment and emotional assessment of the family are needed.

The nursing management of the child with neuroblastoma can encompass the three phases of medical treatment: chemotherapy, surgery, and radiation; see Nursing Management sections earlier in this chapter.

WILMS' TUMOR (NEPHROBLASTOMA)

Nephroblastoma, an intrarenal tumor that is called *Wilms' tumor*, is a common abdominal tumor of childhood and accounts for 6% of all childhood tumors (Dome, Perlman, Ritchey, et al., 2006).

Wilms' tumor is usually an asymptomatic, firm, lobulated mass located to one side of the midline in the abdomen.

Hypertension caused by increased renin activity related to renal damage is reported in 25% of cases; hematuria or abdominal pain is sometimes present.

The diagnosis of Wilms' tumor is based on an ultrasound study of the abdomen and an intravenous pyelogram; CT scanning or MRI of the lungs, liver, spleen, and brain may be performed to identify any metastasis; a complete blood count is obtained, as well as blood urea nitrogen and creatinine levels; liver function tests are performed; histologic examination is performed for tissue typing once the tumor is removed.

Surgery is performed to remove the affected kidney, to examine the opposite kidney, to remove lymph nodes for examination, and to look for other sites of metastasis.

Chemotherapy or radiation therapy, alone or in combination, is sometimes used before surgery to reduce the size of the tumor.

Children with stages III and IV disease often receive vincristine, dactinomycin, and doxorubicin; cyclophosphamide is sometimes added; radiation may also follow surgery, especially in disseminated disease.

Nursing Management

Perform a thorough baseline assessment of the child; **do not palpate** the abdomen because of the potential for spreading the cancerous cells.

Monitor the child's blood pressure carefully, as hypertension is a common finding that may require treatment.

Nursing care during the postrenal surgery phase focuses on pain management and close monitoring of fluid levels; assess daily weight, intake and output (I&O), and urine specific gravity; monitor the function of the remaining kidney; take blood pressure measurements frequently to watch for signs of shock and to assess the functioning of the remaining kidney.

During the chemotherapy phase, monitor the child for side effects of drugs, the potential for infection from the central line site, and the function of the remaining kidney.

Advise parents about home care needs, administration of medications, and monitoring for drug side effects and ongoing needs for health monitoring.

OSTEOSARCOMA OR OSTEOGENIC SARCOMA

Osteosarcoma is a rare, malignant bone tumor that occurs predominantly in 13- to 14-year-old adolescents; the tumor is usually located at the metaphysis of the distal femur, proximal tibia, or proximal humerus (Hartford, Wodowski, Rao, et al., 2006).

Common initial symptoms of osteosarcoma are pain, swelling or mass, and limp or decreased motion; pain can be referred to the hip or back, which can delay diagnosis; deep bone pain with night awakenings, pulmonary metastasis may occur; other metastatic sites include kidney, adrenals, brain, and pericardium (Arndt, 2007).

Diagnosis of osteosarcoma is made through radiographic studies of the affected area and bone scan; CT or MRI scans of involved bone and other potential sites are performed; a complete blood count, liver studies, and renal studies are done for clues to metastases; a blood test is included for serum alkaline phosphatase and lactic dehydrogenase (levels may be elevated), and tumor biopsy is performed to confirm the diagnosis; arteriography may be performed if limb-sparing surgery is contemplated; cardiac assessments are performed to establish baseline function before treatment with doxorubicin.

Treatment involves both surgery and chemotherapy.

Surgery is either a limb-salvage procedure or limb amputation.

Chemotherapy is started before surgery to shrink the tumor, especially in cases where limb-salvage surgery is performed. It is also given postoperatively to treat and prevent metastasis. Drugs commonly used for osteosarcoma include doxorubicin, cisplatin, ifosfamide with mesna, and methotrexate with leucovorin rescue.

Nursing Management

Assess the child's pain or discomfort, mobility, and gait; take vital signs, especially noting temperature and respirations; psychologic assessment of the child and family is needed, especially if amputation is planned; body image disturbances occur when a limb is lost, particularly with school-age children and adolescents; assess the child's understanding of the treatment and of care after surgery; find out what support systems are available for assistance.

Observe the wound postoperatively for infection and hemorrhage; assess circulation above and below the operative site; if edema is found, elevate the limb.

Perform general postsurgical care such as skin care and pain management.

Assess body image and psychosocial adaptation.

Administer chemotherapy if ordered and instruct child and family about the medications.

Ensure that physical rehabilitation is planned and refer appropriately.

Assist the child in transition back into the school system as needed.

EWING'S SARCOMA

Ewing's sarcoma is a malignant, small, round cell tumor usually involving the diaphyseal (shaft) portion of the long bones; the most common sites are the femur, pelvis, tibia, fibula, ribs, humerus, scapula, and clavicle, but any bone may be involved.

Symptoms are similar to those of osteosarcoma and may include pain, swelling, fever, an elevated WBC count, elevated erythrocyte sedimentation rate, and elevated C-reactive protein; a fracture of the affected bone may occur.

Tumor biopsy is necessary for diagnosis, as well as tests described previously for osteosarcoma.

Initial treatment for Ewing's sarcoma is chemotherapy to reduce the tumor, followed by surgical removal of the entire bone or intensive high-dose irradiation of the entire bone; limb-salvage procedures are now commonly performed rather than amputation.

Chemotherapy is always used after initial treatment, as undetectable metastases are commonly present; drugs may include vincristine, doxorubicin, cyclophosphamide, dactinomycin, etoposide, and ifosfamide.

See Osteosarcoma or Osteogenic Sarcoma section for nursing management.

LEUKEMIA

Clinical Manifestations

Leukemia, a cancer of the blood-forming organs, is the most commonly diagnosed pediatric malignancy in children younger than age 14 years; it is characterized by a proliferation of abnormal WBCs in the body.

The main types are acute lymphoblastic leukemia, acute nonlymphoblastic leukemia, and the rare chronic leukemias of childhood.

Leukemia occurs when the stem cells in the bone marrow produce immature WBCs that cannot function normally; these cells proliferate rapidly by cloning instead of normal mitosis, causing the bone marrow to fill with abnormal WBCs; the abnormal cells then spill out into the circulatory system, where they steadily replace the normally functioning WBCs; as this occurs, the protective lymphocytic functions such as cellular and humeral immunity are reduced, leaving the body vulnerable to infections; the malignant WBCs rapidly fill the bone marrow, replacing stem cells that produce erythrocytes (RBCs) and other blood products such as platelets, thereby decreasing the amount of these products in circulation.

Children with acute lymphoblastic leukemia and acute nonlymphoblastic leukemia usually have fever, pallor, overt signs of bleeding, lethargy, malaise, anorexia, and large joint or bone pain.

Petechiae, frank bleeding, and joint pain are cardinal signs of bone marrow failure.

Enlargement of the liver and spleen (hepatosplenomegaly) and changes in the lymph nodes (lymphadenopathy) are common.

If the leukemia has infiltrated the central nervous system (entered it by means of the circulatory or lymphoid system), the child may exhibit signs such as headache, vomiting, papilledema, and sixth cranial nerve palsy (inability to move the eye laterally).

The testicles, spinal cord, and bone marrow are common sites for infiltration.

Diagnostic Tests

Diagnosis is based initially on blood counts and bone marrow aspiration; blood counts reveal anemia, thrombocytopenia, and neutropenia; bone marrow aspiration reveals immature and abnormal lymphoblasts and hypercellular marrow and is the differential test (see common laboratory values in leukemia in Box 19–3).

Percentage of blast cells in marrow is measured, and 25% lymphoblasts is definitive of disease (Brown, 2006).

Levels of serum uric acid and electrolytes such as calcium, potassium, and phosphorus are measured.

Leukemic cells are examined and classified by FAB type; DNA analysis may provide clues about genetic changes.

Clinical Therapy

Treatment of acute lymphoblastic leukemia involves radiation and chemotherapy; radiation is used for central nervous system disease, in T-cell leukemia, and for testicular involvement.

Intensive chemotherapy with several agents is the main treatment.

HSCT transplantation is a treatment option for the child who has a relapse with acute lymphoblastic leukemia and then achieves a second remission; the transplant is given when the child is in remission.

Box 19-3	Laboratory Values in Leukemia	
	Normal	Common values in leukemia
Leukocytes	Less than 10,000/microLiter	Greater than 10,000/microLiter
Platelets	150,000–400,000/microLiter	20,000–100,000/microLiter
Hemoglobin	12–16 g/dL	7–11 g/dL

Transplantation is also used for children with acute nonlymphoblastic leukemia; they do not need to be in remission for the transplant to be performed.

Nursing Management
Assessment
Thorough physical assessment is important to ensure prompt identification of problems without injuring the child who has deficient coagulation and immune function; observe carefully for bruising and other new sites of bleeding as well as fever or other signs of infection.

Once chemotherapy has begun, closely monitor renal functioning through specific gravity, I&O, and daily weight measurement; monitor dietary intake, nausea, vomiting, and constipation; observe for mucosal sores in the mouth.

A central line is usually in place for intravenous infusion of medications, so careful assessment of the line for proper functioning and for signs of infection is needed.

Ask the parents about any behavioral changes; central nervous system infiltration can affect the child's level of consciousness, causing irritability, vomiting, and lethargy.

The intensive treatment involving frequent venipunctures, bone marrow aspirations, and lumbar punctures requires pain assessment and an evaluation of the level of knowledge and coping skills of child and family.

Intervention
Bone marrow suppression necessitates transmission-based precautions.

Perform careful hand hygiene; take temperature frequently; give oral care with antibacterial mouth washes; inspect skin, mouth, rectal area, and central line site for any signs of infection.

Special attention to renal function is needed for certain drugs; hydration with intravenous fluids to attain a specific gravity of less than

1.010 prevents or reduces the severity of hematuria and potential renal damage.

Evaluate the infusion site before and frequently during infusion; although extravasation is not as common with central lines used in cancer treatment as in peripheral lines, it can occur; many chemotherapy agents are extremely toxic to tissues.

Careful monitoring of I&O is required to record intravenous fluids given during chemotherapy infusions, to assess kidney functioning, and to monitor excretion of by-products from destroyed tumor cells; monitor specific gravity every 8 hours as well as before and during administration of the drug and when the intravenous fluids are reduced to maintenance volume levels.

Daily weight measurements are important to assist in planning adequate hydration during chemotherapy, as well as to measure nutritional status.

Drug side effects may necessitate infusion of platelets or packed RBCs.

Provide for management of pain during procedures, treatment, and general care.

Alter the environment to provide for frequent sleep periods, as the child commonly has disturbed sleep patterns.

Facilitate nutritional intake by offering frequent, small feedings of favorite foods and administering antiemetics during treatment that causes nausea.

Inspect oral mucosa and perform gentle oral hygiene.

Record stools and institute methods to prevent and treat constipation as needed.

Facilitate child and family coping; refer to support groups and encourage therapeutic play and recreation.

Recognize that cancer treatment often continues for years and the child requires ongoing assessment, treatment, and health promotion/health maintenance activities.

Patient and Family Education
Instruct parents in the prevention of infection and use nursing care measures to prevent infection.

Instruct in all details of treatment, such as expected effects and side effects of medication or chemotherapy, care of central lines, and fluid needs.

Suggest measures to child and family to enhance physical care:
- Have rest periods each day.
- Avoid areas of exposure to people with illnesses.
- Drink generous amounts of water.
- Eat a healthy diet, using frequent, small, and nutritious meals to obtain enough nutrients.
- Take medicines prescribed to decrease nausea.
- Maintain good oral hygiene with soft toothbrush and water pik.
- Avoid sun exposure and check skin each day for any signs of bruises, pressure areas, cuts, or scratches.
- Promote bowel elimination through regular dietary and toileting practices.
- Report any signs of infection, changes in condition, or other concerns.

Provide emotional care and resources:
- Be prepared for loss of hair with plans for hats, wigs, or other alternatives.
- Continue contact with friends via phone, via Internet, and in person when possible.
- Try relaxation techniques to aid in sleep and management of treatments.
- Talk with clergy, teachers, parents, counselors, friends, or other supportive people about the experience of having leukemia.
- Keep a journal to record feelings and experiences.

Assist in plans for return to school and use of tutors or other methods to provide for educational needs.

HODGKIN DISEASE

Hodgkin disease is manifested by nontender, firm lymphadenopathy, usually in the supraclavicular and cervical nodes but occasionally in the mediastinal area; a mediastinal growth can cause respiratory difficulty because of pressure on the trachea or bronchi.

Fever, night sweats, and weight loss occur in one-third of children with Hodgkin disease and are associated with a more aggressive form of the disease.

The leukocyte count and erythrocyte sedimentation rate may be elevated.

Diagnosis is based on lymph node biopsy; Reed-Sternberg cells (large cells with two nucleoli) are present.

A staging classification is used to determine disease severity; the basis for staging is data obtained from the history, physical examination, chest radiograph study (for metastasis), chest CT scan, CT or MRI scans of the retroperitoneal nodes, lymphangiogram if there is retroperitoneal involvement, laboratory studies (complete blood count, erythrocyte sedimentation rate, serum copper level, liver function tests), positron emission tomography, bone scans, and a radionuclide scan with gallium.

Bone marrow biopsy, bone scan, or a staging laparotomy may be performed in certain situations.

Chemotherapy using a four-drug combination has been found to be the most effective drug treatment. Drugs commonly used include Adriamycin (doxorubicin), bleomycin, cyclophosphamide, dacarbazine, etoposide, mechlorethamine, methotrexate, prednisone, procarbazine, and vinblastine.

Radiation is commonly added, with low doses for children who are still growing and larger doses for those who are physically mature or those whose disease is more advanced at diagnosis.

HSCT is a treatment option in children with advanced disease or relapse.

Nursing management for all soft tissue tumors is found in the Retinoblastoma section.

NON-HODGKIN LYMPHOMA

There are three types of pediatric non-Hodgkin lymphoma: (1) lymphoblastic lymphoma (30%–40%), (2) small noncleaved cell (Burkitt's) lymphoma (40%–50%), and (3) large cell lymphoma (15%; Mann, Attarbaschi, Steiner, et al., 2006).

Children with non-Hodgkin lymphoma present with fever, weight loss, and night sweats less often than those with Hodgkin disease.

The lymph glands are usually enlarged or nodular, with the most frequent sites being the cervical, axillary, inguinal, and femoral nodes; the disease may be diffuse, without nodular glands.

The anterior mediastinum is the primary site for T-cell lymphomas; tumors that occur in this area may compress the airway (causing breathing difficulty) or superior vena cava (leading to swelling of the face, neck, or arms) and can cause pain.

Jaw involvement is common in Burkitt's lymphoma.

An abdominal mass may cause pain, nausea, and vomiting.

CBC is performed; additional blood tests include renal and liver function, electrolytes, uric acid, and lactic dehydrogenase.

Bone marrow aspiration and lumbar puncture are performed.

Chest radiograph, bone scan, gallium scan, CT, and MRI can help to isolate affected body organs.

Diagnosis is confirmed by tissue biopsy.

A staging system is used to describe the tumor mass and extension to other body areas; treatment is tailored to the type of cancer and its stage.

Stages I and II may be treated with drugs such as vincristine, cyclophosphamide, prednisone, and methotrexate for several months; intrathecal medication is added if head and neck cancers are present.

Stages III and IV are treated with additional drugs (up to nine total) for longer periods of time (1–2 years).

HSCT is a treatment option in children with advanced disease or relapse.

Nursing management for all soft tissue tumors is found in the Retinoblastoma section.

RHABDOMYOSARCOMA

Rhabdomyosarcoma is a soft tissue cancer that occurs most often in the muscles around the eyes (extraorbital), in the neck, and less commonly in the abdomen, genitourinary tract, and extremities; genitourinary, bladder, and prostate cancers are more common in children younger than age 5 years, whereas paratesticular and extremity cancer is more common among adolescents.

Tumors occurring close to the eye produce swelling, ptosis, visual disturbances, and eye movement abnormalities.

When the tumor occurs in the genitourinary tract, the result can be urinary obstruction, hematuria, dysuria, vaginal discharge, and a protruding vaginal mass.

Rhabdomyosarcoma occurring in the abdomen may be asymptomatic; there is rapid metastasis to the lungs, bones, bone marrow, and distant lymph nodes, with resultant multiple clinical manifestations.

Diagnosis of the mass is confirmed by CT, MRI, positron emission tomography, bone marrow aspiration, and biopsy of tumor and regional lymph nodes.

CBC, renal and liver studies, and urinalysis are performed.

Lumbar puncture may be used in head and neck tumors.

A useful biologic marker, Desmin, allows differentiation of rhabdomyosarcoma from other round cell tumors.

Chest and lung CT scans are performed.

Treatment involves surgical removal of the tumor when possible.

Surgery is followed by wide-field radiation and chemotherapy with a combination of drugs such as actinomycin, cyclophosphamide, and vincristine.

Nursing management for all soft tissue tumors is found in the Retinoblastoma section.

RETINOBLASTOMA

Retinoblastoma is an intraocular malignancy of the retina.

The first sign of retinoblastoma is a white pupil, termed *leukokoria* or *cat's eye reflex*.

The red reflex is absent, asymmetric, or of a differing color in the affected eye.

Other symptoms may include a fixed strabismus (a constant deviation of one eye from the other), orbital inflammation, glaucoma, and heterochromia (irises of different colors).

Children at risk for retinoblastoma due to family history can be tested for the RB1 gene.

Diagnostic tests for the cancer include full ocular examination and CT or MRI scans of the eye orbit.

All children with a history of retinoblastoma in the family should be examined by an ophthalmologist after birth, at 6 weeks, every 2 to 3 months until 2 years and then every 4 months until 3 years, and then annually (de Andrade et al., 2006) to aid in early diagnosis.

Tumors are classified according to a staging system, from a very small, localized tumor (group I) to tumors involving more than half the retina and with seeding into the vitreous (group V).

Treatment for retinoblastoma may include removal of the eye (enucleation) when there is permanent retinal damage or failure to respond to other treatment.

Other surgical treatments involve cryotherapy or photocoagulation (argon laser therapy).

Radiation is nearly always used, either as the sole treatment or before surgery to shrink the tumor.

Chemotherapy is sometimes used but is often ineffective, as the drugs often fail to penetrate sufficiently into the eye; chemotherapy drugs include carboplatin, etoposide, vincristine, and cyclosporine.

Nursing Management
Assessment

Careful family histories can sometimes identify children at risk who need frequent physical examinations—for example, if a family history of retinoblastoma is present, the child should receive frequent eye examinations.

Physiologic assessment of the child with a soft tissue tumor, such as Hodgkin disease, non-Hodgkin lymphoma, rhabdomyosarcoma, and retinoblastoma, focuses on the child's general condition; accurate height and weight measurements are essential to provide a baseline against which to measure the child's growth during treatment, as well as for calculation of chemotherapeutic drug dosages.

Observe the area of the tumor, such as the face, neck, and abdomen, and describe any changes.

Monitor respiratory status if the tumor is on the face or neck; report any changes in respiratory pattern to the oncology specialist.

Avoid palpation of any tumor site or enlarged area; metastasis can be influenced by injudicious palpation and manipulation of a tumor site.

Notify the oncology specialist of a change in any lymph node or any other area of the body.

Gastrointestinal and genitourinary function can be altered by the presence of a tumor and by treatment such as chemotherapy and radiation; careful monitoring of the child's I&O measurement is essential.

Abdominal and pelvic tumors may affect defecation, so charting of all bowel movements is important; explain to the family and child why keeping accurate records is necessary.

Observe wounds closely for lack of healing as a result of chemotherapy or radiation.

Examine the mouth and extremities for wounds or ulcers.

Nutritional changes caused by treatment affect the body's ability to support healthy cells and heal wounds.

Assessment of the family's psychosocial status and coping mechanisms is an essential component of nursing care.

Assessment of body image is needed when the child has a soft tissue tumor affecting appearance of the head and neck.

Ask about symptoms of depression such as loneliness, lack of interest, anxiety, and suicidal thoughts in school-age children and adolescents.

Intervention

Children with lymphoma affecting the mediastinum may need respiratory support; position the child so that the head is elevated; administer chemotherapy drugs as ordered, maintaining adequate fluids to facilitate excretion of the resultant breakdown products; monitor the central line used for chemotherapy administration; and teach parents care of the central line when the child is at home.

For the child with a rhabdomyosarcoma involving the bladder, monitor urinary output carefully; report hematuria and painful urination; monitor the changes that occur during therapy; administer pain medications as needed, and use distraction and other techniques to decrease the child's discomfort; emphasize to parents the need for follow-up CT and MRI scans after completion of treatment.

When the child with retinoblastoma undergoes removal of the eye, the parents and child need detailed instructions on postsurgical care; demonstrate to the parents care of the socket and use of a conformer to maintain the eye socket shape; when healing is complete and the child receives a prosthetic eye, instruct parents about its insertion and care; the child can gradually be taught to take over this care when old enough; encourage periodic healthcare visits to monitor for signs of a tumor in the other eye.

Adapt developmental interventions as needed to accommodate for sensory alterations.

Attention is directed at the body changes of the cancer and its treatment; children and adolescents may need suggestions to deal with hair loss, disfigurement, and living with serious illness; referral to other children and teens with similar concerns may be helpful.

Parents of all children need help to encourage normal development in the child with cancer.

Nursing management during chemotherapy and radiation is discussed earlier in this chapter in the general sections on these treatment measures.

Patient and Family Education

Teach the family about the chemotherapy drugs and their side effects.

Teach about the care of surgically placed venous access devices.

Provide written and illustrated information about the chemotherapy protocol(s).

Provide the family with radiation and surgery education specific to the tumor treatment.

Refer the family to nutrition resources such as dietitians for ways to promote the child's adequate intake of food and fluid.

Reinforce with families the importance of long-term follow-up after treatment for a soft tissue tumor; increased risk for secondary cancers for two to three decades is possible, and early identification can help with prompt diagnosis.

Partner with other healthcare providers to provide instructions to families as the child transitions from oncology treatment back to the pediatrician so they understand the importance of telling all care providers about the cancer and treatment.

As children grow into teen and young adult years, help them to take over this important task in their care; recommended annual examinations include the following:
- CBC
- Physical examination with special attention to skin, abdomen, and thyroid
- Monitoring for signs of hypothyroidism and hyperthyroidism
- Neurologic and developmental examinations and monitoring of school performance
- First mammogram at 25 years for those with chest radiation
- Pap and pelvic examinations for teen and young adult women; testicular examinations for males
- Mental status assessment

20 Alterations in Gastrointestinal Function

STRUCTURAL DEFECTS

Cleft Lip and Palate

Description and Etiology

Cleft lip with or without cleft palate results from a failure of the maxillary processes to fuse with the elevations on the frontal prominence during the sixth week of gestation; normally, union of the upper lip is complete by the seventh week; fusion of the secondary palate occurs between 5 and 12 weeks of gestation. Failure of the tongue to move downward at the correct time will prevent the palatine processes from fusing.

The cause is believed to be multifactorial, involving a combination of environmental and genetic influences:

- Family history of the condition, presence of other malformations, maternal use of tobacco, the use of anticonvulsants or steroids during pregnancy (Carinci et al., 2007; Merritt, 2005a).
- Higher intake of folate appears to be protective against the defect (Yazdy, Honein, & Xing, 2007).

Clinical Manifestations

Cleft lip may be a simple dimple in the vermilion border of the lip or a complete separation extending to the floor of the nose; the defect may be unilateral or bilateral and may occur alone or in combination with a cleft palate defect.

Cleft palate defects are less obvious when they occur without a cleft lip and may not be detected at birth unless a thorough examination of the oral cavity is performed; clefts of the hard palate form a continuous opening between the mouth and nasal cavity and may be unilateral or bilateral, involving just the soft palate or the soft and hard palate.

Diagnostic Tests

Cleft lip and palate are generally diagnosed prenatally, at birth, or during the newborn assessment.

Because the defects are sometimes associated with other defects, diagnostic studies to detect ear deformities, skeletal deformities, heart defects, and genitourinary defects are conducted.

Clinical Therapy

Because speech, hearing, and dentition may be affected, coordinated care by specialists in plastic and oral surgery, audiology, speech, otolaryngology, and orthodontics is necessary.

The cleft lip is usually repaired around 3 months of age (Merritt, 2005b).

The lip is sutured together using either a diagonal incision or a staggered suture line (Merritt, 2005b). After surgery, soft elbow immobilizers are used to prevent flexion of the arms. Distraction and pain medication are needed to prevent crying, as prolonged crying may disrupt the suture line.

Timing of the cleft palate repair varies among surgeons and depends on the size and severity of the cleft defect. Most surgeons perform closure operations before the child reaches 18 months of age (Merritt, 2005b).

Postoperative feeding protocols vary from the use of special nipples or syringes to breastfeeding.

Infants with cleft lip and cleft palate are prone to recurrent otitis media, which can lead to hearing problems. Ear infections should be promptly evaluated by a health professional with expertise in ear care and treatment.

The child who has had cleft palate repair will require orthodontic care. Early visits will permit assessment of tooth eruption and the need for future orthodontic work.

Nursing Management

Assessment

Assessment of the family's reactions is an integral part of the overall nursing assessment.

Assess the infant's ability to feed adequately.

Perform thorough and ongoing assessments of all body systems, remaining alert for any other abnormalities.

Perform frequent growth measurements.

Assess developmental progression.

Implementation

Facilitate feeding of the infant, assisting the mother to breastfeed or providing a special nurser if needed.

Promote parent–infant bonding by explaining the nature of the structural defect and the procedure for correction.

Interact and speak to the infant in the parents' presence, and point out positive attributes, such as alertness, soft skin, or active movements.

Parents can also be referred to the Cleft Palate Foundation for information about the disorder.

Postoperative care for the infant includes frequent vital signs, respiratory assessment, maintenance of suture line as prescribed, soft elbow immobilizers, and pain medication and distraction to minimize crying. Avoid use of metal utensils and straws after cleft palate surgery.

Ongoing care after surgery involves growth and developmental monitoring, careful assessment of ear infections, and referral for early dental and orthodontic care when needed.

Esophageal Atresia and Tracheoesophageal Fistula
Description and Etiology
Esophageal atresia is a malformation that results from failure of the esophagus to develop as a continuous tube during the fourth and fifth weeks of gestation.

In esophageal atresia, the foregut fails to lengthen, separate, and fuse into two parallel tubes (the esophagus and trachea) during fetal development. Instead, the esophagus may end in a blind pouch or develop as a pouch connected to the trachea by a fistula (tracheoesophageal fistula).

Esophageal atresia is often associated with a maternal history of polyhydramnios. Associated anomalies may include congenital heart defects, gastrointestinal or urinary tract anomalies, and musculoskeletal abnormalities (Orenstein et al., 2007).

Clinical Manifestations
Symptoms in the newborn include excessive salivation and drooling often accompanied by the three classic signs—cyanosis, choking, and coughing.

During feeding, fluid returns through the nose and mouth. Aspiration places the infant at risk for pneumonia. Depending on the type of defect the abdomen may become distended.

Diagnostic Tests
Diagnosis is usually confirmed by attempting to pass a nasogastric or orogastric tube into the stomach. In most cases the tube meets resistance and can be advanced only minimally.

Specific defects and associated anomalies are determined by radiologic examination.

Echocardiogram and abdominal ultrasound are performed.

Careful examination of the lungs is needed.

A delay in diagnosis can be fatal because ingested fluid or secretions may enter the lungs and lead to pneumonia.

Clinical Therapy

A nasogastric tube is inserted to suction the upper pouch.

Intravenous antibiotics and fluids are begun, and surgery is performed as soon as the infant is stable; the first stage usually involves ligation of the fistula and insertion of a gastrostomy tube. In the second stage, the two ends of the esophagus are reconnected, if possible.

Nursing Management

Assessment

The nurse should be alert for the signs and symptoms in the immediate newborn period.

Assess for difficulty feeding and excessive drooling.

Assess for the classic signs of choking, coughing, and cyanosis.

Assess for respiratory distress, and assess the lung sounds carefully.

Esophageal atresia is a surgical emergency; the infant requires close observation and intervention to maintain a patent airway in the preoperative period.

Implementation

Surgical intervention for a newborn is a stressful situation for the parents and family; the parents require emotional support throughout the infant's hospitalization.

Eliciting questions and allowing parents to participate in the infant's care, especially feeding (when permitted), can facilitate bonding and help to prepare parents for care of the infant after discharge.

Preoperatively, suction is readily available to remove any secretions that accumulate in the nasopharyngeal airway; place the infant with the head of the bed slightly elevated to minimize aspiration of secretions into the trachea; continuous or low-intermittent suction via a nasogastric tube is used to remove secretions from the blind pouch; oral fluids are withheld, and the infant is maintained with fluids administered intravenously. Constant monitoring of vital signs and the infant's condition is needed.

Postoperatively, gastrostomy drainage is maintained, and intravenous fluids and antibiotics are administered; total parenteral nutrition (TPN) may be required until gastrostomy or oral feedings are tolerated; monitoring and assessment of feeding tolerance are ongoing; feedings are introduced slowly and in small amounts; assess for respiratory difficulty during reintroduction of feedings.

Monitor weight and growth and developmental achievements throughout the entire treatment period.

Collaborate with the parents regarding home care needs, and teach them about gastrostomy tube care and feeding, signs of infection, and how to prevent postoperative complications.

Pyloric Stenosis

Pyloric stenosis (also called *hypertrophic pyloric stenosis*) is a hypertrophy of the circular muscle of the pyloric canal causing obstruction.

The exact cause of pyloric stenosis is unknown, although frequently there is a family history of the disorder.

Hypertrophy of the circular pylorus muscle results in stenosis of the passage between the stomach and the duodenum, partially obstructing the lumen of the stomach; the lumen becomes inflamed and edematous, which narrows the opening until the obstruction becomes complete.

Manifestations usually become evident 2 to 8 weeks after birth, although onset may vary. Most cases are diagnosed by 12 weeks of age (Vajnar, 2007). Initially, the infant appears well or regurgitates slightly after feedings; as the obstruction progresses, the vomiting becomes projectile.

The infant generally appears hungry, especially after emesis; appears irritable and lethargic; fails to gain weight; and has fewer and smaller stools.

On physical examination, visible peristaltic waves across the abdomen and an olive-sized mass in the right upper quadrant may be evident (Vajnar, 2007).

An abdominal ultrasound is the most common study performed to confirm the diagnosis of pyloric stenosis.

Serum electrolyte and acid–base measurements are used to determine the degree of dehydration, electrolyte imbalance, and anemia; they reveal hypochloremia, metabolic alkalosis. Early diagnosis will decrease the frequency with which infants present with an alteration in electrolytes (Colletti, 2004; Vajnar, 2007).

Surgical correction (pyloromyotomy) is the treatment of choice; open pyloromyotomy is performed through a periumbilical incision or a small, transverse upper abdominal incision; laparoscopic pyloromyotomy is currently used in many cases, and has been shown to be equally as successful as open pyloromyotomy (Wyllie, 2007). With both procedures, the pyloric muscle is split to allow the passage of food and fluid.

Nurses assess for signs and symptoms that may indicate the disorder; observe the infant's abdomen for the presence of peristaltic waves and auscultate bowel sounds that may be hyperactive; palpation reveals an olive-shaped mass in the right upper quadrant of the abdomen, especially when the stomach is empty such as after a vomiting episode.

Preoperatively, assess the infant's history of vomiting, vital signs, weight, and nutritional status; assess skin turgor, fontanels, urinary output, capillary refill, and mucous membranes and weigh diapers to determine whether hydration is adequate; measure vomitus and describe vomiting episodes; be alert for signs of an electrolyte imbalance, particularly low levels of serum chloride, sodium, potassium, and an elevated pH.

Maintain nothing-by-mouth (NPO) status, and administer intravenous fluids preoperatively.

Monitor intake and output (including vomitus), and urine specific gravity; maintain patency of nasogastric tube, and measure aspirated content.

Postoperatively, maintain hydration status, monitor the surgical site for signs of infection, provide pain relief, initiate feedings as ordered, and support the family in learning about the disorder and home care needed on discharge.

Gastroesophageal Reflux and Gastroesophageal Reflux Disease
Description and Etiology
Gastroesophageal reflux (GER) is the return of gastric contents into the esophagus and is the result of relaxation of the lower esophageal sphincter.

Gastroesophageal reflux disease (GERD) is a more serious manifestation of GER; it is a pathologic process in infants manifested by poor weight gain, recurrent vomiting, generalized irritability, refusal to feed, arching, and respiratory symptoms such as wheezing (Gold & Gremse, 2006).

Three mechanisms allow reflux of the gastric contents across the esophagogastric junction and into the esophagus (Arguin & Swartz, 2004, p. 45).

1. Transient lower esophageal sphincter relaxations
2. Hypotensive or incompetent lower esophageal sphincter
3. Anatomic disruption of the esophagogastric junction

Clinical Manifestations

Regurgitation after feeding is the most common sign of GER in infants. The infant may spit a small amount or may have episodes of forceful vomiting (Arguin & Swartz, 2004). Children with GERD are frequently hungry and irritable; they lose weight and experience failure to thrive; there may be a history of vomiting and frequent upper respiratory infections; child is at risk for aspiration and episodes of apnea (Arguin & Swartz, 2004).

Diagnostic Tests

Diagnosis is confirmed by a thorough history of the child's feeding patterns and by diagnostic evaluation using contrast upper GI series (barium fluoroscopy), pH probe monitoring (insertion of a small catheter into the esophagus through the nose that is left in place for 18 to 24 hours to measure pH and thus determine number of reflux episodes), or nuclear medicine scintiscan (gastric emptying study) (Henry, 2004). The child should be tested for cow milk protein allergy since there is an association between gastroesophageal reflux and cow milk allergy. Testing includes cutaneous tests, eosinophil smears of the nasal mucosa, IgG antilactoglobulin levels, and intestinal biopsy (Arguin & Swartz, 2004).

Clinical Therapy

Treatment depends on the severity of the condition; generally, feeding modification, thickened feeds, and positioning are effective management for milder cases. A smaller feeding volume may prove beneficial to avoid overdistention of the abdomen and subsequent reflux. The infant should be burped after every 1 to 2 ounces (Arguin & Swartz, 2004).

Infants should be held upright for 20 to 30 minutes following feedings. Feedings may be thickened by adding rice or the infant may be fed a prethickened formula such as Enfamil AR, which contains rice and is nutritionally balanced.

Medications, such as histamine 2 (H_2) receptor antagonists, proton pump inhibitors, and antacids, may be helpful for some infants and children.

Treatment for severe cases of GERD such as those with recurrent life-threatening aspiration, failure to thrive, and esophagitis may include surgery to create a valve mechanism by wrapping the greater curvature of the stomach (fundus) around the distal esophagus (Nissen fundoplication) (Arguin & Swartz, 2004). A gastrostomy tube is usually inserted during surgery to serve as a vent for trapped gas (Henry, 2004). The gastrostomy tube may be removed after a few weeks or may be left in long term if needed for feedings.

Nursing Management

Assessment

Obtain a thorough history of the child's feeding patterns.

Observe vomiting episodes and document amount, color, and consistency of emesis. Monitor the infant's weight and plot progress on a growth chart.

Observe for any signs of respiratory distress and keep the infant's nose and mouth clear of emesis.

Implementation

Adequate nutrition must be maintained in order for the child to achieve normal growth and development. Infants receiving oral feedings are administered smaller feedings. Elevate the head of the bed to prevent aspiration if vomiting should occur. If the child has a gastrostomy tube, maintain skin integrity around the stoma site.

Administer medications as ordered, remaining alert for expected side effects.

Prepare the child for diagnostic tests.

Provide postoperative care for the child undergoing surgery.

Family Education

Instruct parents how to feed and position the infant, and provide comfort and emotional support.

Partner with parents, and encourage them to hold and cuddle the infant during all feedings.

Show parents how to keep the upper body elevated, and discourage use of infant seats.

Caution the family that the enlarged nipple now has the capacity to deliver too much formula too fast for the infant and may produce a choking hazard.

Providing the infant with a pacifier helps to meet nonnutritive sucking needs.

Teach parents how to suction the nose and mouth if vomiting occurs.

Teach administration and side effects of any medications.

Abdominal Wall Defects

The two most common congenital defects of the anterior abdominal wall are gastroschisis and omphalocele.

Omphalocele is a congenital malformation in which intra-abdominal contents herniate through the umbilical cord. An omphalocele results when the intestines fail to return to the abdomen when the abdominal wall begins to close by the tenth week of gestation. The size of the sac varies depending on the extent of the protrusion. Large defects may contain intestines, stomach, liver, and the spleen (Zimmerman, 2007). Omphalocele occurs at the base of the umbilical cord. The abdominal contents are covered with peritoneum and amniotic membrane (Doughty, 2004). Rupture of the sac results in evisceration of the abdominal contents. Thirty percent of infants with omphalocele will have an associated chromosomal anomaly, and 30% to 50% will have congenital heart defects (Lund, Bauer, & Berrios, 2007).

Gastroschisis is a congenital defect of the ventral abdominal wall, characterized by herniation of abdominal viscera outside the abdominal cavity through a defect in the abdominal wall to the side (most often to the right) of the umbilicus. The most common abdominal organs involved are the small intestine and ascending colon. Unlike the omphalocele, no membrane covers the organs. Approximately 10% to 20% of infants with gastroschisis have an associated anomaly, most often intestinal atresias. Anomalies outside of the gastrointestinal tract are uncommon in infants with gastroschisis (Lund et al., 2007).

Elevated maternal serum alpha-fetoprotein (MSAFP) levels are seen in both gastroschisis and omphalocele. Routine prenatal determination of MSAFP and ultrasonography lead to early diagnosis and coordination of the team of specialists needed to manage these congenital anomalies, including neonatologists and pediatric surgeons (Zimmerman, 2007).

The immediate action upon birth is to protect the sac (in omphalocele) or exposed abdominal contents (in gastroschisis) from injury by placing the infant feet first into a bowel bag that extends to the nipple line and is secured with ties. The bowel bag decreases heat loss and allows for visualization of the defect. The child with gastroschisis should first have the exposed abdominal contents covered with moist sterile gauze.

Temperature regulation is needed for the newborn due to heat loss through exposed viscera. Fluids are required to replace those lost through viscera. Blood cultures are performed before administering antibiotics. An orogastric or nasogastric tube may be inserted to prevent distention. A thorough examination is performed to rule out cardiac and other abnormalities.

Surgical repair of omphalocele and gastroschisis may occur in one or two stages depending on the severity of the defect. For small defects, one surgery may be all that is needed to repair the defect. For larger defects, the first stage of repair may involve nonoperative placement of the abdominal contents or sac into a silastic silo. Once the abdominal cavity can accommodate the intestinal contents, the child will have surgery to close the abdominal wall (Lund, et al., 2007; Zimmerman, 2007).

Preoperative nursing care centers on frequent vital signs, protecting the sac or protruding organs, preventing hypothermia, preventing and identifying infection, and maintaining fluid and electrolyte balance with intravenous fluids. Postoperative care includes measures to control pain, prevent infection, maintain fluid and electrolyte balance, and ensure adequate nutritional intake. Attainment of bowel motility and function varies and is often delayed for weeks after surgery; parenteral nutrition for the infant is used during this period (Lund et al., 2007). Support of the family before and after surgery is essential and includes explanations about the infant's condition and treatment plan, emotional support, and an opportunity for expression of feelings.

Intussusception

Intussusception occurs when one portion of the intestine prolapses and then invaginates or telescopes into another; the most common site of intussusception is the ileocecal valve. The etiology of intussusception is multifactorial; while the exact cause is unknown, intussusception is frequently preceded by a viral infection of the gastrointestinal tract (Hackman, Newman, & Ford, 2005).

Telescoping of the intestine obstructs the passage of stool. The walls of the intestine rub together, causing inflammation, edema, and decreased blood flow. This can lead to necrosis and loss of a significant portion of the intestine if not treated promptly (Fagerman & Farber, 2007).

Onset of symptoms is usually abrupt; a previously healthy infant or child suddenly experiences acute abdominal pain with vomiting and passage of brown stool; the infant may experience periods of comfort between acute episodes of pain. As the condition worsens, painful episodes increase; stools become red and resemble currant jelly because of the mixture of blood and mucus (Fagerman & Farber, 2007). A palpable mass may be present in the upper right quadrant or mid-upper abdomen; rectal bleeding may also occur (Klein, Kapoor, & Shugerman, 2004).

A nasogastric tube is placed for decompression. Diagnosis is made on the basis of the history and confirmed by radiographs and ultrasound of the abdomen. A contrast enema using barium or air can be both diagnostic and therapeutic. In 70% to 90% of cases the hydrostatic pressure from the contrast moves the bowel back into place (Fagerman & Farber, 2007). Surgery to reduce the invaginated bowel is necessary in those not corrected with this procedure.

Preoperative nursing assessment includes vital signs, monitoring for abdominal distention, and auscultating for bowel sounds every 4 hours; monitor intravenous intake, urine output, and measure any vomitus; assess for number and characteristics of stools. Monitor fluid and electrolyte status; maintain patent nasogastric tube; prepare the child and family for diagnostic and surgical procedures.

Postoperative care focuses on monitoring for early signs of infection, managing the child's pain, and maintaining nasogastric tube patency; feeding protocols usually include clear liquid feeding or breastfeeding after normal bowel function returns. Feedings are then advanced to half-strength milk and other foods as the infant or child tolerates them.

Volvulus

During the seventh to twelfth week of gestation the small intestine undergoes rapid growth. In normal development, the intestine rotates counterclockwise as it settles into its permanent position inside the abdominal cavity. If the bowel does not rotate normally during this process, the child is at risk for **volvulus**, a twisting of the intestine (Doughty, 2004). Volvulus disrupts blood flow in the intestines and can lead to necrosis of the bowel, short bowel syndrome, and death. Volvulus is considered a surgical emergency (Aiken & Oldham, 2005). Early diagnosis and treatment is necessary to preserve the bowel and to save the child's life.

Symptoms of volvulus in the infant include bilious vomiting, firm abdomen with distention, irritability secondary to pain, and passage of bloody stools. Confirmation of malrotation of the intestine through upper GI series or contrast studies supports a diagnosis of volvulus. Emergency exploratory surgery to untwist the bowel is essential (Diana-Zerpa & Shapiro-Stolar, 2007). If a portion of the bowel is necrotic, that portion of the bowel is removed. An ostomy may need to be created, depending on the amount of bowel removed (Aiken & Oldham, 2005). The child is at risk for developing short bowel syndrome if a significant amount of bowel is removed.

The infant or child who presents to the emergency room with bilious vomiting and a firm and distended abdomen should be assessed quickly to determine the cause of the symptoms. Once volvulus has been diagnosed, nursing management focuses on keeping the child NPO, administering intravenous fluids, assessing vital signs, and reporting symptoms of a worsening condition. The child who has had surgery to correct uncomplicated volvulus will need care similar to that described for the child with intussusception. If the child had necrotic bowel removed, he or she may have an ostomy for a period of time.

Hirschsprung Disease

Hirschsprung disease, also known as *congenital aganglionic megacolon*, is a congenital anomaly in which inadequate motility causes mechanical obstruction of the intestine.

It is now known that the RET protooncogene is a major gene for the disease. The absence of autonomic parasympathetic ganglion cells in the colon prevents peristalsis at that portion of the intestine, resulting in the accumulation of intestinal contents and abdominal distention; in most cases, the area lacking ganglion cells is limited to the rectosigmoid region of the colon (Kessman, 2006).

In newborns, symptoms include failure to pass meconium in the first 48 hours after birth, abdominal distention, and bilious vomiting (Klar, 2007). If Hirschsprung disease is not treated, the condition can lead to fever, bloody diarrhea (frequent, watery stools), abdominal distention, and enterocolitis (inflammation of the intestines) (Biggs & Dery, 2006).

The older infant or child may have a history of failure to gain weight, malnutrition, chronic progressive constipation (difficult and infrequent defecation with passage of hard, dry stool), and recurrent fecal impaction (Kessman, 2006).

The child may have a history of passage of pencil-thin stools (Biggs & Dery, 2006).

Diagnosis is made on the basis of the history, bowel patterns, anorectal manometry, radiographic contrast studies, and rectal biopsy for presence or absence of ganglion cells.

Anorectal manometry demonstrates absence of relaxation of the internal sphincter, an expected response to rectal distension. Normally, distension of the rectum produces relaxation of the internal sphincter. Abdominal radiograph and contrast studies reveal a distended small bowel and proximal colon with an empty rectum. Rectal biopsy has proven to be the most reliable test for confirmation of the diagnosis; the absence of ganglionic cells and the presence of hypertrophic nerve trunks confirms the diagnosis (Kessman, 2006).

Treatment in infancy involves surgical removal of the aganglionic bowel through an endorectal pull-through procedure. In mild cases in otherwise healthy infants, the affected portion of the bowel can be removed in the newborn period. In severe cases or in ill infants, a temporary colostomy is created. Timing of closure of the colostomy and reanastomosis varies among surgeons, with the procedure generally being performed sometime between 2 and 6 months of age (Black, 2005; Kessman, 2006). For children not diagnosed in infancy, treatment should be implemented as soon as possible after diagnosis.

Nursing assessment in the newborn period includes careful observation for the passage of meconium.

When the disease is diagnosed later in infancy or in childhood, obtain a thorough history of weight gain, nutritional intake, and bowel elimination habits; assess the child's growth and developmental achievements.

Assess the child for abdominal distention, severe constipation alternating with diarrhea (frequent, watery stools), and vomiting; note the appearance of the stool.

Teach parents the need for chronic care over time; regular bowel movements are important to promote adequate elimination and prevent obstruction.

Teach parents how to prevent skin breakdown in the rectal area by changing diapers frequently, cleansing the area carefully, and applying protective ointment at each diaper change.

If surgical correction is necessary, nursing care includes monitoring for infection, managing pain, maintaining hydration, measuring abdominal circumference to detect any distention, and providing support to the child and family.

Parents require instruction in ostomy care in those cases when the child has a colostomy.

Anorectal Malformations

The term *imperforate anus* (absence of the anal opening) is frequently used to refer to anorectal malformations and is classified according to the specific defect. Males with imperforate anus frequently have a rectourethral fistula and females generally have a rectovestibular fistula (Levitt & Peña, 2005). See Table 20–1 for the most recent classification of anorectal malformations. Additional minor defects that may occur include anal stenosis (narrowing of the anus) and imperforate anal membrane (skin covering the anal opening).

Perineal inspection at birth reveals the absent anal opening. Failure to pass meconium within the first 24 hours of birth may be indicative of imperforate anus. Stool in the urine usually indicates the presence of a fistula between the colon and urinary tract. Cloacal malformations in females, in which the urinary tract, vagina, and rectum drain through a common channel, may occur (Levitt & Peña, 2005). Ultrasound and lower gastrointestinal radiographic studies are used to confirm the diagnosis and demonstrate the extent of the anomaly; anorectal manometry may be performed.

Anal stenosis may be treated with dilation alone; an imperforate anal membrane is excised surgically, followed by daily manual dilations. A single operation anoplasty may be used to repair rectoperineal defects; higher defects require a three-stage procedure. A temporary colostomy in the newborn period provides for bowel decompression and for protection of the surgical site when the anomaly is repaired. Reconstructive surgery is generally performed via posterior sagittal anorectoplasty (PSARP).

Table 20–1   Classification of Anorectal Malformations

Male	Female
Cutaneous (perineal fistula)	Cutaneous (perineal fistula)
Rectourethral fistula (bulbar or prostatic)	Vestibular fistula
Rector-bladderneck fistula	Imperforate anus without fistula
Imperforate anus without fistula	Rectal atresia
Rectal atresia	Cloaca
	Complex malformation

Source: From "Outcomes from the Correction of Anorectal Malformations," by M. A. Levitt & A. Peña, 2005, *Current Opinion in Pediatrics, 17*, 394–401.

Nursing care focuses on newborn assessment of anal patency, preoperative and postoperative care, and supporting the family. During the initial newborn assessment, the perineal area is inspected for a poorly developed anal dimple or sacral anomalies; observe and record passage of meconium.

Once the diagnosis is made, monitor the child's intake, output, and cardiorespiratory functioning.

Postoperatively, observe the operative area for signs of infection. Avoid taking rectal temperatures in children who have had anorectal surgery. The child should have a sign posted on the bed that reads "Nothing per rectum." Accurate intake and output is essential. Assess vital signs at least every 4 hours. Assess the child for evidence of pain.

If a temporary colostomy is performed, teach parents how to care for the ostomy site.

HERNIAS

Congenital Diaphragmatic Hernia

In a *diaphragmatic hernia*, abdominal contents protrude into the thoracic cavity through an opening in the diaphragm; sites of herniation include the substernal space, posterolateral region, and the esophageal hiatus.

A diaphragmatic hernia is a life-threatening condition. Severe respiratory distress occurs shortly after birth; as the infant cries, abdominal organs extend into the thorax, decreasing the size of the thoracic cavity; the infant becomes dyspneic and cyanotic.

Characteristic findings include a barrel-shaped chest, sunken abdomen, and diminished or absent breath sounds on affected side; bowel sounds may be auscultated over the chest; heart tones may be auscultated on the right side of the chest; pneumothorax may occur.

Congenital diaphragmatic hernia may be diagnosed in utero by ultrasound; if not identified prenatally, the condition is first identified postnatally by physical signs and symptoms; confirmation is made by chest radiologic examination; magnetic resonance imaging is helpful in confirming the diagnosis and in determining the position of organs in the chest and abdomen (Hedrick, Crombleholme, Flake, et al., 2004).

Immediate respiratory support is essential in an NICU. Extracorporeal membrane oxygenation (ECMO) may be used to provide cardiopulmonary bypass to rest the lungs. Alternatively, inhaled nitric oxide (iNO) and high-frequency oxygen ventilation (HFVO) preoperatively may improve survival outcomes and decrease morbidity associated with congenital diaphragmatic hernia (Bagolan et al., 2004).

The infant is positioned with the head and thorax higher than the abdomen to facilitate downward movement of abdominal organs; a nasogastric tube is inserted to decompress the stomach; ventilator support is necessary to manage respiratory compromise; intravenous fluids are administered through an umbilical artery catheter.

Once the infant's condition is stabilized, the defect is corrected surgically.

Nursing care centers on maintaining ventilatory support of the infant, preoperative preparation, postoperative care, and supporting the family during this life-threatening event.

Place the child on a cardiorespiratory monitor and note the infant's vital signs every 30 minutes.

Observe for worsening of respiratory compromise.

Maintain intravenous fluid administration.

Promote decreased stimulation to keep the infant calm and thus maintain low abdominal pressure.

Keep parents informed about the infant's condition, and provide emotional support before and after surgery.

Postoperative care includes positioning the infant on the affected side to facilitate expansion of the lung on the unaffected side, observing closely for signs of infection, maintaining respiratory support, and carefully monitoring fluid and electrolyte balance.

Partner with parents to encourage their participation in the infant's care to promote parent–infant attachment.

Before discharge, instruct parents in care of incision, prevention of infection, and feeding techniques.

Umbilical Hernia

An umbilical hernia results from imperfect closure or weakness of the umbilical muscle ring; the hernia appears as a soft swelling covered by skin.

Omentum and small intestine herniates or protrudes through the opening with coughing, crying, or straining during a bowel movement. It is easily reduced by pushing the bowel back through the fibrous ring. The size of the defect is determined by measuring the diameter of the muscular ring (Stoll, 2007b).

Most defects that appear prior to 6 months of age will resolve spontaneously by age 1.

Surgery is indicated in cases of strangulation (closure of the umbilical ring around a portion of the bowel, preventing it from moving back into the abdomen) and if the defect does not resolve 3 to 4 years of age or if the defect becomes larger after 1 to 2 years of age (Stoll, 2007b).

Nursing management is generally supportive.

Instruct parents not to apply tape, straps, or coins to reduce the hernia, as these methods have not proven to be effective.

If surgery is required, it is usually performed in an outpatient surgery unit.

Postoperatively, teach parents how to care for the surgical site, to monitor for bleeding, and to recognize signs of infection; reinforce the importance of returning for follow-up evaluation.

Ostomies

An *intestinal ostomy* is an opening, or stoma, into the small or large intestine that diverts fecal matter to provide an outlet when a distal surgical anastomosis, obstruction, or nonfunctioning structure prevents normal elimination.

Depending on the integrity and function of anatomic structures, the ostomy may be temporary or permanent.

Infants and small children with imperforate anus, necrotizing enterocolitis, Hirschsprung disease, volvulus, or intussusception may require a temporary or permanent colostomy or ileostomy; ostomies may also be indicated for children with inflammatory bowel disease, intestinal tumors, or abdominal trauma.

When assessing the family and child approaching ostomy surgery, it is important for the nurse to determine their ability to understand and accept the physical changes that occur. Preoperative education focuses on educating the child and family and preparing them for postoperative management.

Discuss how the ostomy pouch will look and explain the purpose of the appliance in developmentally appropriate terms.

Encourage the parents and child to touch and manipulate all equipment; a younger child can be shown how to place a pouch on a doll; older children can practice placing a pouch on their skin.

Postoperative care of a child with an ostomy is similar to that for any child who undergoes abdominal surgery, including pain management, monitoring for signs of infection, skin inspection, and careful assessment of vital signs and respiratory function.

Management of the stoma may be coordinated by an ostomy nurse or nurse case manager.

Once healing has occurred, assess the stoma, quality and amount of fecal matter, skin condition, and adherence of the pouch; evaluate the understanding and ability of the family to care for the ostomy.

INFLAMMATORY DISORDERS

Appendicitis

Description and Etiology

Appendicitis is an inflammation of the vermiform appendix, the small sac near the end of the cecum.

Appendicitis almost always results from an obstruction in the appendiceal lumen, and can be caused by a fecalith (hard fecal mass), parasitic infestations, stenosis, hyperplasia of lymphoid tissue, or a tumor.

Continued secretion of mucus after acute obstruction of the lumen increases pressure, causing ischemia, cellular death, necrosis, and ulceration.

The appendix may perforate or rupture, resulting in fecal and bacterial contamination of the peritoneum. Peritonitis spreads quickly and if untreated can result in small bowel obstruction, electrolyte imbalances, septicemia, hypovolemic shock, and death. Early diagnosis and treatment of appendicitis is essential to minimize complications related to rupture (Kwok et al., 2004).

Clinical Manisfestations

At onset, symptoms include periumbilical cramps, abdominal tenderness, and fever.

As the inflammation progresses, pain in the right lower abdomen becomes constant. Pain is often most intense at McBurney's point, halfway between the anterior superior iliac crest and the umbilicus.

Symptoms progress to include guarding, rigidity, nausea, vomiting, onset of pain before vomiting, anorexia, and rebound tenderness after palpation over the right lower quadrant.

Vomiting, diarrhea, or constipation may be present; as appendicitis progresses, the child remains motionless, usually in a side-lying position with knees flexed.

Sudden relief of abdominal pain usually means that the appendix has ruptured.

Diagnostic Tests

The presence of elevated white blood cell count (above 10,000/mm^3) generally occurs in appendicitis. While an abdominal ultrasound can be helpful in the diagnosis of appendicitis, computed tomography (CT) is preferred and has been found to be most reliable (Jaffe & Berger, 2005; Tamburrini et al., 2007).

Clinical Therapy

Treatment of acute appendicitis involves immediate surgical removal (appendectomy), either through laparoscopic or open method (Vegunta, Ali, Wallace, et al., 2004).

Preoperatively, the child is kept NPO. Intravenous fluids, electrolytes, and antibiotics are administered. Postoperatively, the child with uncomplicated appendicitis has an abdominal incision; intravenous antibiotics may be administered to prevent infection. The child with uncomplicated appendicitis will generally be discharged the next day.

Postoperatively, the child with ruptured appendix will receive intravenous fluids and antibiotics for several days. A drain may be placed; the wound is closed or left open and packed with saline-soaked gauze.

Nursing Management

Assessment

Preoperatively, the nurse performs a detailed assessment of the child's pain to differentiate appendicitis from other illnesses. Note onset, location, and intensity of pain, precipitating factors, and relief measures tried. During abdominal assessment, auscultate for bowel sounds. Perform palpation last to avoid causing additional pain. Deep palpation of the left side of the abdomen followed by removing the hand quickly can lead to pain in the area of the appendix (rebound tenderness).

Assess vital signs to determine baseline values and monitor at least every 4 hours thereafter. Ask about the last food and fluid intake and any vomiting that has occurred. Assess history of previous surgeries or abdominal conditions.

Postoperatively, assess fluid-volume status every 2 hours; assess skin turgor, eyes, and mucous membranes for signs of dehydration; monitor intake and output; and assess vital signs at least every 4 hours. Assess for signs of return of bowel function. Assess for pain using the appropriate scale. Careful attention should also be paid to the wound site for signs of infection such as increased redness or drainage.

Implementation

Preoperatively, allow the child to assume any position that promotes comfort; administer analgesics routinely as ordered, and note results of medications; ask the family what might be comforting for the child, such as music, gently stroking the back, or having family present.

For many children, appendicitis may be the reason for their first hospitalization and only experience with healthcare personnel beyond their usual provider; the nurse must elicit a history, perform a physical examination, coordinate diagnostic tests, and prepare the child for surgery in a short period of time; emotional support is essential for the child and parents. Good preoperative education can reduce anxiety. Answer any questions the child or parents may have.

Postoperatively, the child should be placed in a semi-Fowler's or side-lying position on the right side. If the appendix has ruptured, lying on the right side facilitates drainage from the peritoneal cavity and facilitates comfort. The child with a ruptured appendix will require intravenous pain medication frequently and prior to scheduled dressing changes if the wound was left open. The child who has an appendectomy for uncomplicated appendicitis will need oral or intravenous pain management for postoperative pain control.

If a nasogastric tube is in place, measure the amount of output from the tube so that adequate fluid replacement can be given. Once bowel function returns and after the nasogastric tube has been removed, offer water in small amounts followed by other clear fluids and advancing to a regular diet as tolerated.

Encourage the child to deep breathe postoperatively by blowing bubbles or use of incentive spirometry.

If the wound was left open, wet-to-dry dressing changes are needed two to three times a day, depending on physician orders.

Administer antibiotics as prescribed.

Necrotizing Enterocolitis
Description and Etiology

Necrotizing enterocolitis (NEC) is a potentially life-threatening inflammatory disease of the intestinal tract that occurs primarily in premature infants. The etiology is multifactorial; causes include intestinal ischemia, bacterial or viral infection (a result of the premature infant's decreased immune response and greater risk for infection), and immaturity of the gastrointestinal mucosa (a result of the premature infant's decreased amount of gastric acid and proteolytic enzymes and underdeveloped protective intestinal mucin layer) (Kliegman & Willoughby, 2005).

Vascular compromise, leading to hypoxia and ischemia, causes a reduced blood flow to the bowel, leading to necrosis of the bowel mucosa; the damaged bowel stops secreting protective enzymes, allowing gas-forming bacteria to invade the necrotic tissue; this bacterial invasion further damages the intestinal mucosa by releasing bacterial toxins and gas, causing abdominal distention.

Necrosis of the bowel can lead to intestinal perforation and sepsis. NEC carries high mortality rates.

Clinical Manifestations

Manifestations generally occur between 3 and 14 days of life but can occur as early as the first day of life and as late as 3 months of age.

Symptoms may include poor feeding, increased gastric residuals prior to feeding, bilious emesis, abdominal distention, temperature instability, lethargy, and irritability; infant may also have bloody stools (Kasson, 2007).

Long-term complications of necrotizing enterocolitis may include short bowel syndrome, strictures, cholestasis, impaired nutrition and growth, and delayed developmental performance.

Diagnostic Tests

Diagnosis is made on the basis of characteristic clinical findings and the presence of free peritoneal gas, dilated bowel loops, bowel distention, and bowel-wall thickening on abdominal radiographs.

Stools and emesis are monitored for occult blood.

Laboratory data reveal anemia, leukopenia, leukocytosis, thrombocytopenia, electrolyte imbalance, and metabolic or respiratory acidosis.

Blood cultures are positive for organism present.

Clinical Therapy

Requires prompt intervention.

Therapy begins with discontinuation of all enteral feedings.

A nasogastric or orogastric tube is inserted and maintained on low suction to prevent gastric distention, and intravenous fluids are started.

TPN may be initiated through a central line.

Antibiotics are administered prophylactically or to treat sepsis.

Perforation or necrosis of the bowel necessitates surgical resection of the bowel; an ileostomy or colostomy may be performed in some cases.

All cases of necrotizing enterocolitis are treated with strict enteric precautions to prevent the spread of infection to other premature infants on the unit.

Early aggressive enteral formula feedings of premature infants are avoided because of the increased incidence of the disease in these cases; human milk has been shown to be protective against the disease, so breastfeeding or feeding the mother's expressed milk is the feeding method of choice for all premature infants.

New treatments are being attempted with probiotics—live and beneficial microorganisms that promote normal gut flora; *Lactobacillus acidophilus* and *Bifidobacterium infantis* are examples of organisms that can be administered by special formula (Kliegman & Willoughby, 2005).

Nursing Management
Assessment
Observe for feeding intolerance by aspirating gastric residual (if the infant is receiving enteral feedings).

Measure abdominal circumference, and assess bowel sounds in the premature or high-risk infant every 4 to 8 hours; even minimal changes in circumference can indicate necrotizing enterocolitis and should be reported to the primary care provider.

Careful monitoring of vital signs, intake, and output is essential to detect any complications.

Careful assessment for infection and maintenance of skin integrity is essential.

Implementation
Maintaining fluid and electrolyte balance is essential; provide intravenous fluids, probiotics, or feedings as ordered.

Provide comfort by holding and cuddling an infant who is NPO, and offer a pacifier to meet nonnutritive sucking needs.

Because the symptoms of necrotizing enterocolitis do not appear until approximately 5 to 7 days after feedings begin, parents may not be prepared for the infant's decline. Recovery is slow and can be complicated.

Give clear explanations and encourage parents to ask questions and express their fears and concerns.

Once the infant is discharged, frequent follow-up care is needed; regular and thorough physical assessments are needed to check weight gain, assess development, and identify signs of complications.

Educate parents regarding feedings, medications, and any other treatments prescribed.

If the infant required an ostomy, teach parents proper care of the stoma.

Meckel's Diverticulum

Meckel's diverticulum results when the omphalomesenteric duct, which connects the midgut to the yolk sac during embryonic development, fails to atrophy; instead, an outpouching of the ileum remains, usually located near the ileocecal valve; the pouch contains gastric or pancreatic tissue, which secretes acid, causing irritation and ulceration. Meckel's diverticulum is one of the most common GI malformations and occurs in 2% of the population. Many people are asymptomatic and do not know they have the disorder (Otten & Stoops, 2007).

The most common sign is painless dark or bright red rectal bleeding, which results from the obstruction or ulceration; often blood is passed without stool; child may have symptoms of intussusception, incarcerated hernia, volvulus, or intestinal obstruction. If untreated, diverticulitis may progress to perforation and peritonitis.

Diagnosis of Meckel's diverticulum is based on the history; radionuclide imaging and scanning can usually detect the gastric tissue, confirming the diagnosis.

Treatment is surgical excision of the diverticulum and removal of any involved bowel; prognosis is good following surgical excision.

Preoperatively, the nurse maintains an intravenous infusion to correct fluid and electrolyte imbalances.

Monitor intake and output.

Observe for rectal bleeding, and test stools for occult blood.

Maintain the child on bed rest.

Assess vital signs every 2 hours, and monitor for signs of shock.

Perform postsurgical abdominal care, including pain relief; administration of intravenous solutions; and monitoring of abdominal sounds, respiratory system, and skin.

At discharge, parents need instructions on caring for the surgical site, preventing infection, providing an adequate diet, and administering prescribed medications.

Recurrent Abdominal Pain

Recurrent abdominal pain is a frequent problem among young children and adolescents, particularly girls of school age.

The pain is generally located in the periumbilical area and occurs on a regular basis.

A thorough history and physical examination are necessary to rule out organic causes.

Laboratory studies, such as a complete blood count, may be ordered to rule out other illness; gastrointestinal studies may be performed in an outpatient setting.

When no organic cause can be identified, treatment of recurrent abdominal pain focuses on providing outlets for the release of stress within the family and in other settings in the child's life, enhancing the child's coping methods, and promoting dietary changes that encourage regular bowel movements.

Cognitive behavioral therapies, such as relaxation techniques, have proven effective because they reduce muscle tension and autonomic arousal (Hyman & Danda, 2004).

Inflammatory Bowel Disease

Inflammatory bowel disease encompasses two distinct chronic disorders, Crohn's disease and ulcerative colitis, that have similar symptoms and treatment.

See Table 20–2 for contrasts in manifestation of the two disorders.

Genetic and environmental factors are involved in the development of IBD. Onset of both of these disorders is most common in adolescence and young adulthood, but either disease can begin in early childhood (Hyams, 2007).

Diagnosis centers on evaluating the cause and identifying the extent of involved bowel and differentiating an infectious process (organisms, e.g., *Shigella* and *Salmonella*) from inflammatory bowel disease.

Table 20–2 Comparison of Ulcerative Colitis and Crohn's Disease

	Ulcerative Colitis	Crohn's Disease
Type of lesions	Continuous, superficial involvement	Segmental, transmural (through the wall) involvement
Clinical manifestations		
Anal or perianal lesions	Rare	Common
Anorexia	Mild to moderate	Can be severe
Diarrhea	Often severe	Moderate
Growth retardation	Mild	Significant
Pain	Present	Common
Rectal bleeding	Present	Absent
Weight loss	Moderate	Severe
Risk of cancer	Slightly increased	Greatly increased

Laboratory and bone age studies help to identify related nutritional, electrolyte, and blood abnormalities.

Anemia is common; an elevated erythrocyte sedimentation rate, elevated C-reactive protein, hypoalbuminemia, and thrombocytosis are other possible findings. Stools are positive for occult blood (Hyams, 2005).

Antineutrophil cytoplasmic antibodies may be detected in serum studies.

Perinuclear highlighting of those autoantibodies (perinuclear antineutrophil cytoplasmic antibodies) is associated with ulcerative colitis and Crohn's disease.

An upper GI series with small bowel follow-through is essential in the diagnosis of Crohn's disease; endoscopy and colonoscopy with biopsy are essential in determining the extent of disease (Hyams, 2005; Silbermintz & Markowitz, 2006).

Treatment for both diseases includes pharmacologic interventions, nutrition therapy, and, in severe cases, surgery.

Nursing management occurs mainly in the community and home and focuses on helping the child and family adjust to the emotional impact of a chronic disease, administering medications and diet therapy, monitoring nutritional status, monitoring growth status, and providing appropriate referrals.

Assess for abdominal distention, tenderness, and pain; monitor bowel sounds and stool pattern; measure abdominal girth.

Body image is a major concern for children and adolescents with inflammatory bowel disease because of disease effects and medication side effects; offer referrals for counseling, and help the child identify his or her own strengths.

Providing adequate stress reduction may be helpful in control of inflammatory bowel disease; collaborate with the parents to teach young children relaxation techniques, such as deep breathing, progressive tensing and relaxing of muscles, and visualization of favorite places; encourage busy school-age children and teens to have quiet and restful times each day, in addition to physical activity periods.

Peptic Ulcer

A *peptic ulcer* is an erosion of the mucosal tissue in the lower end of the esophagus, in the stomach (usually along the lesser curvature), or in the duodenum.

Many cases of ulcer, in both adults and children, are caused by *Helicobacter pylori*, a gram-negative rod that is transmitted by the fecal–oral or oral–oral route (Vaira et al., 2005).

Primary ulcers occur in previously healthy children, whereas secondary ulcers occur in those with a preexisting illness or injury such as a burn and in children receiving medications, such as salicylates, corticosteroids, and nonsteroidal anti-inflammatory drugs.

The most common symptom is abdominal pain (burning) associated with an empty stomach, which may awaken the child at night; vomiting and pain after meals, anemia, occult blood in stools, and abdominal distention may also be present.

Diagnosis is based on the history and radiologic studies. *H. pylori* can be diagnosed by culture of the organism taken via gastroscopy and by measuring urea in the urine and on the breath, since the organism hydrolyzes urea.

When *H. pylori* is the causative agent, antimicrobial agents, such as bismuth salts, tetracycline, and metronidazole combination, are given.

Other drug combinations, such as antacids in liquid form (Maalox, Mylanta) and histamine antagonists (ranitidine, cimetidine, and famotidine), are also used.

The nurse assesses the child for abdominal pain, vomiting, and abdominal distention.

Partner with the family and explain that antibiotics must be administered as scheduled.

Caution parents to avoid aspirin products, which irritate the gastric mucosa; if an antipyretic or pain medication is needed, acetaminophen is administered.

Because psychological stress can contribute to peptic ulcer disease, parents and child should be assisted to identify sources of stress in the child's life.

Assess coping mechanisms and provide referral for psychological counseling, if appropriate.

Teach relaxation techniques, and recommend community classes on yoga or other stress reduction.

DISORDERS OF MOTILITY

Gastroenteritis

Gastroenteritis (acute diarrhea) is an inflammation of the stomach and intestines that may be accompanied by vomiting and diarrhea.

Viral and bacterial infections are the most common cause of gastroenteritis.

Dehydration is the most common serious outcome of gastroenteritis in children; see chapter 14 for a thorough discussion of dehydration treatment and nursing care.

Constipation

Constipation is characterized by a decrease in the frequency of stool passage; the formation of hard, dry stools; or the oozing of liquid stool past a collection of hard, dry stool and no evidence of structural, endocrine, or metabolic disease.

Constipation may be caused by an underlying disease, diet, or psychological factor. Constipation may result from defects in filling, or more commonly emptying, of the rectum. Pathologic causes of defective filling include ineffective colonic propulsive activity, caused by hypothyroidism or use of medication, and obstruction; other causes include a structural anomaly (stricture or stenosis) or an aganglionic segment (Hirschsprung disease).

If the rectum fails to fill, stasis leads to excessive drying of the stools; emptying of the rectum depends on the defecation reflex; lesions of the spinal cord, weakness of the abdominal muscles, local lesions blocking sphincter relaxation, and a desire to avoid painful stools all may impede attempts to defecate.

Constipation in the newborn can indicate an obstructed large bowel, such as with Hirschsprung disease or anorectal anomaly with anal stenosis (Biggs & Dery, 2006). Constipation during infancy is commonly seen as a result of mismanagement of diet; however, the disorder is generally easily managed with dietary changes.

Dietary management is the treatment of choice for constipation that has no underlying pathologic cause.

Constipation in young infants can usually be corrected by increasing the amount of fluids or adding 2 oz of pear or apple juice to daily intake; increasing physical activity and fluid intake may be effective for some children.

Removing constipating foods (bananas, rice, and cheese) from the child's diet often decreases the constipation; increasing the child's intake of high-fiber foods (whole-grain breads, raw fruits, and raw vegetables) and fluids also promotes bowel elimination. In older infants, increasing the intake of fluids, cereals, fruits, and vegetables in the diet should correct the problem.

A single glycerin suppository or enema may be required to remove hard stool.

The nurse assesses the child's diet history; obtain a description of bowel patterns and habits from parents.

Palpate the abdomen, and assess the child's abdomen for firmness or tenderness and the presence of palpable mass (retained stool); auscultate for bowel sounds.

If a digital rectal examination is performed, assess for presence of stool in rectum; assess for hemorrhoids, anal fissures, or other abnormalities of the abdomen or perineum.

Partner with the family and teach parents dietary measures to promote regularity of bowel movements; children can be given a high-fiber diet that includes fruits and vegetables and adequate fluids.

INTESTINAL PARASITIC DISORDERS

Intestinal parasitic disorders occur most frequently in tropic regions; outbreaks take place in areas where water is not treated, food is incorrectly prepared, or people live in crowded conditions with poor sanitation.

In the United States, outbreaks of diseases caused by protozoa or helminths (worms) are increasing.

Young children, especially those in child care, are most at risk of infection; they often lack good hygiene practices and are more likely to put objects and their hands into their mouths.

The most common intestinal parasitic disorders are summarized in Table 20–3 and common medication treatments are outlined in Table 20–4.

DISORDERS OF MALABSORPTION

Celiac Disease

Description and Etiology

Celiac disease, or gluten-sensitive enteropathy, is a chronic malabsorption syndrome; a genetic factor is believed to play a role in etiology (Nehring, 2004).

Celiac disease is an immunologic disorder (Zelnik, Pacht, Obeid, et al., 2004) characterized by intolerance for gluten, a protein found in wheat, barley, rye, and oats.

Inability to digest glutenin and gliadin (protein fractions) results in the accumulation of the amino acid glutamine, which is toxic to mucosal cells in the intestine; damage to the villi ultimately impairs the absorptive process in the small intestine.

Clinical Manifestations

In the early stages, celiac disease affects fat absorption, resulting in excretion of large quantities of fat in the stools (steatorrhea); stools are greasy, foul smelling, frothy, and excessive.

As changes in the villi continue, the absorption of protein, carbohydrates, calcium, iron, folate, and vitamins A, D, E, K, and B_{12} become impaired.

The classic features of celiac disease in infancy include chronic diarrhea, growth impairment, and abdominal distention. The child also demonstrates poor appetite, lack of energy, and muscle wasting with hypotonia (Gelfond & Fasano, 2006). Atypical features are present in children diagnosed with delayed-onset celiac disease around 5 to 7 years of age; symptoms include nausea, vomiting, recurrent abdominal pain, and bloating; the child may also demonstrate delayed growth, iron deficiency, defects in tooth enamel, and abnormal liver function tests (Gelfond & Fasano, 2006).

Table 20–3 Clinical Manifestations of Common Intestinal Parasitic Disorders

Parasitic Infection	Transmission, Life Cycle, Pathogenesis	Clinical Manifestations	Clinical Therapy	Comments
Giardiasis Organism: protozoan *Giardia lamblia*	Transmission is through person-to-person contact, unfiltered water, improperly prepared infected food, and contact with animals. Cysts are ingested and passed into the duodenum and proximal jejunum, where they begin actively feeding. They are excreted in the stool.	May be asymptomatic *Infants*: diarrhea, vomiting, anorexia, failure to thrive *Older children*: abdominal cramps; intermittent loose, foul-smelling, watery, pale, and greasy stools.	Available medications include furazolidone and quinacrine. Furazolidone has fewer side effects than quinacrine but is more expensive. Metronidazole is also effective but is not licensed in the United States for treatment of giardiasis.	Most common intestinal parasitic organism in the United States. Infection may resolve spontaneously in 4–6 weeks without treatment. Parents or caregivers should wear gloves when handling diapers or stool of parasite-infected infant or child.

Alterations in Gastrointestinal Function **385**

Table 20–3 Clinical Manifestations of Common Intestinal Parasitic Disorders (Continued)

Parasitic Infection	Transmission, Life Cycle, Pathogenesis	Clinical Manifestations	Clinical Therapy	Comments
Enterobiasis (pinworm) Organism: nematode *Enterobius vermicularis* Pinworm	Transmission is from discharged eggs inhaled or carried from hand to mouth. Eggs hatch in the upper intestine and mature in 15–28 days. Larvae then migrate to the cecum. After mating, the female migrates out of the anus and lays up to 17,000 eggs. Movement of worms causes intense itching. Scratching deposits eggs on the hands and under the nails.	Intense perianal itching, irritability, restlessness, and short attention span; in females, can migrate to the vagina and urethra to cause infection. Itching intensifies at night when the female comes to the anal opening to lay eggs.	Available medications include mebendazole, pyrantel pamoate, and piperazine citrate. The child and all household members should be treated at the same time. Treatment may be repeated in 2–3 weeks.	Most common helminthic infection in the United States. Transmission is increased in crowded conditions such as housing developments, schools, and childcare centers.

Ascariasis (type of roundworm)

Organism: nematode
Ascaris lumbricoides

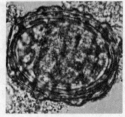

Roundworm (ascariasis)

Transmission is from discharged eggs carried from hand to mouth. Adult lays eggs in small intestine. Eggs are excreted in stool, where they incubate for 2–3 weeks. Swallowed eggs hatch in the small intestine. Larvae may penetrate intestinal villi, entering the portal vein and liver, then moving to the lung. Larvae that ascend to upper respiratory tract are swallowed and proceed to the small intestine, where they repeat the cycle.

Mild infection may be asymptomatic. Severe infection may result in intestinal obstruction, peritonitis, obstructive jaundice, and lung involvement.

Available anthelminthic medications include mebendazole, pyrantel pamoate, or piperazine citrate. Stools should be examined 2 weeks after treatment and monthly for 3 months. Family members and contacts of the child should be treated if indicated. If the child has intestinal obstruction, treatment may include administering piperazine through a nasogastric tube and duodenal scion. Obstructing worms sometimes have to be surgically removed.

Most common in warm climates. Primarily affects children 1–4 years of age.

Table 20–3 Clinical Manifestations of Common Intestinal Parasitic Disorders (Continued)

Parasitic Infection	Transmission, Life Cycle, Pathogenesis	Clinical Manifestations	Clinical Therapy	Comments
Hookworm disease Organism: nematode *Necator americanus* Hookworm	Transmission is through direct contact with infected soil containing larvae. Worms live in the small intestine and feed on villi, causing bleeding. Eggs are deposited in the bowel and excreted in feces. Eggs hatch in damp, shaded soil. Larvae attach to and penetrate the skin and then enter the bloodstream, migrating to the lungs. Larvae then migrate to the upper respiratory passages and are swallowed.	In healthy individuals, mild infection seldom causes problems. More severe infection may result in anemia and malnutrition. Presence of larvae on the skin may cause burning and itching, followed by redness and papular eruption.	Available medications include mebendazole and pyrantel pamoate. Stools should be examined 2 weeks after treatment and monthly for 3 months. Family members and contacts of the child should be treated if indicated.	Children should wear shoes when outdoors, although other unprotected areas of the skin may still come in contact with larvae.

Strongyloidiasis (type of roundworm)

Organism: nematode *Strongyloides stercoralis*

Transmission is from the ingestion of discharged larvae in the soil. Life cycle is similar to that of the hookworm, except this roundworm does not attach to the intestinal mucosa, and feeding larvae (rather than eggs) may be deposited in the soil.

Mild infection may be asymptomatic. Severe infection may result in abdominal pain and distention, nausea, vomiting, and diarrhea. Stools may be large and pale, with mucus. Severe infection may lead to a nutritional deficiency.

Available medications include thiabendazole or mebendazole. Treatment may need to be repeated if symptoms recur after treatment. Family members and contacts of the child should be examined and treated if indicated.

Most common in older children and adolescents.

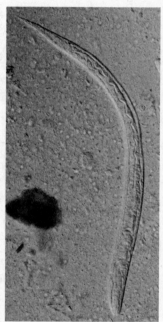

Table 20–3 Clinical Manifestations of Common Intestinal Parasitic Disorders (Continued)

Parasitic Infection	Transmission, Life Cycle, Pathogenesis	Clinical Manifestations	Clinical Therapy	Comments
Visceral larva migrans (toxocariasis) Organism: nematode *Toxocara canis* or *T. cati*, commonly found in dogs and cats 	Transmission through the ingestion of eggs in the soil. Ingested eggs hatch in the intestine. Mobile larvae then migrate to the liver and eventually to all major organs (including the brain). Once migration is complete, they encapsulate in dense fibrous tissue.	Most cases are asymptomatic. Affected children may have a low-grade fever and recurrent upper airway diseases. Severe symptoms include hepatomegaly, pulmonary infiltration, and neurologic disturbances. In all cases there is a hypereosinophilia of the blood.	There is no specific treatment. Corticosteroids have been used in severe cases. Thiabendazole has been recommended, but efficacy is not established (infection usually resolves spontaneously).	Most common in toddlers. Deworm household pets monthly if indicated. Keep children away from areas contaminated with animal droppings.

Source: *Giardia lamblia*, Strongyloidiasis, Hookworm, and Toxocariasis courtesy of the Centers for Disease Control and Prevention, Atlanta, GA. Ascariasis and Enterobiasis from: "Infectious Diseases," by D. L. Murray, 2003, in C. D. Rudolph & A. M. Rudolph (Eds.). *Rudolph's Pediatrics* (21st ed., pp. 1102, 1106). New York: McGraw Hill.

Table 20–4 Medications Used to Treat Intestinal Parasitic Infections

Medication and Indication	Nursing Management

Furazolidone
Used in treatment of:
  Giardiasis
  Enterobacter aerogenes
  Escherichia coli
  Proteus
  Salmonella
  Shigella
  Staphylococcus
  Vibrio cholerae
	Protect medication from heat and light exposure
	Monitor for side effects:
	  Abdominal pain
	  Nausea, vomiting
	  Diarrhea
	  Fever
	  Hypotension
	  Headache
	  Dizziness
	  Hypoglycemia

Mebendazole
Used in treatment of:
  Pinworms
  Roundworm
  Hookworm
  Whipworm
	Tablets may be chewed and swallowed or crushed and mixed with food
	Monitor for side effects:
	  Abdominal pain
	  Diarrhea
	  Fever

Pyrantel pamoate
Used in treatment of:
  Pinworms
  Roundworm
  Hookworm
	Oral suspension should be shaken well before administration
	Administer with milk or fruit juices
	Monitor for side effects:
	  Headache
	  Anorexia
	  Nausea
	  Vomiting
	  Diarrhea

Thiabendazole
Used in treatment of:
  Pinworm
  Roundworm
  Hookworm
	Administer after meals
	Chewable tablets must be chewed thoroughly
	Shake suspension well
	Monitor for side effects:
	  Dizziness
	  Anorexia
	  Nausea
	  Vomiting
	  Diarrhea
	  Pruritis
	  Hematuria
	  Diarrhea

Source: Data from Pediatric Drug Guide by R. M. Bindler & L. B. Howry, 2005, Upper Saddle River, NJ: Prentice Hall Health.

Diagnostic Tests

Diagnosis is confirmed through measurement of fecal fat content, duodenal biopsy, and improvement with removal of gluten products from the diet.

Serum screening tests for IgA antiendomysial antibodies and IgA antitissue transglutaminase antibodies are commonly used in diagnosis (Murdock & Johnston, 2005).

Clinical Therapy

Management of the disease is total exclusion of gluten from the diet for life; barley, wheat, and rye are completely eliminated (Allen, 2004) and symptoms generally improve within a few days to weeks.

The intestinal villi return to normal in approximately 6 months.

Growth should improve steadily, and height and weight should reach normal range within 1 year.

Vitamin supplementation may be needed for a period of time if the child has become malnourished.

Nursing Management

Assessment

Assess the child for vomiting, irritability, anemia, hypotonia, and ulcers of the mouth.

Assess growth pattern and developmental achievements.

Ask the family about the child's bowel elimination patterns.

Observe stools for amount and characteristics.

Implementation

Partner with the parents to establish a nutritional plan for the child.

Offer the parents a thorough explanation of the disease process, and emphasize that celiac disease requires lifelong dietary modifications that must be continued even though the child has improved.

Provide the parents and child with a list of foods that can be consumed, including fruits, meats, rice, and vegetables,

Arrange periodic visits to a dietitian.

Perform regular physical assessments, nutritional monitoring, growth measurement, and developmental screening.

Assist the family to work with the school so that the diet can be successfully integrated into that setting.

Short Bowel Syndrome

Short bowel syndrome is a decreased ability to absorb and digest a regular diet because of a shortened intestine; loss of intestine may result from extensive bowel resection for treatment of necrotizing enterocolitis or from a congenital bowel anomaly (Baron & Blaber, 2005; Jackson & Buchman, 2004).

The extent and location of the involved bowel determine severity of the disorder. Because specific types of absorption occur primarily in certain parts of the bowel, the section lost determines the particular vitamins and other nutrients that are inadequate.

During the first 3 months after bowel resection, watery diarrhea is common; in the transition period, the remaining bowel usually increases its absorptive surface area and partially compensates for the absent intestine.

The infant or young child requires nutritional support initially to provide sufficient nutrients for adequate growth and development, initially receiving TPN only.

Once the bowel begins to recover, in addition to TPN, feedings by mouth or by tube may be started in small amounts. Feedings by this method stimulate the bowel and prevent atrophy of the mucosa (Baron & Blaber, 2005).

Nursing care focuses on meeting the child's nutritional and fluid needs and teaching parents how to care for the child at home during the lengthy recovery period.

HEPATIC DISORDERS

Hyperbilirubinemia of the Newborn
Description and Etiology

The lifespan of the RBC is shorter in newborns than in adults. This increased RBC destruction and the fact that the newborn's liver is immature can lead to physiologic jaundice in the newborn (Cohen, 2006).

Hyperbilirubinemia, an abnormally elevated serum bilirubin level, requires timely assessment and appropriate intervention to prevent central nervous system injury (AAP, 2004).

Physiologic jaundice is described as jaundice in the newborn without any other signs of illness (Cohen, 2006). Jaundice occurs in approximately two out of every three newborns (Maisels, 2005). Jaundice is usually visible 2 to 4 days after birth and lasts until day 6. Peak bilirubin concentration reaches 6–7 mg/dL; however, near-term newborns of 37 weeks' gestation may reach or exceed levels of 13 mg/dL. Preterm infants are more susceptible to the abnormal bilirubin levels of hyperbilirubinemia, with 63% reaching bilirubin levels of 10–19 mg/dL (Shaw, 2003).

Clinical Manifestations

Jaundice in the infant is first evident on the face and then progresses to the trunk and finally to the extremities.

Jaundice may be difficult to see in babies with dark skin color. Symptoms of hyperbilirubinemia include (AAP, 2004b):

- Visible jaundice (yellow/orange hue) head to toe, including the sclera
- Lethargy or irritability
- Poor breastfeeding or bottle-feeding

Diagnostic Tests

A blood test, performed by heel stick or venipuncture, measures total serum bilirubin (TSB) in the newborn. A transcutaneous bilirubin (TcB) measurement device is a noninvasive method for estimating serum bilirubin in infants. This method for measuring bilirubin is generally within 2–3 mg/dL of the total serum bilirubin (TSB) and can be performed instead of the TSB in many cases, especially those infants in which the TSB is less than 15 mg/dL (AAP, 2004b).

Clinical Therapy

Phototherapy most effectively reduces serum bilirubin in newborns with nonhemolytic jaundice.

The point at which phototherapy is implemented depends on whether or not the infant is full or preterm and how many hours old the infant is at the time the bilirubin rises; the goal of phototherapy is to keep the TSB below the exchange transfusion level (AAP, 2004b).

Phototherapy is thought to reduce the amount of indirect, or unconjugated, bilirubin in the baby's bloodstream by promoting excretion via the intestines and kidneys; it exposes the infant's skin to blue light at certain wavelengths, which changes bilirubin into water-soluble forms that can be excreted by the intestines and kidneys, facilitates excretion of unconjugated bilirubin through the liver and speeds passage through the bowel (Shaw, 2003), and causes bleaching of the skin; therefore, visual assessment and transcutaneous assessment of jaundice are not reliable once treatment has been initiated (AAP, 2004b).

Sick term infants and premature, or low-birth-weight, infants should receive phototherapy in an open warmer or incubator to ensure temperature stability (Shaw, 2003); a large term infant can be placed nude in an open bassinet during phototherapy (AAP, 2004b). In most cases, the newborn's diaper can stay in place, which makes it easier to manage increased urine output and loose stools; however, if bilirubin levels are at dangerous levels the diaper should be removed to expose more of the infant's skin surface to the effects of the phototherapy light (AAP, 2004b).

The infant's eyes are covered during phototherapy to prevent retinal damage, but eye protection should be removed during feeding and interaction with parents and caregivers. The infant will need total serum bilirubin levels checked periodically during treatment to evaluate response to treatment and possibly 24 hours after discharge to see if the bilirubin increases after treatment is discontinued (AAP, 2004b).

For term infants who develop uncomplicated hyperbilirubinemia, home phototherapy may be appropriate (AAP, 2004b). Serum bilirubin levels must be monitored regularly at the physician's office, neighborhood laboratory, or by the home healthcare worker.

Many newborns with hyperbilirubinemia are also mildly dehydrated; when breast-fed, supplemental fluid intake in the form of milk-based formula may be used to improve hydration and inhibit the enterohepatic circulation of bilirubin; without evidence of dehydration, intravenous fluid or supplementation with dextrose water is not recommended for term or near-term infants receiving phototherapy (AAP, 2004b).

Nursing Management

The nurse in the newborn nursery and the outpatient setting plays a critical role in identifying the newborn at risk, providing parent education and support, and providing nursing care to the newborn undergoing treatment for hyperbilirubinemia; the nurse coordinates communication among all members of the newborn's care team, including physicians, laboratory personnel, and parents.

Assessment

The newborn should be assessed for jaundice at least every 8 to 12 hours by using digital pressure to blanche the skin. Adequate lighting should be used (Blackwell, 2003).

If the nurse suspects the presence of jaundice, a transcutaneous bilirubin measurement or TSB level is indicated and it is reported to the newborn's primary care provider and documented in the chart (Holcomb, 2005).

Assess feeding ability and state of hydration, including number of wet diapers and stools.

Implementation

For the infant undergoing phototherapy, frequent monitoring is essential to ensure that the infant is receiving the phototherapy properly.

Vital signs should be assessed every 4 to 8 hours, especially the infant's temperature.

An accurate measurement of intake and output is essential to make sure the infant is not dehydrated.

Assist the family in breast- or bottle-feeding as appropriate.

Assess adequacy of breastfeeding prior to hospital discharge.

Coordinate with the newborn's care provider in making appropriate referrals to lactation specialists and support groups in the community when necessary.

Biliary Atresia

Biliary atresia results when the extrahepatic bile ducts fail to develop or are closed (Bezerra, 2005; Flanigan, 2007). The disorder leads to cholestasis, cirrhosis, end-stage liver disease, and death by 2 years of age, if left untreated (Bezerra, 2005; Utterson et al., 2005; Weerasooriya, White, & Shepherd, 2004).

It is the most common cause of pathologic jaundice in infants and is the leading indication for pediatric liver transplantation (Bezerra, 2005; Utterson et al., 2005).

The cause of biliary atresia is unknown.

Absence or blockage of the extrahepatic bile ducts results in blocked bile flow from the liver to the duodenum; this altered bile flow soon causes inflammation and fibrotic changes in the liver.

In addition to blockage, the disease can also be caused by hepatocellular dysfunction.

Lack of bile acids interferes with digestion of fat and absorption of fat-soluble vitamins A, D, E, and K, resulting in steatorrhea and nutritional deficiencies.

Jaundice may not be detected until 2 or 3 weeks after birth; bilirubin levels increase, accompanied by abdominal distention and hepatomegaly.

As the disease progresses, splenomegaly occurs.

The infant experiences easy bruising, prolonged bleeding time, and intense itching.

Stools are puttylike in consistency and white or clay colored because of the absence of bile pigments.

Excretion of bilirubin and bile salts results in tea-colored urine.

Failure to thrive and malnutrition occur as the destructive changes of the disease progress.

Diagnosis is based on the history, physical examination, and laboratory evaluation; laboratory findings reveal elevated bilirubin levels, elevated serum aminotransferase and alkaline phosphatase values, prolonged prothrombin time, and increased ammonia levels.

Percutaneous liver biopsy suggests biliary atresia, and cholangiography and an exploratory laparatomy confirms the diagnosis (Roach & Bruny, 2008).

Treatment involves surgery to attempt correction of the obstruction (hepatoportoenterostomy-Kasai procedure). In this procedure, a segment of the intestine is anastomosed to the porta hepatis. The primary purpose of this procedure is to promote bile flow from the liver. Intravenous antibiotics are administered in the postoperative period to prevent cholangitis. Prophylaxis with oral antibiotics is continued for 1 to 2 years after surgery (Flanigan, 2007).

Additional treatment includes administration of intramuscular vitamin K prior to invasive procedures and surgery to decrease the risk of bleeding afterward; ursodeoxycholic acid to promote bile flow; and vitamins A, D, E, and K to provide supplementation since absorption of these vitamins is impaired.

The infant is breastfed or is given Pregestimil or Nutramigen, formulas that contain medium-chain triglycerides. As the liver disease worsens the child may need cholestyramine and antihistamines to help decrease itching. Enteral feedings and TPN may be needed as well (Flanigan, 2007).

Liver transplantation may be required for survival.

Assess the abdomen for distention. Monitor stool pattern and assess for clay-colored, puttylike stools. Assess skin for jaundice and ecchymosis.

Nursing care includes preoperative and postoperative care, supporting the family, educating the family about home care, and preparing the family for organ transplantation.

Weigh the infant daily; administer TPN, intralipids, and fat-soluble vitamins A, D, E, and K as prescribed.

Diagnosis of this potentially fatal disorder can be devastating to parents; provide emotional support, and offer frequent explanations of tests during the initial diagnostic evaluation.

Posttransplant care includes immunosuppressant drugs and close monitoring for vascular complications. For the child who has received a transplant, teach parents how to identify signs of rejection (nausea, vomiting, fever, jaundice), as well as the administration and side effects of immunosuppressant medications.

Viral Hepatitis
Description and Etiology
Hepatitis is an inflammation of the liver caused by a viral infection.

Hepatitis may occur as an acute or chronic disease.

Acute hepatitis is rapid in onset and, if untreated, may develop into chronic hepatitis.

The most frequently diagnosed causative organisms are hepatitis A virus (HAV), hepatitis B virus (HBV), and hepatitis C virus (HCV). A lesser known type is hepatitis D virus (HDV). This type of hepatitis only occurs in individuals who have HBV infection (Holloway & D'Acunto, 2006). Hepatitis E (HEV) occurs primarily in developing countries and is rarely seen in the United States (CDC, 2005a).

The liver's response to injury by the viruses that cause hepatitis leads to invasion of the parenchymal cells by the virus, resulting in local degeneration and necrosis.

Subsequent infiltration of the parenchyma by lymphocytes, macrophages, plasma cells, eosinophils, and neutrophils causes inflammation that blocks biliary drainage into the intestine.

Impaired bile excretion causes a buildup of bile in the blood, urine, and skin (jaundice).

Structural changes in the parenchymal cells account for other altered liver functions.

Clinical Manifestations
Acute hepatitis infection is characterized by two phases: the anicteric (absence of jaundice) phase and the icteric (jaundice) phase.

The anicteric phase usually lasts 5 to 7 days. Signs and symptoms include nausea, vomiting, anorexia, malaise, fatigue, right upper quadrant pain, hepatosplenomegaly, and fever. The child becomes irritable, looks ill, and requires rest.

In the icteric phase, signs and symptoms include darkening of urine, clay-colored stools, and the characteristic yellowing of the skin and sclera.

However, many children with hepatitis do not have jaundice, leading to difficulty in disease diagnosis and management.

Diagnostic Tests

Diagnosis is often made on the basis of a thorough history and physical examination.

A history of exposure to persons with the disease is significant.

Physical examination reveals a tender, enlarged liver; abdominal pain; and flulike symptoms.

Laboratory evaluation includes serologic testing to detect the presence of antigens and antibodies to HAV, HBV, HCV, or HDV and liver function studies.

Clinical Therapy

The spread of viral infections can be interrupted by elimination of the virus from the infected population, institution of proper hygiene, and passive or active immunization (Table 20–5).

Active immunization for hepatitis A, a two-dose series, is recommended for all persons at risk of acquiring infection, for children, and for those who wish to acquire immunity to the illness. The CDC recommends that all children receive the first hepatitis A vaccine at 1 year of age (Fiore, Wasley, & Bell, 2006).

Immunization for hepatitis B, a three-dose series, is recommended for all children and at-risk adults; the first dose is given within 12 hours of birth to the infant born to an infected mother or to a mother with unknown status (CDC, 2007b; see chapter 8). Management of the illness includes bed rest, hydration, and adequate nutrition during the flulike phase; if prothrombin times are increased, vitamin K is administered.

Nursing Management

Nursing care focuses on preventing the spread of infection, providing fluid and nutritional support, promoting growth and development, reducing risk of complications, and supporting the parents and child.

Table 20–5 Comparison of Hepatitis Types

Type	Immunization Available	Prophylaxis	Primary Transmission	Incubation Period
Hepatitis A	Yes	Immune globulin Hepatitis A vaccine	Fecal-oral	15–19 days
Hepatitis B	Yes	Hepatitis B immune globulin Hepatitis B vaccine	Needlesticks or sharps exposure Intravenous drug use During birth Sexual activity	60–180 days
Hepatitis C	No	None	Needlesticks or sharps exposure Intravenous drug use During birth	14–160 days
Hepatitis D	No	Hepatitis B vaccine	Needlesticks or sharps exposure Intravenous drug use During birth Sexual activity	21–42 days
Hepatitis E	No	None	Fecal-oral	21–63 days

Source: Adapted from "Hepatitis A Fact Sheet," Centers for Disease Control and Prevention, 2007a, retrieved October 21, 2007, from http://www.cdc.gov/hepatitis; "Hepatitis B Fact Sheet," Centers for Disease Control and Prevention, 2007b, retrieved October 21, 2007, from http://www.cdc.gov/hepatitis; "Hepatitis D Fact Sheet," Centers for Disease Control and Prevention, 2006, retrieved October 21, 2007, from http://www.cdc.gov/hepatitis; "Hepatitis C Fact Sheet," Centers for Disease Control and Prevention, 2005b, retrieved October 21, 2007, from http://www.cdc.gov/hepatitis; "Hepatitis E Fact Sheet," Centers for Disease Control and Prevention, 2005a, retrieved October 21, 2007, from http://www.cdc.gov/hepatitis; and "Viral Hepatitis," by N. Yazigi & W. F. Balistreri, 2007, in R. M. Kliegman, R. E. Behrman., H. B. Jenson, & B. F. Stanton (Eds.), Nelson Textbook of Pediatrics (18th ed., pp. 1680–1690). Philadelphia: Saunders.

Cirrhosis

Cirrhosis is a degenerative disease process that results in fibrotic changes and fatty infiltration in the liver; it can occur in children of any age as the end stage of several liver disorders such as hepatitis and biliary atresia (A-Kader & Balistreri, 2007; Boamah & Balistreri, 2007).

The diffuse destruction and regeneration of the hepatic parenchymal cells result in an increase in fibrous connective tissue and disorganization of the liver structure.

Progressive scarring that occurs in cirrhosis leads to altered blood flow to the liver, which causes further deterioration of liver function (Boamah & Balistreri, 2007).

Clinical manifestations of cirrhosis vary. Hepatomegaly may be evident on exam. Jaundice occurs as the disease progresses, an indication of hyperbilirubinemia. Jaundice is sometimes the only sign of hepatic dysfunction, so its appearance must be investigated. Pruritus is common in children with cirrhosis, although it is not related to the degree of hyperbilirubinemia. Other clinical manifestations of cirrhosis in children include ascites, portal hypertension, encephalopathy, and variceal hemorrhage (Boamah & Balistreri, 2007). Severe end-stage complications signaling hepatic failure can occur at any time and with little warning.

Diagnostic evaluation is based on the child's history of infection or disease with liver involvement.

Physical examination may reveal jaundice, skin changes, ascites, and hemodynamic changes.

Laboratory evaluation reveals abnormal liver function tests.

A liver biopsy may help to determine the extent of the parenchymal damage.

Medical management focuses on treating the child's symptoms and achieving optimal nutritional status and growth.

Liver transplant is the only treatment for end-stage liver disease.

Nursing care focuses on monitoring physiologic and psychosocial changes to identify early signs of end-stage hepatic failure.

Monitor vital signs every 2 to 4 hours,

Measure weight daily to assess for fluid retention,

Close monitoring of electrolytes and liver function test results helps determine the need for fluid-replacement therapy.

Measure abdominal girth daily.

Careful administration of medications and monitoring for side effects are necessary because drug metabolism is altered in liver disorders.

If ascites is present, provide a low-sodium, low-protein diet and restrict fluids.

Parents of a child with cirrhosis are coping with a life-threatening disorder, and their anxiety and stress are high; the child may be waiting for a liver transplantation that represents the only hope for recovery; provide support to parents, and encourage them to verbalize their fears and concerns.

INJURIES TO THE GASTROINTESTINAL SYSTEM

Abdominal Trauma

Description and Etiology

Abdominal injuries may be caused by blunt or penetrating trauma; the type of injury determines the extent of organ damage.

Falls are the most common cause of abdominal injury in children; however, automobile accidents and pedestrian injuries are the major cause of severe blunt abdominal trauma in children (Potoka & Saladino, 2005).

ATV (all-terrain vehicle) injuries are increasing in the United States as the popularity of these devices increases (Aitken et al, 2004; Brandenberg, 2004).

Child abuse involving kicking or punching the abdomen is another major cause of blunt abdominal trauma.

Penetrating trauma occurs due to impalement on an object, stabbing, or gunshot wounds (Potoka & Saladino, 2005). The type of injury determines the extent of organ damage.

High-velocity blunt trauma, which may occur in motor vehicle crashes, usually involves multiple organs. Solid organs, such as the liver and spleen, can be bruised or lacerated.

Low-velocity trauma usually results in a single-organ injury and includes sports-related abdominal trauma often associated with a direct blow to the abdomen and bicycle crashes that result in abdominal injury if the handlebars hit the child in the abdomen (Potoka & Saladino, 2005).

Clinical Manifestations

Clinical manifestations of abdominal injury include pain, abdominal distention, muscle guarding, decreased or absent bowel sounds, nausea and vomiting, hypotension, hypovolemia, and shock.

Diagnostic Tests

Suspected abdominal trauma in a child necessitates a thorough history and physical examination; the description of the event should be compared with the child's signs and symptoms.

Plain abdominal radiographs may reveal air in the abdomen.

An ultrasound can reveal free fluid in the abdomen.

A CT scan assesses multiple organs for injury and for the presence of free fluid in the abdomen.

Serial hemoglobin and hematocrit evaluation is essential to determine hemodynamic stability.

Type and cross match of blood is also necessary in case the child needs a blood transfustion; electrolytes and enzyme studies (amylase and lipase) to detect liver, spleen, and pancreas injuries are obtained (Pieper, 2007; Potoka & Saladino, 2005; Saxena, 2006).

Clinical Therapy

Treatment of an abdominal, liver, or spleen injury takes place in the pediatric intensive care unit and focuses on preventing or managing hemorrhage and monitoring for signs of shock.

Nonsurgical management is preferred.

An intravenous infusion is initiated for fluid maintenance and to provide access for blood products.

The child is kept NPO, and a nasogastric tube is inserted.

Blood transfusions and pharmacologic management are used to treat blood loss.

The child is maintained on strict bed rest until bleeding is controlled and the hemoglobin and hematocrit are stable.

Exploratory laparotomy is performed to resect hollow organ injuries or to repair liver or spleen lacerations when bleeding is not controlled.

Nursing Management

Assessment

Nursing care includes initial and ongoing assessments of the child's condition.

Initial assessment includes assessing the abdomen for bruising, pain, guarding, rebound tenderness, distention, and absence of bowel sounds (Eckert, 2005).

Monitor hematocrit and vital signs every hour as warranted to detect hypovolemia.

Assess for increasing heart rate, hypotension, dyspnea, and other changes that may indicate shock.

Monitor the respiratory status as abdominal injuries may also have thoracic involvement.

Strict monitoring of intake and output will give information on the child's fluid status.

Implementation

The child and parents are usually fearful and anxious when the child is admitted to the hospital; if the injury was preventable, parents may have feelings of guilt or anger; provide emotional support.

Administer fluids, blood products, and antibiotics as prescribed.

Maintain nasogastric tube, if present.

Prepare the child and parents for surgery, if necessary.

Provide postoperative care, including pain control, vital sign measurement, and respiratory, cardiovascular, and gastrointestinal system evaluations.

Once the child's condition is stabilized, nursing care shifts to preventive teaching; partner with the child and parents to ensure their understanding of safety measures to prevent future injuries.

21 ALTERATIONS IN GENITOURINARY FUNCTION

URINARY TRACT INFECTION

An infection of the upper or lower urinary tract of bacterial, viral, or fungal origin.

- A lower UTI involves the bladder and urethra.
- An upper UTI or pyelonephritis involves the ureters, renal pelvis, and renal parenchyma.

UTIs in newborns and infants may indicate an abnormality of the genitourinary tract. Renal scarring can result from hydronephrosis or the inflammatory and ischemic effects of the infection.

Many first UTIs are caused by *Escherichia coli,* a common gram-negative enteric bacterium. Other causative organisms include *Staphylococcus, Klebsiella, Proteus, Pseudomonas aeruginosa, Enterobacter,* and *Enterococcus* (Dulczak & Kirk, 2005).

An increased risk of UTI occurs with urinary stasis, infrequent voiding, poor hygiene, inadequate cleansing after bowel movements, an irritated perineum, uncircumcised male in the first 6 months of life, constipation, masturbation, sexual abuse, and sexual activity in adolescent females (Dulczak & Kirk, 2005). Vesicoureteral reflux, the backflow of urine from the bladder into the ureters during voiding, is another cause of UTI and is discussed on page 413.

Clinical Manifestations

Symptoms depend on the location of the infection and the age of the child.

Many UTIs are asymptomatic and are discovered incidentally on routine examination.

Lower UTI

- Neonate—unexplained fever, hypothermia, failure to thrive, poor feeding, vomiting and diarrhea, strong-smelling urine, and irritability
- Infant—fever, diarrhea, vomiting, irritability, lethargy, foul-smelling diapers, poor feeding, failure to gain weight
- Preschooler—fever, hematuria, urgency, dysuria, frequency, cloudy urine, foul-smelling urine, dehydration, abdominal pain, enuresis

- School age—dysuria, enuresis, hematuria, strong-smelling urine, diarrhea, urinary frequency or hesitancy, mood changes, abdominal pain, suprapubic or flank pain, dehydration
- Upper UTI (pyelonephritis)—high fever, chills, abdominal pain, nausea, vomiting, flank pain, costovertebral angle tenderness, moderate to severe dehydration
- May be asymptomatic

Diagnostic Testing

Urine culture and sensitivity collected by midstream clean-catch void or sterile catheterization reveal bacteria in the urine.

Urinalysis reveals white blood cells (WBCs) in the urine. A complete blood count reveals an elevated WBC count.

Radiologic studies are performed to detect structural abnormalities and scarring.

Most common tests performed are a renal and bladder ultrasound soon after the diagnosis of a UTI. A voiding cystourethrogram (VCUG) may be obtained to test for vesicoureteral reflux. Ultrasound and a DMSA scan are also used to detect pyelonephritis and renal scarring (Dulczak & Kirk, 2005).

Clinical Therapy

Antibiotic therapy is begun as soon as urine samples have been collected. Antibiotics are selected based on the age of the child, sensitivity of the cultured organism, and the child's signs and symptoms. The antibiotic is changed if necessary after culture sensitivity is determined. Follow-up cultures may be obtained 48 to 72 hours after drug therapy is started if the child is still febrile (Raszka & Khan, 2005). Children with pyelonephritis should be maintained on antibiotic prophylaxis until radiologic tests are performed to detect any structural defects.

If structural defect is identified, surgical correction may be necessary to prevent recurrent infections that could lead to renal damage.

Nursing Management

Assessment

Obtain a history of urinary symptoms. Determine if there is a history of recurrent urinary tract infections. Assess the infant for toxic (very ill) appearance, fever, and poor feeding. Evaluate the child's oral fluid intake. Assess for quality, quantity, and frequency of voiding. Observe the urinary stream, if possible. Assess the infant's or child's vital signs including blood pressure. This is an especially important assessment in infants and toddlers who cannot communicate. Assess for behavioral changes such as bedwetting and loss of bladder control in older age groups.

Palpate the abdomen and suprapubic and costovertebral areas for masses, tenderness, and distention. Assess for abdominal or flank pain, frequency, urgency, and dysuria. Assess bathing and toileting habits (e.g., determine whether the child takes bubble baths, wipes from front to back, and engages in adequate perineal hygiene). Also be alert for signs of sexual abuse such as bruising or scarring of the perineal region.

Implementation

Administer medications, promote rehydration, assess renal function, and partner with parents and older children to minimize the risk of future infection.

Encourage fluid intake to dilute the urine and flush the bladder.

Emphasize the importance of taking the full course of antibiotics.

Toilet-trained toddlers may regress and need diapers temporarily. Enuresis may occur in children who have previously been dry at night. Reassure parents that this is normal and to give support to the child.

Children with renal scarring should have their blood pressure monitored during future healthcare visits.

Parent and Family Education

Provide education to parents and children about strategies to reduce the risk for future UTIs.

Teach proper perineal hygiene. Girls should always wipe the perineum from front to back after voiding.

Encourage the child to drink plenty of fluids, but avoid caffeinated and carbonated beverages that may irritate the bladder.

Caution against tight underwear; children should wear cotton rather than nylon underwear.

Encourage the child to void more frequently and to fully empty the bladder.

Discourage bubble baths and hot tubs, which can irritate the urethra.

Encourage abstinence of sexual activity. Instruct sexually active girls to void before and after sexual intercourse to flush out bacteria introduced during intercourse.

STRUCTURAL DEFECTS OF THE URINARY SYSTEM

Bladder Exstrophy

Failure of the abdominal wall to fuse during fetal development results in extrusion of the bladder wall through the lower abdominal wall. The rectus muscles and symphysis pubis are widely separated. The upper urinary tract is usually normal.

Clinical Manifestations

The bladder mucosa appears as a mass of bright red tissue and urine continually leaks from the ureters onto the skin (Huether, 2006). The defect occurs in varying degrees of severity. Females have a bifid (split) clitoris. Males have a short penis, and the glans is flattened with dorsal chordee and a ventral prepuce. Epispadias and undescended testes (see pages 410 and 439) occur with this disorder in males. Inguinal hernias may develop in both males and females (Leung, Robson, & Wong, 2005). Sometimes genetic testing is advised to determine the infant's sex due to ambiguity of the genitalia.

Diagnostic Testing

Diagnosis by prenatal ultrasound

Diagnosis based on physical appearance at time of delivery

Renal ultrasound to identify hydronephrosis or other renal abnormalities

Clinical Therapy

Exposed bladder tissue is covered with plastic wrap until surgery is performed to keep the bladder mucosa moist (Elder, 2007).

Surgical reconstruction is performed in several stages to address all defects.

- Primary closure of the bladder and abdominal wall is performed, usually within 24 to 48 hours after birth.
- The wound and pelvis are immobilized to promote healing.
- An osteotomy to rotate the innominate bones of the pelvis to approximate the symphysis pubis reduces tension on the closed bladder and abdominal wall to promote healing.
- Epispadias repair is often performed between 1 and 2 years of age or at the same time as a surgical procedure to improve continence.
- Surgery to reconstruct the bladder neck and reimplant the ureters is performed when the bladder has achieved a capacity of at least 80 ml (Elder, 2007).
- Because the bladder epithelium is abnormal, it is prone to neoplasms. Periodic examination and cystoscopy after the age of

20 years is recommended to detect malignancies since symptoms are often ignored or ambiguous.

Nursing Management

Assessment

Before surgery, monitor urine output and serum and urine chemistries to assess renal function and hydration. Weigh the newborn daily.

Assess family support systems and coping mechanisms.

After surgery, routinely record urine output from each tube every 2 to 4 hours; note any signs of tube obstruction (change in urine output, urine or blood draining from the urethral meatus, or increased intensity of bladder spasms). Assess pain.

Assess for wound dehiscence and bladder prolapse. Monitor lower limb peripheral circulation if a spica cast is used.

Implementation

At time of birth, umbilical cord should be tied, not clamped, since a clamp could cause trauma to the bladder mucosa (Metcalf & Schwarz, 2004).

Protect the bladder mucosa with a saline-soaked dressing covered in plastic wrap. Use a skin sealant to protect the skin from leaking urine (Mercy & Brady-Fryer, 2004).

After surgery, use aseptic technique for wound care, and monitor for signs of infection. Avoid abduction of the infant's legs to reduce stress on the surgical area.

Promote comfort by administering pain medications and antispasmodic agents. Administer antibiotics as prescribed.

Provide emotional support to parents, and promote parent–infant bonding through bathing and feeding.

Patient and Family Education

Teach parents to change dressings and to diaper the infant.

Educate parents to identify signs and symptoms of infection (cloudy urine, increased temperature, purulent drainage, foul odor from the incision, increased fussiness, or decreased feeding), and report them to the healthcare provider.

Discuss the need for follow-up visits to assess urinary function and to plan the next stages of surgery.

Teach parents to initiate toilet training at the appropriate age for bowel movements, even if urinary continence is not yet achieved.

Discuss ways to promote the child's self-esteem and self-confidence with sexual identity and function.

Hypospadias and Epispadias

These conditions are congenital anomalies in which the urethral meatus has an abnormal location on the penis resulting from failure of the urethral folds to fuse completely over the urethral groove.

Hypospadias often occurs in conjunction with congenital chordee—a fibrous line of tissue that results in ventral curvature of the penile shaft—and can interfere with sexual function. Associated defects may also include undescended testes and partial absence of the foreskin (Huether, 2006).

Epispadias and exstrophy of the bladder are the same condition, but epispadias is the milder expression of the condition (Huether, 2006).

Clinical Manifestations

Hypospadias—the urethral meatus may be located anywhere along the ventral surface of the penis, from the perineum to the tip of the glans.

Epispadias—the urethral meatus is located anywhere on the dorsal surface of the penis and may be at the level of the bladder neck (Huether, 2006).

Diagnostic Testing

Diagnosis by prenatal ultrasound or by physical examination at birth

Urinalysis and urine culture

Testing for a chromosome abnormality or problem in androgen metabolism when the meatus is located on the perineum or scrotum

Clinical Therapy

Surgical correction of the structural defect is performed during the first year of life. The infant *should not be circumcised* because the foreskin tissue may be used for surgical repair.

A caudal nerve block is often used for initial postoperative pain relief. Anticholinergic medications such as oxybutynin may be prescribed to relieve bladder spasms.

A urethral stent is placed to maintain patency of the new urethral canal. A suprapubic or urethral urinary drainage catheter may be inserted to let urine flow without tension on the urethral sutures.

Nursing Management

Assessment

Assess the newborn for urine stream, exit site, and angle of urination.

Assess family support systems and coping mechanisms when the newborn is diagnosed with this defect. Assess the older child's level of understanding of the procedures and need for surgery.

After surgery, monitor for penile swelling, dysuria, bleeding at the surgical site, infection, and evidence of pain.

Implementation

Educate the parents to reduce anxiety concerning the future appearance and functioning of the penis. Use dolls and pictures to explain the procedure to an older child.

Protect the surgical site from injury, and ensure that the stent or catheter is not removed.

Encourage fluid intake and document intake and output hourly to detect postoperative urinary complications (kinks in the tubing or obstruction by sediment). Notify the physician if there is no urine output for 1 hour.

Administer medication—anticholinergics, antibiotics, and analgesics.

Patient and Family Education

Demonstrate care of the reconstructed area, including catheter or stent care, incision care, penis care, emptying of the drainage bag, and securing the catheter.

Use a double-diapering technique to protect the stent.

Do not bathe the child in the tub until the stent or catheter is removed.

Restrict the infant or toddler from activities (e.g., playing on riding toys) that put pressure on the surgical site. Avoid holding the infant or child straddled on the hip. Limit the child's activity for 2 weeks.

Encourage fluids to ensure adequate hydration. Offer fruit juice, fruit-flavored ice pops, fruit-flavored juices, flavored ice cubes, and gelatin.

Administer the *complete course* of prescribed antibiotics to avoid infection.

Observe for signs of infection—fever, swelling, redness, pain, strong-smelling urine, or change in flow of the urinary stream. The urine will be blood tinged for several days.

Call the physician if urine is seen leaking from any area other than the penis.

Obstructive Uropathy

Obstructive uropathy is a structural or functional obstruction in the urinary tract that interferes with urine flow and results in urine backflow into the kidneys. Obstructions can occur at various sites:

- Ureteropelvic junction—the ureteropelvic junction (UPJ), the tapered point where the renal pelvis transitions to the ureter, is the most frequent site of obstruction of the upper urinary tract in infants and children (Small & Copel, 2004).
- Posterior urethral valves (PUV)—abnormal folds of mucosa in the male urethra are the most common cause of anatomic bladder outlet obstruction (Small & Copel, 2004).
- Narrowing at the ureterovesicular junction, a ureterocele, a ureter that inserts into an abnormal location within the urinary tract, or ureteral hypoplasia are also possible.

Hydronephrosis, an accumulation of urine in the renal pelvis, results from obstruction. It compromises kidney function, resulting in hypertension, metabolic acidosis, inability to concentrate urine, urinary stasis and infection, and chronic renal failure (CRF).

Clinical Manifestations

Abdominal mass, enlarged kidney, palpable bladder

Hypertension

Urinary frequency, poor urinary stream, enuresis

Hematuria, urinary tract infection (UTI)

Pain

Failure to thrive

Diagnostic Testing

Hydronephrosis may be detected by prenatal ultrasound.

Urinalysis

A diuretic-enhanced radionuclide scan and a voiding cystourethrogram

Serial serum creatinine and electrolyte levels

Arterial blood gases may reveal metabolic acidosis due to improper renal function.

Clinical Therapy

For acute obstructions, immediate intervention is required. Short-term management includes immediate placement of a urethral catheter in newborns with suspected PUV to promote urine drainage, thereby decreasing pressure in the kidneys (Delaney, 2005).

In cases of urinary incontinence—clean intermittent catheterization or diversion with a temporary or permanent ostomy.

Antibiotic prophylaxis is indicated to reduce the risk for UTI.

Nursing Management
Assessment
Palpate the abdomen for a mass or distended bladder. Monitor urine output, and observe the force of the urine stream.

Observe for peripheral edema and costovertebral angle tenderness.

Implementation
Prepare the parents and child for the surgical procedure.

After surgery, monitor vital signs, intake and output, and bladder distention.

Administer antibiotics and antispasmodics, such as oxybutynin. An epidural catheter may have been placed for pain management. Once this is removed, provide prescribed pain medication.

Provide instructions on dressing changes, care for catheters, assessing pain and administering analgesics, and recognizing signs of possible obstruction or infection.

Provide guidelines for seeking health care promptly if signs are noted.

Encourage parents to promote growth and development with age-appropriate activities; however, children should avoid contact sports because of their potential to injure the bladder.

Vesicoureteral Reflux
Backflow of urine from the bladder into the kidneys prevents complete emptying of the bladder and creates a reservoir for bacterial growth (Huether, 2006). A renal ultrasound and voiding cystourethrogram reveals the defect and severity of reflux (e.g., to the ureter, renal pelvis, or dilating the ureter and renal pelvis). Sterile reflux does not seem to cause significant renal damage; however, reflux of infected urine may cause pyelonephritis and renal scarring (Huether, 2006). Long-term complications include renal scarring, hypertension, and chronic renal failure (Nelson, 2006).

Clinical Therapy
Prophylactic antibiotics may be prescribed to prevent UTIs.

Surgery to reimplant the ureters may be required.

Nursing Management

After ureteral reimplantation, monitor urine output through the urinary catheter. The urine is initially bloody and may have clots. Follow orders for irrigating the Foley catheter when urine output is diminished.

Intravenous fluids will be administered at a rate sufficient to maintain adequate urine output.

Administer antibiotics, antispasmodics, and analgesics as prescribed.

Discharge teaching includes administration of antibiotics and anti-spasmodics, a high-fiber diet to reduce constipation, and avoidance of active play for 3 weeks. Provide guidelines to call the physician for a fever of more than 38.5°C (101.5°F), abdominal or back pain, or swelling and redness of the incision.

Prune Belly Syndrome

Prune belly syndrome, also known as Eagle-Barrett syndrome, is a congenital defect characterized by failure of the abdominal muscula-ture to develop.

The skin covering the abdominal wall is thin and resembles a wrin-kled prune.

Other characteristics include urinary tract anomalies, poor ureteral peristalsis, enlarged bladder, high risk for recurrent urinary tract infection, vesicoureteral reflux, and bilateral cryptorchidism.

Diagnosis is confirmed with abdominal ultrasound. An intravenous pyelogram is useful in assessing structural defects.

Abdominal wall reconstruction and correction of genitourinary de-fects, including orchiopexy, are performed to repair defects. Approx-imately 30% of children with prune belly syndrome will develop end-stage renal disease in childhood or adolescence because of inad-equate renal function (Elder, 2007).

Nursing Management

Nursing management for the infant with prune-belly syndrome is the same as for other defects of the genitourinary system, including pre-operative and postoperative management.

Additional management includes psychosocial support for the child and family related to the numerous congenital anomalies, body image concerns, and long-term consequences of the defect.

DISORDERS AFFECTING URINARY ELIMINATION

Enuresis

Enuresis is repeated involuntary voiding by a child who has reached age 5 or 6 years, at which time day and night bladder control is expected.

Enuresis can occur either at night (nocturnal), during the day (diurnal), or both night and day.

Primary enuresis—child has never had a dry night; due to maturational delay and small functional bladder; not associated with stress or psychiatric cause.

Secondary enuresis—child who has been reliably dry for at least 6 months begins bedwetting; associated with stress, infections, and sleep disorders.

Primary nocturnal enuresis is the most common type of enuresis and occurs more frequently in males than females (Elder, 2007).

Clinical Manifestations

Diurnal enuresis—daytime frequency, urgency, constant dribbling, and involuntary loss of bladder control

Nocturnal enuresis—bedwetting

Diagnostic Testing

Urinalysis and urine culture

Functional bladder capacity and urine flow measurement

Bladder sonogram to measure postvoid residual

Clinical Therapy

A spontaneous cure rate occurs in approximately 15% of children each year, with or without intervention.

A multitreatment approach is most effective. Medications, such as desmopressin acetate, oxybutynin, and imipramine, may be used. See Table 21–1.

Nursing Management

Assessment

Review the child's urine and bowel elimination patterns, developmental milestones, toilet-training history, and urinary symptoms.

Inspect the child's lower spine for signs of occult spina bifida (fistulas, sacral dimples, or tufts of hair). Identify potential stressors that may contribute to enuresis.

Table 21–1   Treatment Approaches for Enuresis

Approach	Description
Fluid restriction	Fluid intake is limited in the evening and before the child goes to bed.
Bladder exercises	The child drinks a large amount and then holds urine as long as he or she can. The child practices stopping voiding midstream. Exercises should continue for at least 6 months.
Timed voiding	The child with diurnal enuresis is instructed to void every 2 hours and to use a double-voiding pattern; this trains the bladder to empty completely and avoids overdistention.
Enuresis alarms	A detector strip is attached to the child's pants. The alarm sounds a buzzer that alerts the child when wetting occurs, so the child can get up and finish voiding in the bathroom. This works best for children over 7 years old, and takes 3 to 4 months for success.
Reward system	Set realistic goals for the child and reinforce dry days or nights with stars and stickers on a chart.
Medications	Imipramine, desmopressin, and oxybutynin may be used.

Assess the child's and family's feelings and frustrations about the problem of bedwetting and their motivation to implement therapies.

Implementation

Educate the child and parents about bladder control development and the causes and treatment of enuresis. Make sure the parents are aware that the child cannot control the wetting.

Assess the parents' and child's motivation and readiness for interventions. The child needs to be an active participant in the treatment plan for daytime and nighttime wetting.

RENAL DISORDERS

Nephrotic Syndrome

Nephrotic syndrome is an alteration in renal function of unknown cause in which the glomerular basement membrane has increased permeability to plasma protein.

Proteinuria results in decreased oncotic pressure and edema, because fluid remains in the interstitial spaces instead of being pulled back into the vascular compartment (Robinson, 2003).

Immunoglobulins are lost, resulting in altered immunity.

Loss of protein in the urine, as well as insufficient albumin production by the liver and a decreased albumin concentration as a result of salt and water retention by the kidney, contribute to hypoalbuminemia.

Hypercoagulability occurs because of loss of antithrombin III in the urine and reduced levels of factors IX, XI, and XII. Child is at risk for thrombus.

The liver, stimulated perhaps by hypoalbuminemia or decreased osmotic pressure, responds by increasing synthesis of lipoprotein, resulting in hyperlipidemia.

Most children have minimal-change nephrotic syndrome (MCNS).

Acute renal failure is a rare complication of MCNS, most likely due to changes in glomerular permeability (Walle, Mauel, Raes, et al., 2004).

Clinical Manifestations
Edema develops over several weeks, noted with a gradual or rapid weight gain, snug-fitting clothing, and tight-fitting shoes.

Periorbital edema on waking that resolves during day as fluid shifts to abdomen and lower extremities

Pallor, hypertension, irritability, anorexia, hematuria, decreased urine output, frothy or foamy urine, and nonspecific malaise

Parents often do not seek medical treatment until generalized edema develops on the child's extremities, abdomen, or genitals.

Respiratory distress from pleural effusion may occur in some cases.

Diagnostic Testing
Urinalysis, serum albumin, sodium, BUN, cholesterol, and other electrolytes are assessed.

Hypoalbuminemia of less than 25 g/L and urinary protein excretion of greater than or equal to 40 mg/m2/hour are the criteria for diagnosing nephrotic syndrome in childhood (Ruth, Kemper, Leumann, et al., 2005).

Renal ultrasound to detect structural kidney problems; renal biopsy to examine glomeruli and assess for renal failure or other disorders

Clinical Therapy
Corticosteroids are the primary treatment. Urine protein levels usually fall to trace or negative values within 2 to 3 weeks of the start of

therapy, and remission generally occurs. See Table 21–2 for medications used to treat nephritic syndrome.

Table 21–2 Medications Used to Treat Nephrotic Syndrome

Medication	Nursing Considerations
Corticosteroid therapy Prednisone Intravenous high-dose methylprednisolone may be used if unresponsive to oral steroids	Children who respond successfully to therapy continue to take cortico-steroids daily for 6 weeks and 6 weeks of alternate-day treatment. Monitor for infection, changes in blood pressure, and changes in growth and behavior. If long-term courses of corticosteroids are administered, observe for major side effects such as weight gain and moon face, obesity, gastrointestinal bleeding, growth retardation, hyper-glycemia, hypertension, adrenal suppression, and bone demineralization. Educate parents about appetite-stimulating effect of corticosteroids and to limit calorie intake to prevent excessive weight gain. Administration of live vaccines should be delayed until child is no longer immunosuppressed.
Alkylating/cytotoxic agents Chlorambucil Cyclophosphamide	Monitor WBC count. Assess for gastrointestinal bleeding, alopecia, and impaired growth. Serious long-term side effects include carcinogenesis and risk of sterility in males. Administer medications 1 hour before breakfast or 2 hours after evening meal. An antiemetic may be prescribed for nausea while taking medication. Encourage adequate hydration to reduce cystitis. Educate family to report unusual bleeding, bruising, chills, fever, or other signs of infection.

Table 21–2 Medications Used to Treat Nephrotic Syndrome (Continued)

Medication	Nursing Considerations
	Monitor blood pressure for hypertension, and other side effects such as nausea, vomiting, anemia, and abdominal discomfort.
	Monitor electrolytes, cyclosporine serum concentrations, creatinine clearance, and serum creatinine levels to assess renal status.
	Educate family to administer medication with meals to reduce nausea, administer the medication at the same time each day, and use a glass rather than plastic container for mixing. May dilute with orange or apple juice. Do not use grapefruit juice.
Diuretics *Loop diuretics* Furosemide, bumetanide *Thiazide diuretics*	May be administered orally or intravenously. Monitor for intravascular volume depletion (hypovolemia). Assess vital signs for tachycardia and hypotension. Monitor plasma concentration to identify child at risk for hearing loss. Monitor for other potential side effects including hyponatremia, hypokalemia, and other electrolyte imbalances.
Vasotec (enalapril maleate)	Monitor blood pressure. Assess for transient hypotension, lightheadedness. Monitor serum potassium for side effect of hyperkalemia.
Antibiotics	Administer according to prescribed schedule. Monitor WBC count and assess for signs and symptoms of infection.

Table 21–2 Medications Used to Treat Nephrotic Syndrome (Continued)

Medication	Nursing Considerations
Antithrombotic therapy Heparin, followed by oral anticoagulant therapy	Monitor clotting factors and platelet count. Assess for evidence of thrombosis. Assess for abnormal bleeding (oozing intravenous sites, nosebleeds).
NSAIDs	Establish a routine pain assessment schedule using a pain scale. Administer pain medications around the clock rather than prn.

Source: Data from "Management of Nephrotic Syndrome in Children," by R. F. Robinson, M. C. Nahata, J. D. Mahan, & D. L. Batisky, 2003, *Pharmacotherapy, 23*(8), 1021–1036; "Primary Glomerular Disease," by P. H. Nachman, J. C. Jennette, & R. J. Falk, 2008, in B. M. Brenner (Ed.), *Brenner & Rector's The Kidney* (8th ed., pp. 987–1066). Philadelphia: Saunders; "Alterations of Renal and Urinary Tract Function in Children," by S. E. Huether, 2006, in K. L. McCance & S. E. Huether (Eds.), *Pathophysiology: The Biologic Basis for Disease in Adults and Children* (5th ed., pp. 1337–1352). St. Louis: Elsevier Mosby.; and "Conditions Particularly Associated with Proteinuria," by B. A. Vogt & E. D. Avner, 2007, in R. E. Behrman, R. M. Kliegman, & H. B. Jenson (Eds.), *Nelson Textbook of Pediatrics* (18th ed., pp. 2188–2195). Philadelphia: Saunders.

Intravenous administration of albumin followed by furosemide may occasionally be ordered in the child with massive edema who is unresponsive to fluid restriction and parenteral diuretics (Vogt & Avner, 2007a).

A regular-protein, low-salt diet is recommended.

Relapses occur in up to 50% of children with neprhotic syndrome (Ruth, Landolt, Neuhaus, et al., 2004). Relapses may become less frequent during adolescence; however, long-term studies have revealed that many adults continue to have relapses (Ruth, Kemper, Leumann, et al., 2005).

Nursing Management

Assessment

Assess the child for fluid volume excess, including weight gain, facial and periorbital edema, external genitalia edema, and ascites. Monitor intake and output and vital signs at least every 4 hours. Weigh the child daily using the same scale, and measure abdominal girth to monitor changes in edema and ascites.

Assess the child for signs of hypovolemia during periods of diuresis. Assess for skin breakdown.

Assess for respiratory distress associated with pulmonary congestion, pulmonary edema, and pleural effusion. Monitor for hypertension and signs of circulatory overload.

Test urine for proteinuria and specific gravity once each shift. Monitor electrolytes.

Assess for signs of infection. Assess the child's comfort level and activity tolerance.

Implementation

Administer medications, and monitor for adverse effects of corticosteroids. If the child is receiving IV albumin, monitor closely for hypertension or signs of volume overload.

Implement careful hand hygiene and standard precautions. Use strict aseptic technique during invasive procedures.

Reduce exposure to individuals with respiratory infections and communicable diseases. Educate parents on signs of infection.

Meticulous skin care is implemented to prevent skin breakdown and potential infection.

Perform repeated skin assessments, turn the child frequently, and use therapeutic mattresses (e.g., egg crate, airflow mattress) to help prevent skin breakdown. Keep the skin clean and dry.

Meet nutritional and fluid needs. Keep the child's food preferences in mind when planning menus. Encourage the child to eat by presenting attractive meals with small portions. Socialization during meals may improve the child's appetite. Fluids are generally not restricted except during severe edema.

Promote rest with opportunities for quiet play.

Children may have a distorted body image related to sudden weight gain and edema. Encourage the child and parents to express their feelings and concerns.

Patient and Family Education

Explain the disease process, prognosis, medication administration, and the treatment plan.

Educate parents to monitor urine for protein daily and to maintain records. Encourage parents to monitor body weight and use a urine dipstick weekly during remission to identify early signs of a relapse.

Seek home tutoring until the child can return to school. Emphasize the importance of avoiding contact with individuals who have infectious diseases.

Acute Postinfectious Glomerulonephritis

Acute postinfectious glomerulonephritis (APIGN) is an inflammation of the glomeruli of the kidneys.

It is most often a response to a *group A beta-hemolytic streptococcal* infection of the skin or pharynx. An immune complex reaction localizes on the glomerular capillary wall, leading to inflammation and glomerular injury.

Obstructed glomerular capillaries reduce the glomerular filtration rate. Increased vascular permeability allows red blood cells, red cell casts, and eventually protein molecules to be excreted. Sodium and water are retained, resulting in edema. APIGN is a significant cause of acute and chronic renal failure (ARF and CRF) in children.

Clinical Manifestations

Abrupt onset with flank or midabdominal pain, irritability, malaise, and fever

Microscopic hematuria is present in nearly all cases, and gross hematuria, resulting in tea-colored urine, is found in up to 50% of cases and may last for 1 to 2 weeks; oliguria may or may not be present.

Mild periorbital edema occurs early along with dependent edema of the feet and ankles. Edema may progress in severity to cause a pulmonary effusion (dyspnea, cough, and crackles) or ascites (Gray, Huether, & Forshee, 2006). Acute hypertension may cause an encephalopathy that includes headache, nausea, vomiting, irritability, lethargy, and seizures.

Diagnostic Tests

Urinalysis reveals hematuria, proteinuria, and red and white cell casts.

Serum BUN and creatinine concentrations are elevated.

Serum protein is decreased (hypoalbuminemia) due to mild to moderate proteinuria.

The white blood cell count and erythrocyte sedimentation rate may be elevated. Serum lipid levels are increased in approximately 40% of cases.

Hemoglobin and hematocrit levels reveal anemia, which is common in the acute phase and is generally caused by dilution of the serum by the extracellular fluid. Anemia during the late phase is a result of hematuria.

An antistreptolysin O titer and anti-DNAse B titer help document strep throat and skin infections.

Renal biopsy is rarely required unless there is a progressive deterioration of renal function.

Clinical Therapy

Bed rest and supportive therapy are recommended during the acute phase.

Edema and mild to moderate hypertension should be treated with sodium restriction and a diuretic such as furosemide (Lau & Wyatt, 2005).

Immediate emergency care is needed for severe hypertension with cerebral dysfunction; medication such as hydralazine or diazoxide is administered intravenously.

A course of antibiotics may be given to ensure eradication of the original infectious agent.

Clinical signs, proteinuria, and hematuria resolve within several weeks. Most children recover without significant loss of renal function or recurrence of the disorder (Gray, Huether, & Forshee, 2006).

Nursing Management

Assessment

Monitor vital signs and fluid and electrolyte status, weigh daily, and monitor intake and output. Document urine-specific gravity. Assess the urine color to detect hematuria.

Assess for periorbital and dependent edema. Measure the abdominal girth. Auscultate heart and lung sounds every shift and note respiratory effort to detect signs of fluid overload (crackles, dyspnea, and cough).

Monitor blood pressure. Assess for signs of encephalopathy (headache, blurred vision, vomiting, decreased level of consciousness, confusion, and convulsions).

Assess the child's and parents' level of understanding and the availability of support.

Implementation

Carefully plan the child's fluid intake over the entire day. Make sure parents and visitors understand the need to limit fluids.

Monitor for signs of infection, and reduce the child's exposure to infection. Limit visitors, encourage good hand hygiene, and screen visitors for upper respiratory infections.

Bed rest is indicated during the acute phase. Reposition the child frequently. Protect skin over bony prominences. Elevate lower extremities. Maintain proper hygiene and dry skin.

In most cases a no-added-salt and low-protein diet is implemented. Encourage the anorexic child to eat by providing favorite foods in compliance with the diet.

Support parents who blame themselves for not responding more quickly to the child's initial symptoms. Discuss the etiology of the disease and the child's treatment, and correct misconceptions.

Patient and Family Education

Educate parents about the medication regimen, potential side effects, dietary restrictions, and signs and symptoms of complications. It may require 3 weeks for hypertension and gross hematuria to resolve, and longer for complete resolution of the disorder.

Educate parents to accurately assess the child's blood pressure and test urine for blood or protein.

Emphasize avoiding exposure of the child to individuals with upper respiratory tract infections.

Discuss plans for child's return to normal routine and activities, with periods allowed for rest.

Hemolytic Uremic Syndrome (HUS)

HUS is an acute renal disease and is the most common cause of acute renal failure in young children (Huether, 2006). HUS often linked to *E. coli* strain O157:H7, which is found in undercooked meat and unpasteurized milk (Fioirno & Raffaelli, 2006). *E. coli* bacteria have also been linked to petting zoos at fairs and festivals (CDC, 2006a). Ten to 15% of children with this infection will develop HUS (Fiorino & Raffaelli, 2006).

A toxin damages the lining of the glomeruli, collecting ducts, and distal tubules. The toxin damages the lining of the glomerular arterioles, causing the endothelial cells to swell and become occluded with platelets and fibrin clots. This partial occlusion damages the red blood cells, resulting in hemolytic anemia. Glomerular filtration is decreased, resulting in hematuria and proteinuria.

Clinical Manifestations

An episode of gastroenteritis with diarrhea, upper respiratory infection, or UTI precedes HUS onset by 1 to 2 weeks. HUS signs and symptoms include hypertension, pallor, bruising, and oliguria. The child may also be irritable and have fever, anorexia, abdominal pain, vomiting, diarrhea, mild jaundice, and edema or ascites. Neurologic involvement is indicated by irritability, lethargy, and seizures (Huether, 2006).

Diagnostic Testing

Urinalysis is indicated to detect hematuria and proteinuria.

Serum BUN and creatinine are elevated. Serum chemistries often reveal hyperkalemia and metabolic acidosis as a result of renal failure.

A peripheral blood smear with fragments of red blood cells, fibrin fragments, and a decreased platelet count confirms the diagnosis.

The platelet count is generally less than 150,000 per mm^3 (Razzaq, 2006).

The hemoglobin is generally less than 10g/dL (Fiorino & Raffaelli, 2006).

Clinical Therapy

Supportive treatment for the complications of ARF (fluid restriction and a high-calorie, high-carbohydrate diet low in protein, sodium, potassium, and phosphorus) is indicated.

Enteral nutrition may be needed.

Medications may include calcium gluconate or calcium chloride to replace calcium levels, aluminum hydroxide gel to bind to phosphorus, Kayexalate to remove excess potassium, and antihypertensive agents. Transfusions of fresh-packed red blood cells may be ordered to treat severe anemia. Platelets are given if the child is bleeding or if surgery is needed. Transfusions are carefully administered to prevent hypertension caused by hypervolemia.

About 40% of children need dialysis and approximately 3% to 5% of those affected will die (Fiorino, 2006). Peritoneal dialysis is preferred unless the child has severe colitis and abdominal tenderness. Some children may develop chronic renal failure; however, most regain normal renal function (Huether, 2006).

Nursing Management
Assessment
Monitor vital signs, neurologic signs, laboratory values including electrolytes, and blood counts. Monitor daily weights, and assess intake and output. Observe for signs of progressive renal impairment. Monitor for petechiae and ecchymosis. Monitor the child for abdominal discomfort from diarrhea or other gastrointestinal disturbances.

Assess the coping strategies of the child and family and their availability of support.

Implementation
Care is the same as for ARF (see Acute Renal Failure section).

Avoid invasive procedures, when possible, to prevent unnecessary bleeding.

Provide enteral nutrition, as necessary, during acute illness phase. When able to tolerate oral feeding, promote adequate nutritional intake by offering small-portion, high-calorie, high-carbohydrate foods that are low in sodium, potassium, and phosphorus. Monitor bowel sounds and for vomiting and diarrhea.

Encourage parents to participate in the child's care. Encourage parents to monitor siblings for signs of diarrhea or HUS.

Teach parents about medications, dietary and fluid restrictions, and reducing risk of consumption of contaminated beef.

Polycystic Kidney Disease
Polycystic kidney disease is an autosomal recessive and dominant genetic disorder in which cellular hyperplasia of the kidneys' collecting ducts causes dilation of the ducts. Fluid secreted into these ducts enables cyst sacs to form. The cysts become larger and fibrose, slowly replacing much of the kidney's mass and reducing renal function. Tubular atrophy may occur in some children, whereas others have minimal changes in renal function. Polycystic kidney disease is associated with liver abnormalities that progress in severity with age to fibrosis, portal hypertension, and biliary infection.

Newborns with severe PKD die shortly after birth from pulmonary hypoplasia.

Clinical Manifestations
Potter facies (low-set ears, small jaw, and a flattened nose) in children with autosomal recessive PKD.

Hypertension in early infancy, often severe.

Expected urine output or oliguria may occur.

Respiratory distress and feeding intolerance may occur due to enlarged kidneys (Davis & Avner, 2007).

As uremia develops, children have progressive developmental delay, growth failure, and renal osteodystrophy.

Diagnostic Tests

Sonogram or renal biopsy confirms the diagnosis; is often diagnosed on prenatal ultrasound.

Liver function tests are usually normal initially. A liver biopsy may be performed.

Clinical Therapy

Treatment is supportive.

Medications—diuretics for hypertension; antibiotics treat urinary tract infection; growth hormones may be administered to some children to promote growth.

Fluid and electrolyte abnormalities are managed.

Renal osteodystrophy is treated to suppress the parathyroid hormone.

Dialysis or kidney transplant, but liver problems complicate the child's health. Up to 20% to 30% of these children die by 15 years of age (Davis & Avner, 2007).

Other family members are screened for subclinical cases.

Nursing Management

Same as for the child with renal insufficiency and CRF. See Chronic Renal Failure section.

Observe the child for signs of progressive renal impairment.

Establish a home management plan focusing on medications, diet adequate in protein and calories, and management of acute gastrointestinal illnesses.

Refer the family for genetic counseling.

Acute Renal Failure

Acute renal failure (ARF) is a sudden loss of adequate renal function in which the kidneys are unable to clear metabolic wastes and to regulate extracellular fluid volume, sodium balance, and acid–base homeostasis.

ARF occurs in one of three ways:

- Prerenal—decreased perfusion to an otherwise normal kidney may occur in association with a systemic condition. Hypovolemia secondary to dehydration is generally the cause; however, alterations in renal vasculature or cardiac function may also precipitate prerenal ARF. Prerenal ARF is the most common type of ARF in infants and young children (Lum, 2007).
- Primary kidney damage (intrinsic factors) may result from infection, diseases such as hemolytic uremic syndrome or acute glomerulonephritis, cortical necrosis, nephrotoxic drugs, or accidental ingestion of drugs or poisons. Kidney tubule is the structure most susceptible to damage. Injury to the tubule resulting in acute tubular necrosis is the most frequent cause of intrinsic renal failure in children (Lum, 2007).
- Postrenal ARF is caused by obstruction of the urinary flow from both kidneys, such as occurs in posterior urethral valves or a neurogenic bladder. Children may have oliguria, or normal or increased urine output. Renal failure without oliguria usually indicates a less severe renal injury. Children who recover from ARF may have residual kidney damage and compromised renal function.

Clinical Manifestations

Characteristically, a healthy child suddenly experiences nonspecific symptoms that indicate a significant illness or injury (e.g., nausea, vomiting, edema, gross hematuria, oliguria, and hypertension). These symptoms are a result of electrolyte imbalances, uremia, and fluid overload. The child appears pale and lethargic.

Diagnostic Tests

Diagnosis of renal failure is based primarily on urinalysis and blood chemistry results, including BUN, serum creatinine, sodium, potassium, and calcium levels (Table 21–3).

Imaging studies assessing kidney structures, renal blood blow, and renal perfusion and function may be performed to determine whether the child has ARF or chronic renal failure; a renal biopsy may be required to examine the glomeruli.

Clinical Therapy

Treatment depends on the cause of the ARF.

Goal is to minimize or prevent permanent renal damage while maintaining fluid and electrolyte balance and managing complications.

Table 21–3 Diagnostic Tests for Renal Failure

Diagnostic Tests	Findings in Renal Failure
Urinalysis	
Ph	Acidic urine
Osmolarity	Greater than 500 prerenal ARF
	Less than 350 intrinsic ARF
Specific gravity	High prerenal ARF
	Low intrinsic ARF
	Normal: postrenal ARF
Protein	Positive
Serum Chemistry*	
Potassium	Elevated
Sodium	Normal, low, or high; depends solely on the amount of water in the body
Calcium	Low
Phosphorus	High
Urea nitrogen	Increased
Creatinine	Increased
pH	Low acidic

Note: ARF = Acute Renal Failure
*Please refer to chapter 5 for normal values.

IV fluid boluses with normal saline or lactated Ringer's solution are indicated for hypovolemia; albumin may be administered when blood loss is the cause of circulatory depletion.

Children with fluid overload, such as those with pulmonary edema, require diuretic therapy and dialysis if poor response to diuretics; fluid requirements are calculated to maintain zero water balance (intake should equal urine output and insensible fluid loss).

Eliminate all sources of potassium intake until hyperkalemia is controlled. Other electrolyte imbalances are treated.

Antibiotics are indicated for infection.

Nephrotoxic antibiotics such as aminoglycosides (e.g., gentamicin, vancomycin) should be avoided. Extra carbohydrate intake during the catabolic state is indicated.

Nursing Management

Assessment

Assess vital signs, level of consciousness, hydration status, peripheral perfusion, and signs of acute illness or injury. Assess for signs of electrolyte imbalance.

Weigh daily. Monitor urinalysis, urine culture, and blood chemistry studies. Inspect urine for color. Cloudy urine may indicate infection; tea-colored urine suggests hematuria. Assess urine-specific gravity and intake and output.

Assess the child's and parents' stressors, coping abilities, and the availability of support.

Implementation

- Estimate the child's fluid status by daily monitoring of intake and output and blood pressure two or three times daily. Also obtain a weight at least daily on the same scale at the same time of day. Monitor serum chemistry values, especially for sodium and potassium. The aim of maintaining fluid balance is to achieve a stable serum sodium concentration and a decrease in body weight by 0.5% to 1% a day.
- If the child has oliguria, limit all fluid intake, including parenteral nutrition, to replacement of insensible fluid loss, which is about one-third the daily maintenance requirements in afebrile children. Fluid requirements are increased by 12% for each centigrade degree of temperature elevation.
- If serum sodium concentration rises and weight falls, insufficient fluids have been given. If the serum sodium level falls and the weight increases, excessive fluids have been given.

Administer antibiotics and antihypertensive agents as prescribed. Monitor drug levels. Be alert to signs of drug toxicity.

Tailor the child's diet to nutritional need and high-metabolic rate. Parenteral or enteral feeding may be used until oral feeding is possible. Sodium, potassium, and phosphorus may be restricted. See Table 21–4.

Use standard precautions and thorough hand hygiene to prevent infection.

Encourage parents to verbalize fears and assist them in working through feelings of guilt. Explain procedures and treatment measures to decrease anxiety.

Teach parents to administer medications, correctly measure the blood pressure, and identify symptoms of progressive renal failure.

Table 21–4 Nutritional Information for the Child with Kidney Disease

High-Sodium Content Foods	High-Potassium Content Foods	High-Phosphorus Content Foods
Soups and sauces: such as gravy, spaghetti and tomato sauce, barbecue sauce, steak sauce	*Fruit:* apricots, avocados, bananas, citrus fruits, fresh pears, nectarines, dates, figs, cantaloupe and other melons, prunes, and raisins	*Dairy products:* milk, cheese, yogurt, custard, pudding, ice cream
Processed lunch meats: bologna, ham, salami, hot dogs, etc.	*Vegetables:* celery, dried beans, lima beans, potatoes, leafy greens, spinach, tomatoes, winter squash	Dried beans, peas
Smoked meat and fish: bacon, chipped beef, corned beef, ham, lox		Nuts, peanut butter
		Chocolate
		Dark cola
Sauerkraut, pickles, and other pickled foods	*Whole grains:* especially those containing bran	Sausage, hot dogs
Seasonings: horseradish, soy sauce, Worcestershire sauce, meat tenderizer, and monosodium glutamate (MSG)	Sardines, clams	
	Peanuts	
	Dairy products: milk, ice cream, pudding, yogurt	
	Potassium-containing salt substitutes	

Collaborate with a nutritionist to assist the family in appropriate food choices and menu planning, integrating ethnic and cultural food preferences.

Chronic Renal Failure

CRF is a progressive, irreversible reduction in kidney function that leads to end-stage renal disease (ESRD), the most advanced form of CRF. Long-term complications of CRF and ESRD include hypertension, anemia, bone disease, poor growth, and social developmental issues.

In children, CRF usually results from developmental abnormalities of the kidney, obstructed urine flow and reflux, hereditary diseases such as polycystic kidney disease, and infections such as hemolytic uremic syndrome and glomerulonephritis (Lum, 2007).

As renal failure progresses, metabolic acidosis occurs because the kidneys cannot excrete the acids that build up in the body.

Renal osteodystrophy occurs as the kidneys are unable to produce activated vitamin D and to excrete phosphorus, causing phosphorus levels to rise and serum calcium levels to fall.

The parathyroid gland responds by drawing calcium and phosphorus from the bones to maintain the adequate serum calcium and phosphorus levels.

Hypocalcemia may occur as the parathyroid glands become less responsive to vitamin D and lower serum calcium levels (Legg, 2005).

Growth retardation is caused by disturbances in the metabolism of calcium, phosphorus, and vitamin D; decreased caloric intake; and metabolic acidosis.

The healthy kidneys also produce erythropoietin (the growth factor responsible for the production and maturation of red cells); lack of erythropoietin and progressive renal disease are the underlying causes of the anemia of CRF.

Clinical Manifestations

Initially asymptomatic; as progression continues, renal insufficiency occurs with polyuria as the kidneys cannot concentrate the urine. Symptoms such as pallor, headache, nausea, and fatigue develop.

Decreased mental alertness and ability to concentrate may be seen.

The child may have anemia leading to tachycardia, tachypnea, and dyspnea on exertion.

As the disease progresses, the child experiences a loss of appetite and complications of renal impairment, including hypertension, pulmonary edema, growth retardation, osteodystrophy, delayed fine and gross motor development, and delayed sexual maturation.

In ESRD, uremic symptoms develop, including nausea, vomiting, anorexia, unpleasant (uremic) breath odor, progressive anemia, uremic frost (urea crystals deposited on the skin), pruritus, malaise, headache, progressive confusion, tremors, pulmonary edema, dyspnea, and congestive heart failure.

Diagnostic Testing

The child's glomerular filtration rate (GFR) is calculated from prediction equations using the serum creatinine level and the patient's height and gender. Imaging studies are indicated to identify kidney damage. A renal biopsy may sometimes be performed.

Serum electrolyte, phosphate, BUN, creatinine levels, and pH are taken to monitor fluid and electrolyte status; see Table 21–5 for findings related to renal failure.

Table 21–5   Medications Commonly Used by Children with Chronic Renal Failure (CRF)

Medication	Nursing Considerations
Vitamin and mineral supplement (Nephrocaps)	Only prescribed vitamins should be used; over-the-counter brands may contain elements that are harmful.
Phosphate-binding agents: calcium carbonate (Tums), calcium acetate (PhosLo) or sevelamer hydrochloride (Renagel)	Ensure that the phosphate-binding agent is aluminum-free.
Calcitriol (Rocaltrol)	Monitor serum calcium level. Ensure that a calcium supplement is provided.
Epoetin alfa (Epogen, Procrit)	Given by IV or SC injection. Monitor blood pressure, as hypertension is an adverse effect. Monitor hematocrit and serum ferritin level according to facility guidelines.
Iron supplementation	May be administered orally or by IV during hemodialysis.
Growth hormone	Record accurate height measurements at regular intervals.
Antihypertensive agents: angiotensin-converting enzyme inhibitor (enalapril, lisinopril) Loop diuretics	Monitor renal function and electrolyte balance.

Note: ESRD= end-stage renal disease.

Clinical Therapy

Goals of treatment are to slow the progression of kidney disease, prevent complications, and promote growth and development, using a combination of dietary, fluid, and electrolyte management and hypertension control. Treatment is modified as the child's status changes.

- Dietary management focuses on maximizing caloric intake for growth while limiting phosphorus, potassium, and sodium as needed to maintain electrolyte levels in balance (Vogt & Avner, 2007b).

- Adequate calcium needs to be part of the meal plan: Enteral or parenteral feedings may be required to achieve optimal protein intake, especially in children under 1 year of age.
- Complex carbohydrates should be chosen along with vegetables and fruits that are lower in potassium. Vegetable oils, hard candy, sugar, honey, and jelly may be recommended to add calories to the child's diet.
- Growth hormone helps some children achieve their target height.
- Phosphate-binding agents, vitamin D, and calcium supplementation are used to prevent some of the bone demineralization associated with renal osteodystrophy.
- Children who progress to ESRD require renal replacement therapy. See Renal Replacement Therapy section.

Nursing Management

Assessment
Observe for signs of edema, poor growth and development, osteodystrophy, and anemia. Assess vital signs, particularly blood pressure. Observe for signs of electrolyte alterations.

Implementation
Assess for signs of electrolyte imbalance such as weakness, muscle cramps, dizziness, headache, and nausea and vomiting in children who are taking diuretics.

Emphasize to the child and family the importance of good hand hygiene practices.

Monitor for signs of infection.

Provide small, frequent feedings and attractive meals, while adhering to food restrictions. Acknowledge the child's preferences in meal planning.

Plan the child's 24-hour fluid intake so the child has some fluids with meals, to take medications, and when thirsty. Use medicine cups or small cups for fluids given. Ensure that all visitors know and maintain the child's fluid restriction.

The parents and child need opportunities to express and work through their feelings related to the disease, prognosis, and treatment restrictions. Help children express their feelings through drawings or therapeutic play.

Support school-age children and adolescents who are embarrassed about their appearance and perceived differences from peers.

Patient and Family Education

Provide information about the disease process, dialysis treatments, and kidney transplantation as the disease progresses. Stress the importance of long-term treatments.

Identify a consistent time within the family routine for medication administration. Educate the family about side effects of medications and complications associated with the disease.

Emphasize the need for the 23-valent pneumococcal and meningococcal vaccines. Immunization with live-virus vaccines should occur before kidney transplantation.

Promote social development and interaction with other children while attempting to reduce exposure to infection. Schedule dialysis to allow the child to participate in school.

Educate the school nurse and teachers about dialysis treatment and how to assist the child when a peritoneal dialysis exchange needs to occur during the day.

Assist in selecting clothing to cover the dialysis shunt site and to complement and enhance the child's physical appearance.

Refer to the National Kidney Foundation and local support groups.

Develop a plan for adolescents to transition from pediatric to adult services.

Renal Replacement Therapy
Peritoneal Dialysis

The abdominal peritoneum is the membrane through which the body's waste products pass from the blood to the abdominal cavity. The dialysis solution that enters the abdomen through a catheter typically contains dextrose that pulls body wastes and extra fluid into the abdominal cavity. The wastes and extra fluid leave the body with the drained dialysate.

Continuous ambulatory peritoneal dialysis uses gravity to instill prefilled bags of dialysis solution into the peritoneal cavity four or five times a day. The fluid remains in the cavity for 4 to 8 hours and is then drained by hanging the bag lower than the pelvis.

Automated peritoneal dialysis uses an automatic cycler to instill and drain the dialysate approximately five times over a 10-hour period, usually overnight. One additional exchange may be needed during the day. With this method, the number of connections and disconnections is minimized, which reduces demands on the family as well as the risk of infection. Of the peritoneal dialysis types, this method is used most often in children (Warady & Chada, 2007).The primary complications are peritonitis and abdominal hernia. Peritonitis is treated with antibiotics infused in the dialysate.

Nursing Management

Educate the child and family to perform peritoneal dialysis and catheter care using sterile technique to reduce the risk of peritonitis.

Assist the family to develop home routines that minimize disruptions to attending school and daily family life. Reinforce the importance of adhering to the prescribed diet and daily exchanges.

Hemodialysis

- Hemodialysis is a process in which the blood flows from the patient through a machine with a special filter that removes body wastes and extra fluids. Blood is pumped out of the body and through a dialyzer, where waste products and extra fluids diffuse out across a semipermeable membrane, before the blood is returned to the body.

- Hemodialysis for children is offered in a special dialysis center on an outpatient basis, or it can be performed at bedside during hospitalization. Treatment is usually performed three times a week, with each session lasting approximately 3 to 4 hours.

- Vascular access is accomplished with an arteriovenous fistula, a synthetic graft between the arterial and venous circulation, or a double-lumen cannula inserted into a large vein. Two needles are inserted, one to carry blood to the dialyzer and one to return cleaned blood to the body.

- Hemodialysis is more efficient than peritoneal dialysis but requires close monitoring for symptoms related to hypotension or rapid changes in fluid and electrolyte balance. Disequilibrium syndrome (rapid changes in the body's water and electrolyte balance during treatment) may occur during or soon after the dialysis procedure is first initiated. Other complications include access thrombosis and infection. Heparin is used to reduce the risk of thrombosis.

Nursing Management

Monitor vital signs, blood pressure, oral intake, and urinary output every half hour while the child is on the dialysis equipment. Weigh the child before and after the dialysis to determine any fluid imbalances that require adjustment during the next hemodialysis session.

Educate the child and family about the administration of heparin and the control of bleeding from minor trauma.

Reinforce dietary limitations, and review menu planning to assure that the child's daily nutritional needs are met.

Encourage daily care to the catheter site and showering rather than tub baths. Activities such as swimming should be discouraged.

Kidney Transplantation

A kidney transplant is the only alternative to long-term dialysis for children with ESRD. Blood-type compatibility between the donor and recipient is required, and a human leukocyte antigen system match graft improves survival. A living-relative donor kidney has a higher survival rate than a cadaver kidney.

Children and their families are screened carefully prior to transplant in an effort to identify problems that could lead to rejection of the kidney or infection that could be life threatening if the immune system is suppressed.

After transplantation, the child must take immunosuppressive medications such as corticosteroids, azathioprine, cyclosporine, tacrolimus, and monoclonal antibodies to suppress rejection. Immunosuppression regimens use various combinations and sequences of these drugs to reduce the incidence of acute and chronic rejection. Chronic rejection is the most prominent cause of transplanted kidney loss (Benfield, 2003).

Signs of rejection include fever, increased BUN and serum creatinine levels, pain and tenderness over the abdomen, irritability, and weight gain. However, because the size of the kidney transplanted is often large in comparison to the child's size, rejection may be further advanced before symptoms appear, making it more difficult to reverse the rejection process (Benfield, 2003).

Complications of immunosuppressive therapy include opportunistic infection, lymphomas and skin cancer, and hypertension. Nonadherence with therapy is the primary cause of transplanted kidney loss in 10% to 15% of all pediatric kidney transplant recipients.

Nonadherence is highest among families in crises without adequate support and in adolescents who refuse or forget to take their medications, have mild cognitive impairment, or have depression (Feinstein, Keich, Becker-Cohen, et al., 2005). Adherence is higher in adolescents when their parents are knowledgeable and supportive, and when they promote the adolescent to become competent in self-care. Some primary kidney diseases, such as glomerulonephritis and hemolytic uremic syndrome, can also recur in the transplanted kidney.

Nursing Management

Educate the child and family about the transplantation process and protocols for immunosuppression. Emphasize that adherence to treatments is essential for the success of the transplant.

Educate the family about signs of acute rejection and infection and when to call the child's physician.

Evaluate the child's and parents' understanding of and adherence to the prescribed regimen.

Education is ongoing, and requires frequent evaluation of child and parental understanding. Monitor adherence to immunosuppressive treatment at each visit in an effort to identify any issues early.

Families and children need to understand that nonadherence places them at risk for rejection of the kidney and return to dialysis.

STRUCTURAL DEFECTS OF THE REPRODUCTIVE SYSTEM

Phimosis

The foreskin over the glans penis cannot be retracted in infants and young males owing to natural adhesion; however, the foreskin usually separates from the glans during childhood and retracts. Narrowing of the preputial opening may obstruct urine flow and cause balanitis, inflammation, or infection of the glans penis. *Paraphimosis*, inability of the foreskin to return to its normal position over the glans, constricts the penis, is a medical emergency, and must be relieved by surgery.

Circumcision, surgical removal of the foreskin, has long been a common practice performed in some countries and cultures during the newborn period. It is performed to prevent phimosis, for ease of proper male hygiene, and to prevent urinary tract infections and penile cancer. Circumcision is contraindicated in neonates with blood dyscrasias, family history of bleeding disorder, and those that are premature. Anomalies such as hypospadias, epispadias, and chordee are also contraindications since the foreskin may be needed for later reconstruction (Steadman & Ellsworth, 2006).

Betamethasone cream (0.05%) applied twice daily for 4 to 8 weeks to the outer prepuce is an effective alternative to surgery for phimosis and has few side effects. Often the child is able to achieve foreskin retraction without surgery (Steadman & Ellsworth, 2006).

Nursing Management

Educate parents about care of the uncircumcised newborn male, and tell them to avoid forcibly retracting the foreskin. Educate the older child to return the foreskin to its normal position after cleaning to avoid constricting blood flow.

If circumcision is requested by parents of the newborn or it is the method of treatment for phimosis, nursing care focuses on preoperative preparation of the infant, including the advocacy for and assistance in giving the newborn local anesthesia.

Postoperatively, the nurse assesses the infant's vital signs and the operative site for bleeding, and urination. If topical steroids are prescribed as treatment for phimosis, educate the parents about application of the medication.

Patient and Family Education

After circumcision, educate the parents to cover the head of the penis with a small amount of petroleum jelly with each diaper change until the redness goes away.

Pale-yellow, sticky drainage may form on the head of the penis and is a normal part of the healing process.

Squeeze soapy water over the head of penis once a day, rinse with warm water, and pat dry.

The diaper should fit appropriately—not too loose as that may cause rubbing with movement and not too tight as that may cause pain.

Parents should be advised to contact the healthcare provider if there is increased redness, bleeding, or swelling of the head of the penis.

Cryptorchidism (Undescended Testes)

In *cryptorchidism*, one or both testes fail to descend through the inguinal canal into the scrotum. Normally, the testes descend during the seventh to ninth month of gestation. Causes include a testosterone deficiency, an absent or defective testis, a structural problem such as a narrow inguinal canal, a short spermatic cord, or adhesions. This disorder occurs in 3% to 6% of term male infants and in 20% to 30% of preterm infants (Morgan & McCance, 2006).

The higher temperature in the abdomen compared to the scrotum results in morphologic changes to the testis that are apparent by 1 year of age. Complications of cryptorchidism include infertility and malignancy.

Clinical Manifestations

Palpation of the scrotum fails to reveal one or both testes, and an inguinal hernia may also be present. In a majority of cases, the testes descend spontaneously by 3 months of age. An undescended testis may be located in the inguinal canal, abdomen, perineum, or even the thigh.

Diagnostic Tests

Although diagnosis is made on physical examination, diagnostic studies including ultrasound, CT scan, and MRI are utilized to determine the location of the testes. A diagnostic laparoscope may also be needed to locate the testis. When neither testis can be palpated, hormonal and chromosomal evaluation may be performed to detect an intersex disorder.

Clinical Therapy

If the testis does not descend spontaneously, an orchiopexy is performed at 1 year of age before further damage occurs. An incision made at the testicle's location allows blood vessels to be disentangled so the testis reaches the lower scrotum. The testis is stitched to the inside wall of the scrotum to keep it in place.

Nursing Management

Prepare the parents and infant for the outpatient surgical procedure, and address parents' concerns.

Postoperatively, focus on maintaining comfort, monitoring urine output, and preventing infection. Administer prescribed analgesics.

Educate the parents to gently clean the incision site with each diaper change and to identify signs of infection. Provide guidelines for pain medication administration.

Sponge bathe the child for 2 days after surgery, and then a tub bath may be given. No medicine or ointment should be placed over the incision. Teach parents to identify signs of infection such as redness, warmth, swelling, and discharge and to notify the physician if present. Inform parents to avoid straddling the infant across the hip and to permit no strenuous activity or straddle-toy riding for 2 weeks after surgery to promote healing and to prevent injury.

Teach adolescents to perform monthly testicular examinations.

Inguinal Hernia and Hydrocele

An inguinal hernia is a painless inguinal or scrotal swelling that occurs when abdominal tissue, such as bowel, protrudes into the groin.

A hydrocele is a fluid-filled mass in the scrotum that often resolves spontaneously by 1 year of age (Elder, 2007). The major complication of an inguinal hernia is incarceration (intestinal strangulation and testicular ischemia).

Clinical Manifestations

Diagnosis is made by physical examination at birth or in early infancy. Palpation of the scrotum reveals a round, smooth, nontender mass that is noted with either a hernia or hydrocele. Parents may report an intermittent bulge in the groin or swelling in the scrotum. Swelling associated with a hernia may become more apparent with straining and reduced in size when the child is quiet or asleep.

Clinical Therapy

Outpatient surgery for repair of inguinal hernia is performed as an elective procedure at an early age (usually after 3 months of age to reduce anesthesia risks) to avoid incarceration (hernia cannot be reduced and circulation to trapped tissue is impaired), which is a medical emergency. A nerve block may be given in the operating room to reduce postoperative pain. Surgical intervention for a hydrocele is rarely required.

Nursing Management

Before surgery, assess the newborn for signs of incarceration.

Postoperative care includes monitoring of vital signs and inspection of the incision for swelling, bleeding, or drainage. Assess the circulation in the leg on the side of the surgical repair to detect any potential blood flow obstruction resulting from edema of the groin. Assess for pain.

Educate the parents about incision site care, signs of infection, and the expected appearance of the scrotum (often bruised and edematous). Encourage provision of pain medication at home.

Testicular Torsion

Testicular torsion is an emergency condition in which the testis suddenly rotates on its spermatic cord, obstructing its blood supply, leading to vascular engorgement and ischemia. Often the testicles are positioned horizontally in the scrotum, a congenital anomaly known as a bell clapper deformity, which predisposes the male to this condition (Eaton et al., 2005).Testicular torsion most often occurs as a result from trauma to the scrotum, but can occur during sporting activities, exercise, and sexual activity. The affected testis is positioned higher in the scrotum than the unaffected testis because of the shortened vascular pedicle.

Clinical Manifestations

Severe pain and erythema in the scrotum, nausea and vomiting, abdominal pain, and scrotal swelling that is not relieved by rest or scrotal support may be present.

The testes are tender to palpation and become edematous; cremasteric reflex is absent.

Clinical Therapy

Diagnosis is based on signs and symptoms. Doppler ultrasonography and radionuclide imaging are the most commonly used tests used to confirm the diagnosis. One of these tests may be performed to confirm the diagnosis prior to surgery if it can be performed immediately (Ringdahl & Teague, 2006).

When testicular torsion is reduced within 6 hours after onset of symptoms, there is a 90% chance of saving the testis. Manual reduction under intravenous sedation may be attempted, but emergency surgery is more common and is the only way to ensure resolution of the problem (Ringdahl & Teague, 2006). The procedure is usually performed bilaterally to prevent future torsion in the other testis. If torsion was reduced manually, elective orchiopexy is recommended to prevent recurrence (Ringdahl & Teague, 2006).

Nursing Management

Assess the child's symptoms, and recognize that pain and swelling in the scrotum is a true emergency. Provide analgesics, as ordered, and prepare the child for surgery. Educate the adolescent and family about the surgery and the need for rapid intervention. Reassure the child and family that fertility should not be affected because only one testis is affected.

Provide guidelines for home care of the incision, pain management, and avoidance of strenuous activity or lifting heavy objects for 2 weeks after surgery. Teach the adolescent to perform testicular self-examination.

SEXUALLY TRANSMITTED INFECTIONS

Sexually transmitted infections (STIs) are caused by organisms of bacterial, parasitic, and viral origin. Children and adolescents can become infected with sexually transmitted organisms through sexual experimentation, sexual play, molestation, and sexual abuse. Some diseases, such as chlamydia, syphilis, and gonorrhea, acquired after the neonatal period are almost always indicative of sexual contact (Hornor, 2004).

When a child younger than 10 years is infected, consider the possibility of sexual abuse.

See Table 21–6 for clinical manifestations and clinical therapy for STIs.

Nursing Management
Assessment
Key areas to discuss when obtaining a sexual history include information related to partners, pregnancy prevention, protection from sexually transmitted infections, sexual practices, and past history of STIs (CDC, 2006c).

Table 21–6 Clinical Manifestations of Common Sexually Transmitted Infections

Sexually Transmitted Infection	Clinical Manifestations and Complications	Clinical Therapy and Patient Education
Chlamydia *Chlamydia trachomatis*	Adolescent females: yellow mucopurulent endocervical discharge, dysuria, pelvic pain, mild abdominal pain, vaginal spotting, cervicitis, salpingitis, pelvic inflammatory disease (PID); 75% are asymptomatic (Grimshaw-Mulchay, 2006). Adolescent males: urethritis (an infection of the urethra), mucoid gray or clear discharge, dysuria, proctitis, epididymitis; 50% are asymptomatic (Grimshaw-Mulchay, 2006). Complications associated with chlamydia in females include pelvic inflammatory disease (PID) and infertility. Chlamydia is a leading cause of early pneumonia and conjunctivitis in newborns.	Diagnosis by culture or a nucleic-acid-amplified test on the urine. Recommended medication therapy includes doxycyline or erythromycin for 7 days, or single-dose azithromycin. HIV-positive persons with chlamydia receive the same treatment as those who are HIV negative. All sexual partners should be evaluated, tested, and treated. Abstain from sexual intercourse until individual and all sex partners have completed treatment to prevent reinfection. Encourage use of condoms. All sexually active female adolescents should be screened at least annually for chlamydia.

Table 21–6 Clinical Manifestations of Common Sexually Transmitted Infections (Continued)

Sexually Transmitted Infection	Clinical Manifestations and Complications	Clinical Therapy and Patient Education
Genital herpes *Herpes simplex virus 1* (HSV-1) or 2 (HSV-2)	Most infected with HSV-2 are not aware of their infection. Presentation can be variable and ranges from no symptoms to systemic involvement. Common symptoms include dull pain, itching, and small lesions or pimples on genitalia, buttocks, or thighs. Two types of lesions develop, either fluid-filled blisters on an erythematous base or, more commonly, painful papules and ulcers. Ulcers can appear between vaginal folds, in posterior cervix, on glans penis or shaft of penis, in rectum, or in anus. Ulcers heal within 2–4 weeks. Lymph nodes closest to lesions are frequently enlarged. Disease frequently recurs four to five times a year with episodes lasting 5–10 days. Triggers include stress, menses, or trauma.	Diagnosis is confirmed by virology and type-specific serologic tests. There is no permanent cure. Recommended drug therapy is acyclovir given for 7–10 days. Antiviral medications can shorten and prevent outbreaks during the period of time the person takes the medication. Daily suppressive therapy for herpes can reduce transmission to partners. A cesarean delivery is usually performed for infected pregnant women. Discourage oral sex if ulcers are present in mouth, on lips, in vagina, or on penis. Discourage anal sex when lesions are active. Encourage use of condoms, although they may not prevent transmission. Emphasize that the patient remains contagious, even after lesions are healed.
Gonorrhea *Neisseria gonorrhoeae*	Symptoms and severity vary from mild to severe and are different for males and females. In females, areas that can be infected include urethra, cervix, fallopian tubes, and Bartholin and Skene glands.	Diagnosed by culture of vaginal or urethral discharge or nucleic-acid-amplified test on the urine. Recommended drug therapy includes a single dose of ceftriaxone IM or Cefixime orally in one dose.

Table 21–6 Clinical Manifestations of Common Sexually Transmitted Infections (Continued)

Sexually Transmitted Infection	Clinical Manifestations and Complications	Clinical Therapy and Patient Education
	In males, areas include urethra, prostate, seminal vesicles, epididymis, and Littre and Cowper glands. Of females, 51% are asymptomatic (Burstein & Murray, 2003). The classic sign is discharge from the vagina and urethra; however, infections involving conjunctiva, pharynx, and anus area are also seen. Prepubescent girls: heavy, thick, green or creamy vaginal discharge, vulvovaginitis. Pubescent girls: purulent vaginal discharge, cervicitis. Fallopian tube and pelvic inflammatory disease involvement can lead to sterility. Prepubescent and adolescent boys: yellow purulent urethral discharge, erythematous meatus, frequency, dysuria, and painful or swollen testicles. Although many men with gonorrhea may have no symptoms at all, some men have some signs or symptoms that appear 2 to 5 days after infection; symptoms can take as long as 30 days to appear.	Sexual partners should be treated if adolescent has had sexual contact within 60 days of onset of symptoms. Encourage use of condoms or abstinence. Emphasize the importance of taking all of the medication prescribed to cure gonorrhea. The individual and all sex partners must avoid sex until they have completed their treatment for gonorrhea.

Table 21–6 Clinical Manifestations of Common Sexually Transmitted Infections (Continued)

Sexually Transmitted Infection	Clinical Manifestations and Complications	Clinical Therapy and Patient Education
	Signs and symptoms of rectal infection in both genders include discharge, anal itching, soreness, bleeding, or painful bowel movements, though individuals may be asymptomatic. Infections in the throat may cause a sore throat but are usually asymptomatic. Transmission to the neonate during vaginal delivery can cause blindness, joint infection, or sepsis. Gonorrhea is a common cause of PID.	
Human papillomavirus (HPV)	The most common STI in the United States (CDC, 2006b). Warts are small, flat, and fleshy-colored with a cauliflower appearance. Adolescent females: warts clustered or alone on the vulva, perineal area, vagina, or cervix; itching, bleeding, burning, irritation. A subclinical infection may be detected through a Pap smear. Specific types of HPV cause 90% of cervical cancers (AAP, 2006). Adolescent males: may be asymptomatic; warts on the penis, near base of penis on scrotal skin, or near anus.	Diagnosis is based upon physical findings or biopsy. The PAP smear may be abnormal. No cure exists. Treatment for external genital warts may include cryotherapy, topical podophyllin resin, Imiquimod 5% cream, Podofilox 9.5% solution or gel. Encourage abstinence or condom use, but condoms are not sufficient to prevent contact transmission. The disorder is transmissible even after treatment. Encourage females to receive the HPV vaccine (see chapter 19).

Table 21–6 Clinical Manifestations of Common Sexually Transmitted Infections (Continued)

Sexually Transmitted Infection	Clinical Manifestations and Complications	Clinical Therapy and Patient Education
Trichomoniasis *Trichomonas Vaginalis*	Adolescent females: pale yellow to gray-green discharge that may be frothy or have a fishy odor, dysuria, vulvar pruritis, occasional abdominal pain; symptoms worsen during menses; more commonly have symptoms than males. Adolescent males: most common site is the urethra; mucoid or purulent urethral discharge, pruritis, dysuria; however, males are usually asymptomatic.	Diagnosis is made by culture. Recommended drug therapy includes Metronidazole or Tinidazole orally as a single dose or Metronidazole orally twice a day for 7 days. Both partners should be treated at the same time to eliminate the parasite. Alcoholic beverages should be avoided during and for several days after treatment if a single dose is used. Sexual contact should be avoided until both partners are cured. No follow-up test is needed if symptoms resolve after treatment.
Syphilis *Treponema Pallidum*	Appearance of classic signs and symptoms of syphilis depends on stage of disease. *Primary stage* manifests as an ulcer on labia, within vagina, on penis, in anus, or on lips or tongue that appears at invasion site approximately 2 weeks to 3 months after infection. Ulcer has an indurated border and smooth base (chancre), and it is painless. Lymphadenopathy is usually present. Ulcer spontaneously heals within 5 weeks.	Diagnosis is made by serologic tests or direct fluorescent antibody tests of lesion exudates. Due to the risk of fetal death, every pregnant woman should have a blood test for syphilis. Syphilis is easy to cure in its early stages. Recommended drug therapy includes single IM injection of benzathine penicillin G. For children allergic to penicillin, erythromycin PO is prescribed for 15 days.

Table 21–6   Clinical Manifestations of Common Sexually Transmitted Infections (Continued)

Sexually Transmitted Infection	Clinical Manifestations and Complications	Clinical Therapy and Patient Education
	Second stage: appears up to 10 weeks after initial infection with fever, malaise, lymphadenopathy, patchy alopecia, and diffuse rash. Rash can be macular, papular, papulosquamous, or bullous, and appearance on the palms and soles is classic. Flat mucous patches called condylomata latum appear on genitals. *Latent stage:* asymptomatic, follows the second stage by about 6 weeks. It can last for several years or be lifelong. *Tertiary stage:* occurs more than 2 years after onset and manifests as neurosyphillis, cardiovascular disease, or ophthalmic or congenital syphilis.	Saline compresses and a topical antibiotic are often used to treat lesions on the skin. Treat all sexual contacts within the past 90 days to 1 year of diagnosis, depending on stage when diagnosed. During syphilis treatment, abstain from sexual contact with new partners until the syphilis sores are completely healed. Encourage abstinence or the use of condoms plus spermicidal foams, cream, or jelly to prevent infection.

Source: Data from *Red Book: Report of the Committee on Infectious Disease* (26th ed.), American Academy of Pediatrics, 2006, Chicago, IL.; "Diagnosis and Management of Sexually Transmitted Disease Pathogens among Adolescents," by G. R. Burstein & P. J. Murray, 2003, *Pediatrics in Review, 24*(3), 75–81; "HPV and HPV Vaccine Information for Health Care Providers," Centers for Disease Control and Prevention, 2006f, accessed May 27, 2007, from http://www.cdc.gov/std/HPV/hpv-vacc-hcp-3-pages.pdf; "Sexually Transmitted Diseases Treatment Guidelines, 2006," Centers for Disease Control and Prevention, 2006, *Morbidity and Mortality Weekly Report, 55* (RR-11), 1–94; "Chlamydia: Diagnosing the Hidden STD," by L. J. Grimshaw-Mulcahy, 2006, *The Clinical Advisor*, 32–41; and "Update to CDC's *Sexually Transmitted Diseases Treatment Guidelines, 2006*: Fluoroquinolones No Longer Recommended for Treatment of Gonococcal Infections," Centers for Disease Control and Prevention, 2007d, *Morbidity and Mortality Weekly Report, 56*(14), 332–336.

Identify signs and symptoms indicative of STIs during the physical examination. Routine screening of sexually active adolescents is recommended. When a child or adolescent is diagnosed with one STI, screen for the presence of others.

Assess the adolescent's anxiety or concern about an infection or fear that parents will be notified.

Implementation

Educate the adolescent about the specific infection diagnosed, its treatment, the need to complete all doses, potential adverse effects, and recommended follow-up. Reinforce the need to notify all sexual partners for treatment.

Provide psychological support, as the adolescent may be upset, ashamed, embarrassed, or angry about having the infection.

Encourage sexually active adolescents to receive hepatitis B immunization and HPV immunization if not already obtained. Counsel the adolescent on ways to reduce the risk of contracting STIs.

Refer the child with signs of an STI for evaluation of sexual assault by a facility or healthcare provider specializing in collecting evidence and providing specialized care. Similarly, refer any adolescent who has been sexually assaulted to a sexual assault nurse examiner or other healthcare provider who can collect evidence, coordinate medical treatment, and coordinate mental health support.

Patient and Family Education

Educate adolescents about the risk for STIs, potential complications, and methods to prevent an STI.

Abstinence is the best prevention.

Limit the number of sexual contacts; practice mutual monogamy.

Always use condoms and spermicidal gels or foams for vaginal and anal intercourse.

Refrain from oral sex if the partner has active sores in mouth, vagina, anus, or on the penis.

Reduce high-risk sexual behaviors. Use of recreational drugs and alcohol can increase sexual risk-taking.

Seek care as soon as symptoms are noticed, make sure the partner gets treatment, and avoid sexual intercourse until the STI is cured.

Seek annual screening, as some STIs have no symptoms.

Pelvic Inflammatory Disease

PID is an infection of the upper genital tract caused by the ascending spread of organisms in the cervix and vagina. It is usually caused by *Chlamydia trachomatis* or *Neisseria gonorrhea*.

Clinical Manifestations

Mild or dull bilateral lower abdominal pain or right upper quadrant pain.

Dysmenorrhea that is more severe or longer lasting than usual.

Dysuria, vaginal discharge, pain with sexual activity, prolonged or increased menstrual bleeding, nausea and vomiting.

Diagnostic Tests

Clinical findings, such as uterine or adnexal tenderness or tenderness with cervical motion with pelvic examination.

Elevated erythrocyte sedimentation rate, elevated C-reactive protein level, and white blood cells seen on microscopic examination of vaginal secretions, and documented cervical infection with gonorrhea or chlamydia (CDC, 2006f).

A transvaginal sonogram may reveal thickened and fluid-filled fallopian tubes with or without free pelvic fluid.

Clinical Therapy

Parenteral antibiotic therapy is often used for the first 24 hours before converting to oral antibiotics for the remaining 14 days of treatment. Common intravenous antibiotics used include a combination of cefotetan or cefoxitin plus doxycycline. If doxycycline is contraindicated, clindamycin plus gentamycin may be substituted (CDC, 2006f). Oral regimens include ceftriaxone or cefoxitin, plus doxycycline with or without metronidazole (CDC, 2007e). Follow-up physical examination is performed in 72 hours to ensure treatment adherence and to detect improvement in symptoms and reduced tenderness of the uterus, adnexae, and cervix. Rehospitalization and IV antibiotics are initiated if no improvement is noted.

Nursing Management

Identify the risk for STIs and PID in all adolescent females. Administer medications intravenously for the first 24 hours, making arrangements for the adolescent to return for a second dose 12 hours after the first. Provide education for the ongoing treatment with oral antibiotics, ensuring that the adolescent understands the importance of taking all medications on schedule for the full 14 days. Provide signs of adverse effects and actions to take if they occur.

Assist the adolescent to discuss the health problem with the parents.

Provide counseling about methods to reduce the risk for reinfection. Provide information about the potential PID consequences, such as infertility, ectopic pregnancy, and chronic abdominal pain.

Encourage regular health visits with screening for STIs, as future *Chlamydia* and gonorrhea infections may be asymptomatic.

22 ALTERATIONS IN ENDOCRINE FUNCTION

DISORDERS OF PITUITARY FUNCTION

Diabetes Insipidus

Diabetes insipidus is a disorder of the posterior pituitary gland. Two forms of diabetes insipidus occur: central (neurogenic) antidiuretic hormone (ADH) deficiency and familial nephrogenic diabetes insipidus. Both disorders involve ADH, a hormone secreted by the posterior pituitary gland. In normal circumstances, thirst is the regulator for ADH release (Kache & Ferry, 2005). The most important function of ADH is to bind to the collecting ducts of the kidney and promote reabsorption of water back into the circulation.

ADH facilitates concentration of the urine by stimulating reabsorption of water from the distal tubule of the kidney. When ADH is inadequate, the tubules do not resorb water, leading to polyuria (passage of a large volume of urine in a given period) and severe dehydration. The urine cannot be concentrated, no matter how dehydrated the child becomes.

Clinical Manifestations

Both forms of diabetes insipidus have an abrupt onset and similar manifestations:

Central diabetes insipidus—polyuria, polydipsia, hypernatremia, nocturia, enuresis, thirsty at night, irritable if fluids withheld, constipation, fever, and dehydration

Nephrogenic—polyuria, polydipsia, hypernatremia in neonatal period, dilute urine, vomiting, dehydration, fever, and mental status changes

Diagnostic Tests

Serum sodium is elevated; urine osmolality is decreased (less than 300 mOsm/L).

Urine specific gravity is decreased (less than 1.005).

Urine-to-serum osmolatity ratio is less than 1 (Kache & Ferry, 2005).

Diagnosis confirmed by plasma arginine vasopressin level before and after a water deprivation test.

Clinical Therapy

Water replacement therapy is essential to prevent severe dehydration and hypotension.

Central (neurogenic) diabetes insipidus is treated with intranasal, intravenous, oral, or subcutaneous desmopressin acetate (DDAVP); dose must be titered for sufficient coverage of metabolic needs while not high enough to cause water overload (Raine et al., 2006).

Nephrogenic diabetes insipidus is treated with thiazide diuretics and a high fluid intake. The child's sodium and potassium levels must be carefully monitored to prevent hypernatremia and hypokalemia (Kache & Ferry, 2005; Raine et al., 2006).

Nursing Management

Assessment

Assess for signs of fluid volume deficit, monitoring and documenting intake and output and specific gravity.

Weigh daily, assess skin integrity and mucous membranes, assess fontanels in infants.

Monitor vital signs and level of consciousness.

Implementation

Administer replacement fluids, and keep fluids within child's reach at all times.

Notify healthcare team if there are signs of dehydration or no decrease in urine output after administration of desmopressin acetate. Monitor serum osmolality and sodium for increasing values; report decreasing specific gravity.

Patient and Family Education

Educate parents about making fluids available to the child as needed, administering DDAVP, obtaining and recording daily weights, measuring intake and output, and recognizing signs of inadequate fluid intake.

Encourage the family to obtain a medical alert identification for the child.

Growth Hormone Deficiency

Growth hormone deficiency is a disorder in which the pituitary gland fails to produce sufficient growth hormone. The cause may be idiopathic or related to a central nervous system disorder such as infection, infarction, tumor, trauma, or effects of chemotherapy or irradiation. Infants typically have normal birth weights and lengths and by 1 year of age are below the third percentile on the growth chart.

Clinical Manifestations

Primary characteristics include the following:

- Growth retardation, short stature, and delayed bone maturation are observed.
- Growth rate is typically less than 5 cm (2 in.) per year.
- Higher-pitched voices, youthful facial features, and delayed dentition may also be noted as these children become older.

Other characteristics may include hypoglycemic seizures, hyponatremia, neonatal jaundice, pale optic disks, micropenis, and undescended testes.

Diagnostic Tests

Growth hormone levels, growth hormone stimulating tests, and insulin-like growth factor-1 levels are used to confirm the disorder.

Radiographic imaging of the hand or wrist is used to evaluate the bone age (stage of bone ossification). See Table 22–1 for diagnostic tests for short stature.

Table 22–1   Diagnostic Tests for Short Stature

Test	Purpose Related to Short Stature
Insulin-like growth factor-1 and insulin-like growth factor binding protein-3	Screens for growth hormone deficiency
MRI of the pituitary gland	Detects pituitary malformation or tumor
Provocative growth hormone testing	Tests for growth hormone deficiency
Bone age	Identifies other potential causes of delayed growth
Karyotype (girls)	Detects Turner syndrome
Thyroid function studies	Detects hypothyroidism
ACTH and cortisol levels	Detects other pituitary hormonal deficiencies
Urine creatinine, pH, specific gravity, urea nitrogen, electrolytes	Detects chronic renal failure
Complete blood count and erythrocyte sedimentation rate	Screens for inflammatory bowel disease with anemia
Antigliadin antibodies	Screens for celiac disease

Source: Data from "Hormones of the Hypothalamus and Pituitary," by J. S. Parks & E. I. Felner, 2007a, in R. M. Kliegman, R. E. Behrman, H. B. Jenson, & B. F. Stanton (Eds.), *Nelson Textbook of Pediatrics* (18th ed., pp. 2291–2293). Philadelphia: Saunders Elsevier; "Hypopituitarism," by J. S. Parks & E. I. Felner, 2007b, in R. M. Kliegman, R. E. Behrman, H. B. Jenson, & B. F. Stanton (Eds.), *Nelson Textbook of Pediatrics* (18th ed., pp. 2293–2299). Philadelphia: Saunders Elsevier; and "Disorders in Growth," by A. Grimberg & D. D. DeLéon, 2005, in T. M. Moshang (Ed.), *Pediatric Endocrinology: The Requisites in Pediatrics* (pp. 127–167). St. Louis: Elsevier Mosby.

Clinical Therapy

Replacement growth hormone is administered by injection. Replacement therapy is continued until either the child achieves an acceptable height or growth velocity declines to less than 2 cm per year.

Nursing Management

Assessment

Carefully measure and document the child's height and weight on a growth chart, and monitor over time. Assess the child's psychosocial adaptation to short stature. Assess parents' ability to cope with child's short stature and treatment regimen.

Implementation

Provide instructions on site selections and injection administration.

Assist family with establishing techniques to minimize trauma of injections.

Educate family about potential side effects and actions to take if noticed.

Direct family to education resources such as The Magic Foundation (http://www.magicfoundation.org) or Human Growth Hormone Foundation (http://www.hgfound.org).

Growth Hormone Excess (Hyperpituitarism)

Hyperpituitarism, a disorder in which excessive secretion of growth hormone increases the growth rate, is rare in children. If combined with precocious puberty, a tumor of the hypothalamus may be present. Heights of 7 to 8 feet can be attained if oversecretion of growth hormone occurs before the closure of the epiphyseal plates. If oversecretion occurs after closure of the epiphyseal plates, acromegaly occurs.

Increased levels of insulin-like growth factors (insulin-like growth factor-1) establish the diagnosis. Radiographic testing is used to evaluate for presence of a brain tumor. Treatment may include surgical removal of tumor, radiation therapy, radioactive implants, or administration of high doses of sex hormones to close the epiphyseal plates. If the pituitary gland is removed, the child requires lifelong pituitary hormone replacement.

Nursing Management

Early identification is crucial. Monitor and document height on growth chart, and monitor trends. Early referral is necessary for children demonstrating growth rates exceeding expected development. Nursing care focuses on educating patients and families about the disorder and treatment, psychosocial support, and postoperative care (if surgical intervention is required).

Precocious Puberty

Precocious puberty is defined as the appearance of any secondary sexual characteristics before 8 years of age in girls (breast development or pubic hair) and 9 years of age in boys (pubic hair) (Pinyerd & Zipf, 2005). Some practitioners have proposed changing the defining age of precocious puberty for girls to 7 for Caucasians and 6 years of age for African American girls because the onset of puberty in females is occurring at an earlier age in many females.

Clinical Manifestations

Secondary sexual characteristics

Accelerated growth rate

Advanced bone age

Behavioral changes (e.g., mood swings, emotional lability)

Diagnostic Tests

Serum studies: luteinizing hormone, follicle-stimulating hormone, testosterone, estradiol

Provocative testing: gonadotropin-releasing hormone stimulation test

Radiologic imaging of the brain, as well as a bone age test, may be performed.

Clinical Therapy

Treatment may be initiated immediately to slow or stop the progression of sexual development in children below the expected age of puberty. A gonadotropin-releasing hormone analogue (GnRHa) is administered, usually leuprolide acetate (Lupron) injections once a month or nafarelin acetate (Synarel) intranasally twice a day. Treatment often continues until a more normal age for puberty is reached (e.g., 11 years in girls and 12 years in boys). Simple monitoring of growth patterns may be the only intervention for children closer to the lower expected age for puberty to begin.

Nursing Management
Assessment

Assess secondary sexual characteristics and sexual maturity rating (see chapter 2).

Document height and weight and plot on growth curve.

Assess child's psychosocial adaptation to changes in body image.

Assess for parental anxiety related to child's physical changes.

Implementation
Promote positive body image.

Ensure proper medication administration.

Reassure child that friends will experience the same stages of development eventually.

Patient and Family Education
Educate child and parents about treatment and condition.

Teach appropriate administration of medication and adherence to treatment regimen.

Advise parents of need to discuss issues of sexuality at an earlier age than normal.

Encourage parents to dress child to match child's chronologic age.

Syndrome of Inappropriate Antidiuretic Hormone
In the syndrome of inappropriate antidiuretic hormone (SIADH), an excessive amount of ADH is secreted. It is seen in children with central nervous system infections, brain tumors, and brain trauma; in children with pulmonary disorders such as pneumonia, asthma, or cystic fibrosis; and in children receiving positive pressure ventilation. Some medications, including diuretics and chemotherapy, have been associated with SIADH.

Clinical Manifestations
Signs are related to water intoxication and hyponatremia and include the following:
- Elevated blood pressure, distended jugular veins
- Crackles on lung examination
- Intake exceeding output; weight gain without edema; concentrated urine with decreased urine output
- Fluid and electrolyte imbalance
- Lethargy, confusion, headache, altered level of consciousness, seizures, and possible coma if serum sodium levels continue to fall

Diagnostic Tests
Serum sodium and blood urea nitrogen are low.

Serum osmolality is low, and urine osmolality is high.

Specific gravity is high.

Clinical Therapy

Fluid restriction is indicated to prevent further hemodilution.

Diuretics are considered to eliminate excess body weight.

Demeclocycline is used to block action of ADH.

Intravenous hypertonic saline is given to supplement sodium in severe hyponatremia.

Nursing Management
Assessment
Accurately document intake and output; weigh daily.

Monitor serum and urine electrolytes and urine specific gravity as ordered.

Monitor for altered mental status, headache, and seizures.

Implementation
If the patient is discharged with SIADH, teach the importance of daily weights and reporting weight gains to healthcare provider. Help family recognize hidden sources of water and fluids, such as popsicles, to prevent excessive fluid intake. Encourage child to wear medical alert identification.

DISORDERS OF THYROID FUNCTION

Hyperthyroidism

In hyperthyroidism, circulating thyroid hormone levels are increased, resulting in an increased basal metabolic rate, cardiovascular function, gastrointestinal function, and neuromuscular function, as well as weight loss, heat intolerance, and increased metabolism of fats, protein, and carbohydrates. It is rare in children and is almost always due to Graves' disease (LaFranchi, 2007).

Clinical Manifestations
Signs vary based on amount of hyperactivity of the sympathetic nervous system and include:

Palpitations, tachycardia

Eyelid lag, fatigue, irritability, muscle weakness, nervousness, restlessness, pruritis, tremors

Diaphoresis, heat intolerance, increased growth rate, goiter, exophthalmos

Frequent bowel movements, increased appetite, nausea, thirst, weight loss

Urinary frequency, nocturia

Anxiety, behavioral problems, declining school performance, emotional lability, inability to concentrate, insomnia

Diagnostic Tests
Thyroid-stimulating hormone (TSH) level is decreased; T_3 (triiodothyronine) and T_4 (thyroxine) levels are elevated.

A thyroid scan is performed to identify nodules or to confirm the high uptake of radioactive iodine.

Clinical Therapy
The excessive release of thyroid hormones is inhibited with antithyroid medication (methimazole or propylthiouracil), radiation therapy, or surgery (thyroidectomy). See Table 22–2 for medications used.

Nursing Management

Assessment
Assess vital signs. Keep a record of food intake. Perform accurate measurement and recording of height and weight to establish baseline and identify patterns of growth. Observe behavior, activity, and level of fatigue. Assess the family's response to the chronic condition, as well as the family's response to the child's disturbing symptoms.

Implementation
While the child is in hyperthyroid state, promote increased caloric intake, management of child's activity and rest periods, and cool environment. Protect the eyes.

Postoperatively, elevate the head of bed to 30 degrees to promote patent airway. A tracheostomy kit, suction supplies, and IV calcium gluconate should be immediately available for emergency treatment of hypocalcemia and respiratory distress. If thyroidectomy is performed, thyrotoxicosis does not immediately resolve because the half-life is 7 to 8 days. Antithyroid medications should be slowly tapered (Boger & Perrier, 2004).

Emphasize the need for lifelong thyroid hormone replacement if the child has undergone radiation or thyroidectomy.

Recommend medical alert identification.

Reinforce importance of follow-up to monitor thyroid levels and growth and development.

Hypothyroidism
Hypothyroidism is a disorder in which levels of active thyroid hormones are decreased.

Table 22–2 Medications Used for the Management of Hyperthyroidism

Medication	Nursing Considerations

Antithyroid medications
  Methimazole (Tapazole)
  Propylthiouracil (PTU)
	Monitor for side effects, including fever, rash, mild leukopenia, nausea, arthralgia, pruritis, hives, and mild increase in liver enzymes; the more serious side effects include liver and bone marrow failure.

	Emphasize the importance of taking medication as prescribed and to take it at the same time each day.
	Monitor for symptoms of hypothyroidism.
Propranolol (Inderal)	Monitor for side effects, including hypotension.
	Emphasize the importance of taking the medication as prescribed.
Radioiodine (oral, in solution, or capsule)	Assess for allergy to iodine.
	Antithyroid medications should be discontinued 5–7 days prior to treatment.
	Ensure adolescent is not pregnant before beginning treatment.
	Teach family to avoid physical contact with secretions (urine, stool, saliva, sweat) for several days after the treatment.
	Emphasize the importance of monitoring thyroid function.
	Hypothyroidism is a potential complication.

Source: Data from "Advances in Assessment, Diagnosis, and Treatment of Hyperthyroidism in Children," by K. S. Amer, 2005, *Journal of Pediatric Nursing, 20*(2), 119–126; "Disorders of the Thyroid Gland," by S. LaFranchi, 2007, in R. M. Kliegman, R. E. Behrman, H. B. Jenson, & B. F. Stanton (Eds.), *Nelson Textbook of Pediatrics* (18th ed., pp. 2316–2340). Philadelphia: Saunders Elsevier; and "An Optimal Treatment for Pediatric Graves' Disease Is Radioiodine," by S. A. Rivkees & C. Dinauer, 2007, *The Journal of Clinical Endocrinology & Metabolism, 92*(3), 797–800.

Congenital hypothyroidism is usually caused by a spontaneous gene mutation, an autosomal recessive genetic transmission of an enzyme deficiency, hypoplasia or aplasia of the thyroid gland, failure of the central nervous system–thyroid feedback mechanism to develop, or iodine deficiency. Mental retardation (cretinism) is irreversible if the disorder is not treated. A small percentage of these cases is caused by hypothalamic-pituitary hypothyroidism and has thyroid-stimulating hormone resistance. Some children have a transient form of congenital hypothyroidism due to transplacental transfer of maternal thyroid-blocking antibodies or antithyroid medications (Eugster, LeMay, Zerin, et al., 2004).

Acquired hypothyroidism can be idiopathic or result from autoimmune thyroiditis (Hashimoto's thyroiditis), late-onset thyroid dysfunction, isolated thyroid-stimulating hormone (TSH) deficiency due to pituitary or hypothalamic dysfunction, or exposure to drugs or substances such as lithium that interfere with thyroid hormone synthesis.

Clinical Manifestations

Congenital hypothyroidism has few clinical symptoms in the first weeks of life. When untreated, characteristic features—thickened protuberant tongue, thick lips, dull appearance—appear in the first few months of life. Other signs include prolonged neonatal jaundice, hypotonia, respiratory distress, bradycardia, decreased pulse pressure, hypothermia, cool extremities, mottling, pallor, umbilical hernia, a posterior fontanel larger than 1 cm in diameter, difficulty feeding, lethargy, swollen eyelids, constipation, and a hoarse cry (Palma Sisto, 2004).

Children with acquired hypothyroidism have many of the same signs as adults: decreased appetite, dry cool skin, thinning hair or hair loss, depressed deep tendon reflexes, bradycardia, constipation, sensitivity to cold temperatures, abnormal menses, and a goiter (a nontender enlarged thyroid gland). Manifestations unique to children include changes in past normal growth patterns with a weight increase, decreased height velocity, delayed bone and dental age, muscle hypertrophy with muscle weakness, and delayed or precocious puberty.

Diagnostic Tests

Congenital hypothyroidism: usually detected during newborn screening of T_4 and TSH. A thyroid scan or ultrasound of thyroid to confirm presence and position of thyroid gland and radiologic examinations of bone growth may be performed.

Acquired hypothyroidism: T_4, TSH, and antithyroid antibody measurement are indicated.

Clinical Therapy

Lifetime thyroid replacement hormone: levothyroxine (Synthroid).

Nursing Management

Assessment

Perform routine newborn screening when child is discharged from newborn nursery and at first health visit.

Perform periodic monitoring of T_4 and TSH and bone age in affected children.

Measure and record height and weight on growth curve.

Implementation

Educate patient and family about lifelong need for hormone replacement therapy.

Teach side effects of hypothyroidism to patient and family and instruct them to promptly report any of these changes to their healthcare provider.

Reinforce importance of follow-up to monitor growth and thyroid levels.

DISORDERS OF THE PARATHYROID

Hyperparathyroidism

Primary hyperparathyroidism, rare during childhood, is most often the result of a tumor (adenoma) that secretes the hormone without proper regulation (Doyle & DiGeorge, 2007). Secondary hyperparathyroidism is due to disease outside of the parathyroid gland, leading to excessive secretion of parathyroid hormone; it is commonly seen in chronic renal failure when the kidneys are unable to reabsorb calcium, causing low serum calcium levels and stimulating continual secretion of parathyroid hormone to maintain normal serum calcium levels (Molina, 2006).

Symptoms of primary hyperparathyroidism may include bone pain, nephrolithiasis (kidney stones), and pathologic bone fractures. Hypercalcemia may cause symptoms of muscle weakness, peptic ulcer disease, fatigue, volume depletion, and subtle mental disturbance (Viera, 2002). For primary hyperparathyroidism, surgical parathyroid exploration is performed to remove the adenoma. Surgical cure rate is estimated to be 90% (Viera, 2002). Treatment of secondary hyperparathyroidism focuses on prevention of hypercalcemia utilizing vitamin D replacement and phosphorus binders.

Nursing Management

Nursing care centers on fluid management and electrolyte monitoring. In children who require surgery, assess for respiratory distress and a potential airway obstruction due to edema and a potential hematoma around the tracheal space; monitor for signs of infection; educate the child and parents to recognize signs of hypocalcemia and on appropriate calcium supplementation. Follow-up is important to monitor serum calcium and phosphorus levels to detect persistence of hyperparathyroidism.

Hypoparathyroidism

Primary hypoparathyroidism is rare but may result from congenital disorders, from surgical removal of the parathyroid glands, by disease processes that destroy the parathyroid glands, or by medications. Hypoparathyroidism can also be idiopathic. The primary result is hypocalcemia and hyperphosphatemia in the blood.

Infants may display hyperirritability, muscle rigidity, seizures, vomiting, abdominal distention, apneic episodes, intermittent cyanosis, or twitching. Muscle pain and cramps may progress to numbness, stiffness, and tingling of the hands and feet. A positive Chvostek sign reveals hyperreflexia. Life-threatening tetany and convulsions may occur (Doyle & DiGeorge, 2007). Intravenous calcium and calcitriol are administered to treat seizures, tetany, life-threatening hypotension, and cardiac arrhythmis. Oral calcitriol and calcium are given for an indefinite time period (Palma Sisto, 2004). Foods with high phosphorus content (dairy products and eggs) are limited.

Nursing Management
Assess and stabilize the airway, breathing, and circulation; initiate cardiorespiratory monitoring; maintain seizure precautions until normal serum calcium levels are attained; obtain intravenous access; and administer calcium supplementation as ordered.

Ensure that family understands need for calcium supplementation, reduced intake of phosphorus, and periodic monitoring of calcium levels. Inform the family that hypoparathyroidism may require life-long therapy.

DISORDERS OF ADRENAL FUNCTION
Adrenal Insufficiency (Addison Disease)
Adrenal insufficiency, also known as Addison disease, is a rare disorder in childhood characterized by a deficiency of glucocorticoids (cortisone) and mineralcorticoids (aldosterone). The lack of glucocorticoids affects the body's ability to handle stress (Gance-Cleveland, 2003).

Most cases are caused by an autoimmune process, but may also be acquired after trauma, or with tuberculosis, HIV infection, meningococcemia, or fungal infections that destroy the adrenal glands.

Clinical Manifestations
Adrenal insufficiency develops slowly as adrenal glands deteriorate.

Early signs: weakness with fatigue, lethargy, emotional lability, anorexia, salt craving, and poor weight gain or weight loss.

Additional signs: hyperpigmentation at pressure points, lip borders and gingival margins, nipples, palms and soles, body creases, and scarred areas of the body; generalized bronzing of the skin or freckling without tan lines even in winter months; abdominal pain, nausea, vomiting and diarrhea, and symptomatic hypoglycemia.

Addisonian crisis: severe hypotension, weakness, fever, abdominal pain, hypoglycemia, seizures, dehydration, circulatory collapse, shock, and coma.

Diagnostic Tests

Serum cortisol (low) and urinary 17-hydroxycorticosteroid levels measured in early morning

Adrenocorticotropic hormone stimulation (ACTH) test of adrenal gland reserve

Serum electrolytes

Computed tomography scan of abdomen to visualize adrenal glands

Clinical Therapy

Replacement of deficient hormones (hydrocortisone); oral hydrocortisone in lowest therapeutic dose to control symptoms and promote growth; fludrocortisone (Florinef) is administered to replace the missing mineralcorticoid in children with aldosterone deficiency.

Nursing Management

Assessment

Assess vital signs for changes in heart rate or blood pressure. Assess weight, skin turgor, and mucous membranes to determine presence of dehydration. Monitor nutritional intake, elimination patterns, muscle strength, and level of consciousness. Monitor laboratory values, intake and output, and daily weight.

Implementation

Administer intravenous fluids as indicated, and encourage fluid intake as prescribed.

Ensure the family recognizes symptoms that require reporting (bleeding, dizziness, lethargy, weakness, changes in blood pressure or heart rate, and weight gain).

If the child has vomiting within 1 hour of taking oral steroid dose, the dose is repeated. Increase dose of medication with illness.

Double or triple steroid medication is prescribed in anticipation of stressful events.

Injectable form of medication must be available at home and at school for emergencies.

Encourage a medical alert identification for the child.

Congenital Adrenal Hyperplasia

Congenital adrenal hyperplasia is an autosomal recessive disorder causing deficiency of one of the enzymes necessary for the synthesis of cortisol and aldosterone. Increased secretion of adrenocorticotropic hormone occurs in response to low cortisol levels, leading to overproduction of adrenal androgens and virilization of female genitalia.

Seventy-five percent are salt-losing caused by aldosterone deficiency. Twenty-five percent are non-salt-losing with simple virilization.

Clinical Manifestations

Females: pseudohermaphroditism, masculinized genitalia at birth (enlarged clitoris, partial or complete labial fusion), normal uterus and fallopian tubes, vagina and urethra have a common opening (urogenital sinus).

Males: may appear normal at birth, may have slightly enlarged penis and hyperpigmented scrotum, may have an adult-size penis at school age, but testes are appropriately sized.

Precocious puberty, acne, tall stature, and excessive muscle development may be noted as the child grows.

Diagnostic Tests

Diagnosis in infants and children is usually confirmed by laboratory evaluation of serum 17-alpha-hydroxyl progesterone (17-OHP) level. Routine newborn screening for congenital adrenal hyperplasia is performed in 44 states (National Newborn Screening and Genetics Resource Center, 2006). Prenatal diagnosis is available. In instances of ambiguous genitalia, a karyotype determines the infant's gender. Ultrasonography may be used to visualize pelvic structures.

In the salt-wasting form of the disorder, the child may have hyponatremia, hyperkalemia, acidosis, hypoglycemia, a high urine sodium level, and low serum and urinary aldosterone levels. Serum concentrations of testosterone in girls and androstenedione in boys and girls are elevated in affected infants. Measurement of ACTH and 17–hydroxyprogesterone levels reveals high readings, while serum cortisol is inappropriately low in comparison to ACTH (White, 2007). Diagnosis may be delayed in the non-salt-losing form until 3 to 7 years.

Clinical Therapy

Lifelong replacement of deficient hormones with oral glucocorticoids is indicated.

If salt-wasting form, salt is added to the infant's formula and a mineralcorticoid (Florinef) is given to replace the missing hormone.

Hormone dosage must be doubled or tripled during acute illnesses or injury and for surgery; injectable hydrocortisone is administered for severe stress.

Generally there are no side effects to the hormone; however, elevated doses can result in hypertension and growth impairment.

Adrenalectomy is recommended only in cases in which medical therapy is ineffective (Pang, 2003).

Nursing Management

Assessment

Assess the infant and child for signs of dehydration, electrolyte imbalance, and hypovolemic shock in the salt-wasting form of the disease. Monitor airway, breathing, circulation, and responsiveness.

Assess vital signs and assess peripheral perfusion (capillary refill, distal pulses, color and temperature of the extremities) frequently to detect early changes in condition, such as hypovolemia.

Assess the parents' emotional response to a child with ambiguous genitalia and a chronic condition. Explore their values and beliefs with regard to gender roles and sexuality while awaiting karyotype results.

Implementation

Support parents having difficulty accepting that their infant, whose genitalia looks male, is really female. With medication and surgery, the genitalia can assume a female appearance, and females have all of the organs necessary for future child bearing.

Assist parents in educating child's siblings and other family members about the condition.

Refer to infant as "your baby" not "your son" or "your daughter" until gender identity is confirmed.

Provide genetic counseling to parents and to the adolescent with CAH. Prenatal testing can detect congenital adrenal hyperplasia.

Teach family how to administer injectable hydrocortisone, about the need for emergency treatment if hydrocortisone is not available, and to carry an emergency kit with the child.

Inform parents of increased risk of rapid dehydration when child has salt-wasting form and develop an emergency plan for illness.

Encourage use of medical alert identification.

Cushing's Disease

Cushing's disease results from excess levels of glucocorticoids (especially cortisol) in the bloodstream,

During infancy, most cases of endogenous Cushing's disease are due to a functioning adrenocortical tumor. The tumor is usually a malignant carcinoma; however, it may be a benign adenoma (White, 2007).

Other causes include hyperplasia of one or both adrenal glands and benign tumors of the adrenal glands. The increased secretion of cortisol alters metabolism.

Clinical Manifestations

Gradual excessive weight gain, growth retardation, hypertension, and mental and behavior problems may be observed.

Generally, it takes 2 to 5 years for the child to develop typical cushingoid appearance (moon face, buffalo hump).

Other signs include obesity, hirsutism, muscle weakness, growth retardation, mental changes, and delayed puberty.

Diagnostic Tests

Increased 24-hour urinary levels of free cortisol, and 17-hydroxycorticosteroid (17-OHCs); elevated nighttime salivary cortisol level.

Chronic hyperglycemia and an elevated glycosylated hemoglobin concentration.

Adrenal suppression test with an 11-p.m. dose of dexamethasone reveals that adrenal cortisol output is not suppressed overnight as would occur normally in children.

Computerized tomography (CT) and magnetic resonance imaging (MRI) are used to detect the specific location of tumors in the adrenal and pituitary glands.

Clinical Therapy

Surgical resection of pituitary adenoma is indicated.

Replacement glucocorticoid therapy may be needed for several months after surgery.

Irradiation of the pituitary is performed when surgical removal of the adenoma does not substantially reduce cortisol levels.

Lifelong hydrocortisone replacement is needed when both adrenal glands are removed.

Prognosis for children with malignant adrenal tumors is poor.

Nursing Management

Assessment

Monitor the vital signs, weight, fluid status, and nutritional status.

Monitor serum electrolytes.

Implementation

Provide preoperative and postoperative teaching and care. Refer to chapter 19 for care of the child with cancer. Postoperatively, elevate the head of the bed 30 degrees to promote effective breathing.

Patient and Family Education

Ensure that the patient and family understand this disorder and its treatment.

Explain that the child's cushingoid appearance is reversible with treatment.

Offer nutritional guidance for healthy food selections for weight management.

Encourage the child to discuss feelings about physical appearance.

Develop a schedule for administration of hydrocortisone replacement therapy, in the morning or every other day to mimic a diurnal pattern. Give oral preparations with meals to decrease gastric irritation.

Teach parents how to administer injectable hydrocortisone for times when the child cannot take oral medication. Steroid replacement is needed during illness to prevent severe illness or cardiovascular collapse.

Signs of acute adrenal insufficiency may include increased irritability, headache, confusion, restlessness, nausea and vomiting, diarrhea, abdominal pain, dehydration, fever, loss of appetite, and lethargy.

Encourage medical alert identification for the child.

DISORDERS OF PANCREATIC FUNCTION

Diabetes Mellitus Type 1

In the United States, approximately 1 in every 400 to 600 children and adolescents have type 1 diabetes (American Diabetes Association, 2008). Each year approximately 13,000 children under age 18 are diagnosed with type 1 diabetes (CDC, 2005). Peak incidence in childhood is between 7 and 15 years of age; however, type 1 diabetes can present at any age (Alemzadeh & Wyatt, 2007).

Type 1 diabetes is a multifactorial disease caused by autoimmune destruction of insulin-producing pancreatic beta cells in genetically predisposed individuals (Sepa, Wahlberg, Vaarala, et al., 2005). Type 1 has familial tendencies but no pattern of inheritance.

Insulin helps transport glucose into cells for use as an energy source. Without insulin, the serum glucose level rises and the glucose level inside the cells decreases.

When glucose is unavailable to the cells for metabolism, free fatty acids provide an alternate source of energy. The liver metabolizes fatty acids at an increased rate, producing acetyl coenzyme A (CoA). The by-products of acetyl CoA metabolism (ketone bodies) accumulate in the body, resulting in a state of metabolic acidosis, or ketoacidosis.

Clinical Manifestations

Classic signs of polyuria, polydipsia, and polyphagia (excessive appetite) with significant weight loss

Fatigue/lethargy

Headaches

Stomachaches

Occasional enuresis in previously toilet-trained child

Symptoms develop gradually over a month or shorter time period

Diagnostic Tests

Diagnosis is based on the presence of classic symptoms and one of the following plasma glucose values (American Diabetes Association, 2008):

- Fasting plasma glucose greater than or equal to 126 mg/dL (7 mmol/L), no caloric intake for at least 8 hours.
- Two-hour plasma glucose greater than or equal to 200 mg/dL (11.1 mmol/L) during an oral glucose tolerance test.

- Plasma glucose concentration greater than or equal to 200 mg/dL (11.1 mmol/L) taken at any time of day regardless of time of last meal.

Ketones may be found in the blood or urine.

Autoantibodies can indicate an autoimmune dysfunction.

Plasma c-peptide levels and fasting insulin levels will be low in type 1 diabetes (Berry, Urban, & Grey, 2006).

Clinical Therapy

Multiple approaches to insulin therapy are available for children and adolescents:

- Basal-bolus therapy—basal insulin is administered once a day using glargine, and then a bolus of rapid-acting insulin is administered with each meal and snack based on the carbohydrate grams consumed and the blood glucose level. See Table 22–3 for action times of different insulin types.
- Continuous subcutaneous insulin infusion (CSII) pump therapy is increasingly used by children and adolescents, as the technology makes it possible to more closely match the plasma insulin levels in normal children.

The goal of insulin therapy is to maintain a range of blood glucose levels that varies by the child's age. Glycemic goals for children

Table 22–3   Action Times by Insulin Type Administered Subcutaneously

Type	Onset	Peak	Duration
Rapid-acting			
Insulin lispro, insulin glulisine, or insulin aspart	5–10 min	0.5–2hr	3–4 hr
Short-acting			
Regular	0.5–1.0 hr	2–5 hr	6–8 hr
Intermediate-acting			
NPH	1–3 hr	5–8 hr	12–18 hr
Very Long-acting			
Glargine or Detemir	1.5–4 hr	None	20–24 hr

Source: Adapted from "Insulin Analogues in Children and Teens with Type 1 Diabetes: Advantages and Caveats," by M. Rachmiel, K. Perlman, & D. Daneman, 2005, *Pediatric Clinics of North America, 52*, 1651–1675.

younger than 6 years old are generally less stringent since they lack the cognitive capacity to recognize and respond to hypoglycemic symptoms (Silverstein et al., 2005).

Insulin dose is adjusted according to frequent serum glucose monitoring, at least four times per day, and delivered by multiple subcutaneous injections or insulin pump.

Nutrition planning—counting carbohydrates, number of calories individualized to child for growth and activity

Exercise program

Nursing Management
Assessment
Assess physiologic status: vital signs, hydration, and level of consciousness.

Monitor blood glucose, electrolytes, and blood gases as ordered.

Monitor growth and developmental milestones.

Assess the adolescent's problem-solving skills.

Assess family strengths and coping for disease management.

- Do both parents or does the single parent work? Who else cares for the child?
- What is the child's daily schedule? Does it vary daily or on the weekend?
- Does the child have other chronic conditions or behavioral, cognitive, or visual problems?
- What other stressors exist in the family?
- Assess adolescent's willingness and challenges in adhering to treatment plan.

Implementation
Teach the family survival skills when child is newly diagnosed: blood glucose monitoring, drawing up and injecting insulin, urine testing for ketones, record keeping, survival food guidelines, and when to call the healthcare provider.

Coordinate care with diabetic nurse educator for disease management focusing on the following:
- Signs and symptoms of hypoglycemia and hyperglycemia
- Goals of insulin therapy, correct administration of insulin, rotation of sites

- Washing hands before pricking finger for blood
- Keeping a rapid-acting source of sugar readily available
- Planning a balance of food intake, exercise, and insulin
- Healthy foot habits

Sick-day guidelines to help prevent diabetic ketoacidosis:
- Monitor serum glucose levels more often than routine.
- Do not skip doses of insulin; insulin dose may need to be increased.
- Work to maintain food and fluid intake.
- Monitor urine for ketones.
- Call healthcare provider if fever or infection is present.

Coordinate with nutritionist to develop the food plan; use Food Guide Pyramid to identify correct portions of food, carbohydrate counting, and consistent intake of carbohydrates.

Encourage medical alert identification.

Provide emotional support and refer family to support groups and sources of information.

Assist family in coordinating with the school to develop an individualized health plan.

Diabetic Ketoacidosis

Diabetic ketoacidosis (DKA) is a common and potentially life-threatening condition that occurs primarily in children with type 1 diabetes, but can occur in type 2 diabetes (Ummpierrez, 2006).

The muscle cells break down protein into amino acids that are then converted to glucose by the liver, leading to hyperglycemia. The adipose tissue releases fatty acids that are transformed by the liver into ketone bodies. Their accumulation leads to ketoacidosis. The hyperglycemia causes an osmotic diuresis, resulting in dehydration, acidosis, and hyperosmolarity. The rising ketones lead to metabolic acidosis. DKA is associated with severe metabolic, electrolyte, and fluid imbalances.

Clinical Manifestations

Characteristic signs of DKA include polyuria, polydipsia, weight loss, abdominal pain, nausea and vomiting, tachycardia, signs of dehydration, and flushed ears and cheeks.

Kussmaul respirations, acetone breath (fruity smell), altered level of consciousness, and hypotension may be observed.

Hyperglycemia, glycosuria, and ketonuria are also present.

Abdominal or chest pain, nausea, and vomiting may also be present.

May progress to electrolyte disturbances, arrhythmias, altered consciousness, pupillary changes, irregular respirations, inappropriate slowing of the heart rate, and widening pulse pressure.

Diagnostic Tests
See Table 22–4 for laboratory findings.

Computed tomography of brain is indicated if cerebral edema develops.

Clinical Therapy
Child is hospitalized and receives isotonic intravenous fluids and electrolytes for dehydration and acidosis.

Short-acting insulin is given by continuous intravenous infusion to lower serum glucose at a rate no greater than 100 mg/dL/hour.

Mannitol is indicated if cerebral edema is suspected.

Nursing Management
Assessment
Monitor vital signs, respiratory status, perfusion, and mental status continuously.

Table 22–4 Laboratory Findings in the Child with Diabetic Ketoacidosis

Laboratory Study	Results
Serum glucose	Greater than 200 mg/dL
Serum ketones	Positive
Arterial blood gas pH	Acidotic: pH 7.3 or below and bicarbonate less than 15 mEq/L
Potassium	Elevated
Chloride	Elevated
Sodium	Decreased
Phosphate	Decreased
Calcium	Decreased
Magnesium	Decreased
Blood urea nitrogen and creatinine	Elevated due to dehydration
White blood cell count	Generally elevated due to presence of infection or dehydration
Serum osmolality	Greater than 350 mOsm/kg (normal is 275–295 mOsm/kg)
Urine	Positive for glucose and ketones

Assess for changes in neurologic status, respiratory pattern, blood pressure, and heart rate. Monitor for cardiac arrhythmias associated with hypokalemia.

Assess for signs of dehydration, including dry skin and mucous membranes, and depressed fontanels in infants.

Implementation
Monitor blood glucose levels hourly or as indicated.

Monitor electrolyte, acid–base balance, urine glucose, and ketone levels.

Monitor urine output hourly.

Assess for signs of hypoglycemia, which may occur during insulin infusion.

Adequate fluids are given to reverse the fluid deficit.

The insulin infusion must be carefully titrated to control the gradual reduction in hyperglycemia.

Provide support to the family.

Patient and Family Education
Signs that could indicate progression to DKA and should be reported to healthcare provider include the following (Bismuth & Laffel, 2007; Boland & Grey, 2004; Masharani, 2007):

- Abdominal pain
- Nausea and vomiting that persists for over 6 hours
- More than five diarrheal stools in 1 day
- 1- or 2-day history of polyuria and polydipsia
- Has illness (e.g., viral or other) and is unable to eat
- Change in mental status
- Temperature over 102°F (38.9°C) for 12 hours
- Blood glucose 400 mg/dL on two separate readings, or greater than 200 mg/dL and moderate to large ketones
- Large ketones present
- Fruity breath odor
- Evidence of a bacterial infection (e.g., fever, drainage, dysuria, or other evidence of a urinary tract infection)
- Difficulty breathing
- Decreased urine output

Hypoglycemia in the Child with Diabetes
Hypoglycemia can develop within minutes in children with type 1 diabetes mellitus. Severe hypoglycemia episodes may occur at night

in children who are treated with two to three injections per day. Other common causes include an error in insulin dosage, errors in injection technique, inadequate calories because of missed meals, or exercise without a corresponding increase in caloric intake. Severe hypoglycemia can cause seizures.

Signs occur with a serum glucose reading of approximately 70 mg/dL or less and include sudden onset of irritability, nervousness, tremors, shaky feeling, difficulty concentrating or speaking, behavior change, confusion, or repeating something over and over. Delirium, loss of consciousness, and seizures can occur if not promptly managed.

Nursing Management

Prompt recognition is essential to quickly manage symptoms and prevent further reduction in glucose level.

Ensure that parents understand recognition and treatment of hypoglycemia. Include the following guidelines:

If the child shows signs of hypoglycemia, test the blood glucose level.

Assist the child to perform the test, as skills needed to get an accurate reading deteriorate with the child's altered mental status.

If the blood glucose reading is less than or equal to 70 mg/dL, give glucose rapidly. Give 1/2 cup orange juice, 3/4 cup of sugar-sweetened beverage, 1 small box of raisins, or 3 or 4 glucose tablets.

Wait 15 minutes and recheck the blood glucose level. Repeat the glucose if it is still less than or equal to 70 mg/dL. Recheck the blood glucose level in another 15 minutes.

Once blood sugar has returned to at least 80 mg/dL, give a more substantial snack such as cheese and crackers if the next meal will be more than 30 minutes later or an activity or exercise is planned.

If the child is unconscious, administer IM or SQ glucagon or spread glucose paste on the gums.

Diabetes Mellitus Type 2

Type 2 diabetes is associated with insulin resistance. While it is sometimes connected to an insulin secretory defect in the pancreas caused by a decrease in the beta cell weight and number and insulin deficiency (Gungor, 2004), it is more commonly associated with decreased insulin receptors at the cellular level. Significant risk factors for type 2 diabetes include obesity, low levels of physical activity, a diet high in fat, race, and family history of diabetes (Alemzadeh & Wyatt, 2007; Berry, Urban, & Grey, 2006).

Insulin fails to transfer glucose into the cells. The pancreas produces more insulin to facilitate glucose transfer and overcome insulin resistance, resulting in hyperinsulinemia. As insulin resistance worsens, the pancreas is unable to hypersecrete enough insulin.

Clinical Manifestations

Obese

Acanthosis nigricans

Polyuria, polydipsia may be mild or absent

Lipid disorders, hypertension

Androgen-mediated problems such as acne, hirsutism, menstrual disturbances, polycystic ovary disease

Excessive weight gain and fatigue due to insulin resistance

Some children (5%–25%) are in ketoacidosis at the time of diagnosis (Berry, Urban, & Grey, 2006).

Diagnostic Tests

Serum glucose levels of 200 mg/dL or greater without fasting, or a fasting glucose of 126 mg/dL or greater, are diagnostic of diabetes.

Urine ketones are found in about 50% of children with type 2 diabetes.

Hemoglobin A1c will be elevated.

Fasting lipid profile (dyslipidemia—primarily low HDL-C and elevated triglycerides) is usually present.

Autoantibodies and fasting C peptide are used to differentiate between type 1 and type 2 diabetes.

Clinical Therapy

Nutritional education for gradual sustained weight loss and metabolic control of blood glucose levels

Exercise

Oral medication (e.g., metformin) if diet and exercise efforts are inadequate

Insulin may be required at time of presentation and may ultimately be needed long term for glycemic control if weight and exercise goals are not met.

Nursing Management
Assessment
Assess child with body mass index above 85th percentile for signs of insulin resistance (acanthosis nigricans, hypertension, dyslipidemia).

Perform blood glucose and blood pressure monitoring.

Assess diet and activity patterns.

Consider evaluating siblings.

Implementation
Provide emotional support to child and family.

Teach the child and family about the disease and its management.

Help family plan strategies for daily management of condition, blood glucose monitoring, and medications.

Work with a nutritionist to help the family substitute high-calorie and high-fat foods for allowable foods matching the family's resources and ethnic preferences.

Encourage exercise and reduction of sedentary computer and television time.

Encourage annual evaluation for complications of diabetes.

GONADAL FUNCTION DISORDERS

Amenorrhea

Primary: Absence of menarche by 14.5 years with no growth or development of secondary sexual characteristics. Primary amenorrhea is most often caused by structural defects of the reproductive system, chromosomal abnormalities (such as Turner syndrome), or hypothalamic or pituitary tumors, thyroid dysfunction, or polycystic ovary disease. No underlying pathologic condition is identified in some adolescents; may occur in competitive athletes.

Secondary: Absence of three or more consecutive menstrual periods after menstruation has begun. Most often due to pregnancy; may also occur in competitive athletes.

Diagnostic testing may include a pregnancy test, bone age, hormone levels (estrogen, luteinizing hormone, follicle-stimulating hormone, and prolactin), and a vaginal examination (to determine vaginal patency). Therapy is dependent on etiology. The most common approach is birth control pills containing estrogen and progesterone.

Nursing Management

Explain that irregular and variable-duration cycles are common for 1 to 2 years after menarche.

Provide education about safe sexual practices to the adolescent who is or is considering being sexually active. Offer birth control.

Provide emotional support.

Encourage athletes to eat a well-balanced, high-calorie diet and to take calcium supplementation. Teach about medications prescribed.

Dysmenorrhea

Dysmenorrhea is menstrual pain or cramping during the menstrual cycle due to an increased secretion of prostaglandins during the ovulatory cycle that causes uterine muscle contraction, leading to ischemia and pain. Endometriosis or pelvic inflammatory disease may cause secondary dysmenorrhea.

Pain usually occurs after the beginning of ovulation and ends on the second day of the menstrual cycle. Cramping in the lower abdomen and pelvic regions may radiate to the back. Other symptoms may include nausea, vomiting, headache, diarrhea, urinary frequency, or fatigue.

A gynecologic examination may detect tenderness and identify any abnormalities. Cultures are taken if a sexually transmitted infection (STI) is possible. Treatment includes nonsteroidal anti-inflammatory drugs and oral contraceptives.

Nursing Management

Educate adolescents to begin taking nonsteroidal anti-inflammatory drugs 2 to 3 days before the onset of the menstrual cycle and to take with food to avoid gastrointestinal upset.

Guided imagery, hypnosis, meditation, chiropractic massage, and reflexology are nonpharmacologic methods that may be useful in the relief of dysmenorrhea. Application of a heating pad may also be helpful. Intake of vitamin B_6 with B-complex vitamins, vitamin E, calcium, and magnesium may help relieve symptoms of dysmenorrhea (Shuler, Huebscher, Miller, et al., 2004).

DISORDERS RELATED TO SEX CHROMOSOME ABNORMALITIES

Klinefelter Syndrome

Klinefelter syndrome is a chromosomal disorder in which males have an extra X chromosome, usually 47,XXY, causing hypogonadism, androgen deficiency, and infertility in males.

Clinical Manifestations

Males appear normal at birth.

Disruptive behavior in school and emotional problems often occur due to auditory processing problems and speech delay.

Intelligence quotient (IQ) scores may be similar to those of siblings, but academic difficulty is common because of memory, data retrieval skills, and verbal processing problems (Misra & Lee, 2005).

Tall and thin appearance with disproportionately long legs and normal arm span for height may be observed. Gynecomastia is generally present.

Delayed onset of puberty with abnormal progression, decreased testicular size. Less facial and body hair may develop.

Associated complications of Klinefelter syndrome include cardiac abnormalities, pulmonary disease, dental abnormalities, and scoliosis.

Diagnostic Tests

Chromosomal analysis revealing one or more extra X chromosomes confirms the diagnosis.

Clinical Therapy

Testosterone replacement is begun at puberty, when the male is 11 or 12 years of age; testosterone is given by intramuscular injection every 3 to 4 weeks to maintain serum testosterone levels within the normal range.

Dose is increased gradually until an adult dose is reached between 15 and 17 years of age; treatment does not improve fertility. Hormone treatment helps improve psychological well-being and social functioning (Misra & Lee, 2005). It also helps to promote normal body proportions and prevent gynecomastia.

Nursing Management

Assess secondary sexual characteristics, height, and weight.

Assess patient and family coping.

Support parents to work with the school to provide education tailored to needs.

Refer for speech therapy if needed.

Help parents identify child's strengths and promote success and self-esteem.

Turner Syndrome

Turner syndrome is the most common sex-chromosome abnormality in females and is caused by a complete loss, partial absence, or other abnormality of one X chromosome.

Conditions that may be associated with Turner syndrome include congenital heart defects, hypertension, structural abnormalities of the kidney, autoimmune thyroiditis, celiac disease, hearing loss, orthodontic anomalies, strabismus, congenital hip dysplasia, and scoliosis (Morgan, 2007).

Clinical Manifestations

Short stature (less than fifth percentile)

Short, webbed neck with low posterior hairline

Cubitus valgus (increased angle at the elbow), scoliosis, broad chest with widely spaced nipples

Lymphedema of the hands and feet

Hyperconvex fingernails

Dark, pigmented nevi

Delayed puberty, amenorrhea, underdeveloped ovaries, infertility

Few girls have all of these features (Misra & Lee, 2005).

Diagnostic Tests

Diagnosed definitively by a karyotype, which reveals the classic 45,X chromosome pattern or a combination 45,X/46,XX pattern (Morgan, 2007).

May be suspected prenatally based on results of maternal serum screening and ultrasound. The diagnosis must be confirmed by chorionic villus testing or amniocentesis (Loscalzo, Bondy, & Biesecker, 2006).

Clinical Therapy

Growth hormone therapy may be prescribed to promote growth during childhood, and the therapy can begin at age 2 (Halec & Zimmerman, 2004). Low-dose estrogen therapy is usually begun at around 12 years of age, with a gradual dosage increase to mimic natural puberty (Tyler & Edman, 2004). Progesterone is added to the estrogen therapy to initiate cyclic menstrual periods.

Nursing Management

Assess for signs and symptoms of cardiac, renal, gastrointestinal, vision, hearing, musculoskeletal, or thyroid dysfunction.

Assess growth and plot on growth curve. Educate parents to administer growth hormone and to monitor for side effects.

Promote the girl's self-esteem.

INBORN ERRORS OF METABOLISM

Fatty Acid Oxidation Defects

Mitochondrial oxidation of fatty acids is an imperative energy-producing pathway during periods of starvation, when the body metabolizes fat for fuel. Autosomal recessive gene defects occur in almost every stage in the fatty acid oxidation pathway, leading to many subclasses of fatty acid oxidation defects.

Clinical Manifestations

Most commonly, acute life-threatening coma and hypoglycemia induced by a period of fasting are observed.

May be asymptomatic except for times of illness or stress.

Other signs may include cardiomegaly, hepatomegaly, and muscle weakness.

Diagnostic Tests

Routine newborn screening may identify some disorders.

Most cases are identified during an acute presentation of symptoms when laboratory evaluation may include blood gases, electrolytes, hepatic profile, plasma lactate, plasma amino acids, urine organic acids, acylcamitine profile, quantitative carnitine levels, and urine for ketones.

Hypoglycemia is usually present and ketone levels are unusually low (Thomas & Van Hove, 2007).

Liver function tests demonstrate elevated transaminases, urea, and ammonia.

Plasma and tissue concentrations of total carnitine are reduced. Skin biopsies are often obtained for fibroblast analysis.

Physical examination may reveal hepatomegaly due to fatty infiltration.

Clinical Therapy

Acute condition is treated with 10% dextrose.

Frequent feedings and avoidance of fasting (no more than 8–12 hours without food) are indicated.

Carnitine supplementation may be required in some disorders (Thomas & Van Hove, 2007).

Nursing Management

Educate parents to feed the infant around the clock every 2 to 4 hours.

Do not let children or adolescents go longer than 8 to 12 hours without food. Encourage several low-fat and high-carbohydrate snacks throughout the day.

If the infant or child is unable to sustain oral intake during acute illness, refer to the hospital for intravenous dextrose supplementation. Simple infections can become life-threatening.

Refer family to genetic counseling. Test siblings even if asymptomatic.

Galactosemia

Galactosemia is an autosomal recessive disorder of carbohydrate metabolism that results from a deficiency of the liver enzyme galactose 1-phosphate uridyltransferase, one of three enzymes needed to convert galactose to glucose. Galactose metabolites accumulate in the eyes, liver, kidney, and brain, rapidly damaging the organs and causing life-threatening problems. Children become susceptible to gram-negative sepsis.

Clinical Manifestations

Early manifestations: poor sucking, failure to gain weight due to vomiting followed by diarrhea, hypoglycemia, and an enlarged liver

Late signs: mental retardation, jaundice, ascites, sepsis, lethargy, seizures, hypotonia, cataracts, and coma

Diagnostic Tests

Routine newborn screening for galactosemia is performed in all U.S. newborn screening programs (March of Dimes, 2007).

Physical examination and laboratory tests (galactose, AST, and ALT are abnormally high) are indicated. Urine specimens are checked for reducing substances.

Clinical Therapy

Elimination of galactose from diet, lactose-free formula (e.g., Nutramigen, meat-based, or soybean) *or*

Lifetime galactose-free diet (no milk, cheese products, foods with dry milk products)

Nursing Management

Educate the family about the disorder and required diet.

Assess coping mechanisms and provide needed emotional support.

Teach families to screen foods for added milk solids and to avoid antibiotics with lactose fillers.

Calcium supplementation is often required.

Advise parents that several galactose-free cheeses are sold commercially.

Refer family for genetic counseling.

Maple Syrup Urine Disease

Maple syrup urine disease (MSUD) is a disorder of amino acid metabolism that has an autosomal recessive inheritance pattern.

In MSUD, three essential amino acids (leucine, isoleucine, and valine) cannot be metabolized because of absent or defective enzyme branched-chain alpha-ketoacid dehydrogenase (Simon, Flaschker, Schadewaldt, et al., 2006).

All three amino acids are essential to form normal structures such as the hair, skin, and muscle. Leucine has the potential to accumulate in the brain and cause cerebral edema, progressive neurologic impairment, and death (Bodamer & Lee, 2006).

Clinical Manifestations

Within 4 to 7 days of life, the newborn develops symptoms of poor appetite, lethargy, vomiting, variable muscle tone, irritability, seizures, high-pitched cry, severe ketoacidosis, and a sweet odor of maple syrup in bodily fluids. The symptoms may quickly progress to coma and death if not treated (Bodamer & Lee, 2006; March of Dimes, 2006).

Diagnostic Tests

Routine newborn screening; however, not performed in all states

Urine for ketones

Blood tests for elevated leucine, isoleucine, alloisoleucine and valine

Clinical Therapy

Acute treatment: Remove branched-chain amino acids and their metabolites from tissues and body fluids by hydration or dialysis. Provide sufficient intravenous calories to reverse the infant's catabolic state.

Chronic treatment: Provide specially formulated medical formulas rich in amino acids, calories, vitamins, and minerals with the three amino acids removed; provide special low-protein foods for growth and adequate calories to support twice the child's basal metabolic rate; and perform daily urine testing for ketones to detect a catabolic state.

Nursing Management

Educate the family about the disorder and dietary requirements.

Ensure family understands how to mix the infant's formula.

Help parents develop a "sick-day" plan that ensures food and formula when ill to prevent ketoacidosis.

Refer to nutritionist for diet counseling.

Permit moderate exercise only to prevent increase in leucine levels.

Help family identify support groups and sources of information.

Phenylketonuria

Phenylketonuria (PKU) is an autosomal recessive disorder of amino acid metabolism that affects the body's use of protein caused by a mutation of the phenylalanine hydroxylase gene. It results in phenylalanine accumulation in the blood or phenylalanine metabolites in the urine. Severe mental retardation, seizures, and death result if untreated.

Clinical Manifestations

Phenylalanine accumulates in the blood, causing a musty or mousey body and urine odor, irritability, vomiting, hyperactivity, hypertonic, hyperreflexive deep tendon reflexes, seizures, and an eczema-like rash (Rezvani, 2007). Persistence of elevated phenylalanine leads to disruption of cellular processes of myelination and protein synthesis and results in a seizure disorder and untreatable mental retardation.

Microcephaly, prominent maxilla and widely spaced teeth, enamel hypoplasia, and growth retardation are other common findings in untreated children (Rezvani, 2007).

Diagnostic Tests

Screening for phenylketonuria is required by law in all 50 states.

If the test shows elevated levels of plasma phenylalanine, a repeat quantitative test is performed. If the second test is positive, the family is referred to an outpatient treatment center.

Serum levels of phenylalanine should be measured periodically throughout life.

Clinical Therapy

Special formulas and a diet low in phenylalanine (e.g., Lofenalac, Minafen, Albumaid XP) are indicated.

Breastfeeding is possible if infant's serum phenylalanine levels are monitored.

Elemental medical foods with modified protein hydrolysates are substituted for high-protein foods (meats and dairy products).

The low-phenylalanine diet should be maintained for life. If dietary control is lost before 6 years of age, there is a significant impact on IQ. The low-phenylalanine diet is especially important for adolescent females and women prior to conception and during pregnancy to prevent congenital anomalies (low birth weight, microcephaly, mental retardation, and congenital heart defects) in the fetus (Rouse & Azen, 2004).

Nursing Management

Assess child for consequence of PKU (neurologic signs, atopic dermatitis, cognitive and behavioral problems).

Assess child's adherence to diet. If dietary control is lost before age 6 years, there is significant impact on IQ.

Teach patient/family to avoid high-protein foods (meats and dairy products) and aspartame because they contain large amounts of phenylalanine.

Support parents. Identify financial issues associated with purchase of elemental medical foods and assist with insurance coverage negotiations for those expenses.

23 ALTERATIONS IN NEUROLOGIC FUNCTION

ALTERED STATES OF CONSCIOUSNESS

An altered level of consciousness (LOC) is an important indicator of neurologic dysfunction. *Consciousness* is the brain's responsiveness to sensory stimuli and involves alertness and cognitive power. *Unconsciousness* is depressed cerebral function, or the inability of the brain to respond to stimuli. Categories of altered LOC are confusion, delirium, obtunded, stupor, and coma. Causes of altered LOC include hypoxia, trauma, infection of brain or meninges, poisoning, seizures, metabolic disturbance, electrolyte or acid–base imbalance, intracranial tumor, stroke, and congenital structural defect. Increased intracranial pressure (ICP) results from these conditions.

Clinical Manifestations

Signs of progressive alteration in LOC:

- Slight disorientation to time, place, and person
- Restless or irritable
- Drowsy but responds to loud verbal commands, withdraws from painful stimuli
- Response to pain progresses from purposeful to nonpurposeful
- Nonresponsive, decorticate or decerebrate posturing

Some children may have signs of increased intracranial pressure (ICP). See Table 23–1.

Newborns may have lethargy, irritability, or hyperalertness.

Diagnostic Testing

Laboratory tests performed to identify potential cause of altered LOC: complete blood cell count, blood chemistry, clotting factors; assessment of cerebrospinal fluid (CSF) for protein, glucose, and blood cells; culture of blood, urine, CSF toxicology assessments of blood and urine.

Electroencephalogram; computed tomography (CT), magnetic resonance imaging (MRI), skull radiographs; ICP monitoring

Clinical Therapy

Oxygen and assisted ventilation (when gas exchange is inadequate)

Metabolic, acid–base, or electrolyte imbalance correction

Antibiotics for suspected infection

Table 23–1   Signs of Increased Intracranial Pressure

Timing of Signs	Signs
Early signs	Headache
	Visual disturbance, diplopia
	Nausea and vomiting
	Dizziness or vertigo
	Slight change in vital signs
	Pupils not as reactive or equal
	Sunsetting eyes
	Seizures
	Slight change in level of consciousness
Additional signs in infants	Bulging fontanel
	Wide sutures, increased head circumference
	Dilated scalp veins
	High-pitched, cat-like cry
Late signs	Significant decrease in level of consciousness
	Cushing's triad
	Increased systolic blood pressure
	Bradycardia
	Irregular respirations
	Fixed and dilated pupils

Intravenous (IV) fluids for hypovolemia; management of increased ICP; maintenance of cerebral perfusion pressure (CPP)

Nursing Management
Assessment

Identify a potential cause of altered LOC from history.

Assess the child's physiologic status: responsiveness, ability to maintain the airway, vital signs, head circumference, breathing patterns, air exchange. Monitor pulse oximetry and arterial blood gases.

Neurologic assessment includes cranial nerves (see Table 2–3), pupil size, reaction to light, consensual reaction, eye movements, and motor function. A modification of the Glasgow Coma Scale may be used at specific intervals to monitor changes in LOC and neurologic functioning in infants and young children (Table 23–2).

To rapidly assess responsiveness in infants, the acronym AVPU helps:
- Alert, responsive to parents, cuddles, coos or babbles, smiles
- Verbal, responsive to verbal stimulation

Table 23–2   Glasgow Coma Scale for Infants and Young Children

Category	Score*	Preverbal Child Criteria	Older Child and Adult Critieria
Eye opening	4	Spontaneous opening	Spontaneous opening
	3	To voice	To voice
	2	To pain	To pain
	1	No response	No response
Verbal response	5	Smiles, coos, babbles, cries to appropriate stimuli	Oriented to time, place, and person; uses appropriate words and phrases
	4	Irritable; cries	Confused
	3	Cries to pain	Inappropriate words or verbal response
	2	Moans to pain	Incomprehensible words
	1	No response	No response
Motor response	6	Spontaneous movement	Obeys commands
	5	Purposeful, localizes pain	Localizes pain
	4	Withdraws to pain	Withdraws to pain
	3	Flexor posturing	Flexor posturing
	2	Extensor posturing	Extensor posturing
	1	No response/flaccid	No response/flaccid

*Add the score from each category to get the total. The maximum score is 15, indicating the best level of neurologic functioning. The minimum is 3, indicating total neurologic unresponsiveness.

Source: From Jankowitz, B. T., & Adelson, P. D. (2006). Pediatric traumatic brain injury: Past, present, and future. Developmental Neuroscience, 28, 264–275.

- *P*ain, responsive to painful stimulation only
- *U*nresponsive to painful stimulation

Implementation

Maintain airway patency, endotracheal tube or tracheostomy management, suctioning. Provide supplemental oxygen. Assist ventilation as needed.

Prepare for seizures, and protect child from injury.

Perform routine care and oral care; protect eyes.

Provide nutrition.

Provide sensory stimulation, talk, or play music or tapes of stories; stroke and touch the child in a soothing manner; orient child to time, place, and person.

Provide emotional support to parents, involve them in care, encourage them to express feelings.

Plan for transition to long-term care or home.

CEREBRAL PALSY

Cerebral palsy (CP), a group of permanent disorders of movement and posture development causing activity limitation, results from insult to the fetal or infant brain (e.g., infection, intraventricular hemorrhage, hyperbilirubinemia). CP is primarily a motor disorder, but sensory, perceptual, cognitive, communication, and behavioral disturbances occur in some children (Rosenbaum, Paneth, Leviton, et al., 2007). CNS infection and brain trauma are the major sources of CP in young children. Four types of motor dysfunction seen include spastic, dyskinetic, ataxic, and mixed. The prognosis for infants and children with CP depends on the level of physical involvement and on the presence of intellectual, visual, or hearing deficits. Functional consequences increase even though the brain injury itself does not progress (Pellegrino, 2007).

Clinical Manifestations

Wide variability in symptoms, related to area of the brain involved.

Abnormal muscle tone, lack of coordination with spasticity, delayed developmental milestones; mental retardation or learning disabilities; hearing, speech, and language impairments; seizures.

Spastic (Cerebral Cortex or Pyramidal Tract Injury): persistent hypertonia, rigidity, leads to contractures and abnormal curvature of the spine; exaggerated deep tendon reflexes; persistent primitive reflexes.

Dyskinetic (Extrapyramidal, Basal Ganglia): muscle tone abnormalities in entire body; involuntary movements; tremors, difficulty with fine and purposeful motor movements; exaggerated posturing; inconsistent muscle tone that may change during the day.

Ataxic (Cerebellar, Extrapyramidal): abnormalities of voluntary movement involving balance and position of the trunk and limbs; difficulty controlling hand and arm movements during reaching; increased or decreased muscle tone; muscle instability and wide-based, unsteady gait; hypotonia in infancy.

Mixed (Multiple Areas): no dominant motor pattern; unique compensatory movements and posture to maintain control over specific neuromotor deficits; combination of characteristics from other types.

Diagnostic Testing

Ultrasonography to detect fetal and neonatal brain abnormalities, such as intraventricular hemorrhage

Neuromotor tests of movement patterns, tone, and primitive reflexes.

CT scans and MRI to view anatomic structures; positron emission tomography (PET) to evaluate brain metabolic functioning

Clinical Therapy

Physical and occupational therapy to promote improved muscle tone and better motor control for function; braces and splints to prevent contractures or to manage scoliosis; tone-reducing casts to keep spastic muscles in stretched position; static positioning devices; mobility devices (tricycle, walker, wheelchair).

Surgery to lengthen tendons, reduce spasticity, balance muscle power, and stabilize uncontrollable joints.

Medications are used to control seizures, to control spasms, and to minimize gastrointestinal side effects (cimetidine or ranitidine). Baclofen is administered orally or by intrathecal pump to decrease muscle spasticity. Injection of botulinum toxin into specific muscles helps to temporarily control spasticity. See Table 23–3.

Assistive devices, technology, and speech therapy may also be indicated.

Nursing Management
Assessment

Identify child at risk for CP. Assess for developmental delays and orthopedic, visual, auditory, and intellectual deficits; assess for abnormal muscle tone or abnormal posture, persistence of primitive reflexes beyond the expected age (see chapter 2). Identify asymmetric or abnormal crawling by using two or three extremities; identify hand dominance before the preschool years.

Monitor growth, development, and nutrition.

Provide screening for hearing and vision impairments.

Implementation

Provide adequate nutrition—high-calorie diets or supplements needed due to chewing and swallowing difficulties. Teach techniques to promote swallowing. Give small amounts of soft foods at a time in back of mouth. Use feeding utensils with large, padded handles. Ensure adequate fiber in diet to reduce constipation risk.

Table 23–3 Medications Used to Treat Cerebral Palsy

Medication	Nursing Management
Diazepam, lorazepam, clonazepam *Oral*	Can cause drowsiness and excessive drooling, which can interfere with feeding and speech. Taper drug when discontinued, as physiologic dependence develops.
Dantrolene *Oral*	Can cause drowsiness, muscle weakness, and increased drooling. Perform liver function testing periodically.
Baclofen *Intrathecal* *Oral*	Oral drug can cause drowsiness, nausea, headache, and low blood pressure. Intrathecal route allows lower continuous dosing, reducing side effects (hypotonia, increased seizures in children with known epilepsy, sleepiness, and nausea and vomiting). Monitor for intrathecal pump failure and signs of infection.
Botulinum toxin type A *Injection*	Used to improve walking in children with equinus gait; may be used in hip adductors and hamstrings to improve positioning. May have stumbling, leg cramps, leg weakness, and calf atrophy. Repeated injections needed to continue effect.

Note: Data from "Cerebral Palsy," by L. Pellegrino, 2007, in M. L. Batshaw, L. Pellegrino, & N. J. Roizen (Eds.), *Children with Disabilities* (6th ed., pp. 387–408). Baltimore: Paul H. Brooks Publishing Co.

Maintain skin integrity—protect the skin over bony prominences and under splints and braces.

Maintain proper body alignment—in the bed or in a chair. Use splints and braces to support the child and reduce the risk for contractures.

Promote physical mobility—perform range-of-motion exercises to maintain joint flexibility and to prevent contractures. Position the child to foster flexion to enhance interaction with the environment. Encourage use of child's adaptive appliances during hospitalization. Refer parents to get help with the acquisition of adaptive devices, such as customized wheelchair.

Promote safety—use safety belts in strollers and wheelchairs. Determine if an adaptive car safety seat is needed.

Promote growth and development—plan activities to promote fine and gross motor skills; refer to early intervention programs; foster cognitive learning opportunities.

Promote communication—if hearing impaired, refer to learn sign language or other communication methods; a computer may help communication.

Provide emotional support—listen to parents' concerns, encourage them to ask questions and share feelings. Refer to support group.

Provide referral to social services for financial resources for adaptive equipment or for special transitions in the child's life, such as plans for adult living.

Patient and Family Education

Educate about the disorder and the child's special needs.

Teach administration, desired effects, and side effects of medications prescribed.

Encourage regular dental care, as enamel defects and malocclusion are common, along with hyperplasia when anticonvulsants are prescribed.

Prepare parents for possible seizure when pertussis and measles-mumps-rubella vaccines are given, when child has coexisting seizure disorder.

Prepare parents to become the child's case manager when appropriate.

Provide guidance for development of an individualized education plan (IEP) to address mobility and educational support for behavior problems, perceptual problems, and speech difficulties. Explore vocational training options and provide guidance for development of individualized transition plan during adolescence.

CONDITIONS CAUSED BY INFECTION

Bacterial Meningitis

Bacterial meningitis is an inflammation of the meninges most often caused by *Neisseria meningitides* in U.S. children between 2 months and 12 years (Prober, 2007, p. 2514); *Haemophilus influenzae* type b and *Streptococcus pneumoniae* are less common causes. Group B streptococcus and gram-negative enteric bacilli are more common causes in the newborn (Chávez-Bueno & McCracken, 2005). Inflammation causes the brain to swell, causing headache and increased ICP. Inflammation of the spinal nerves and roots causes a stiff neck. Potential complications include hearing loss, seizures, subdural effusion, hydrocephalus, septicemia, and septic arthritis.

Clinical Manifestations

In infants: fever; change in feeding pattern; vomiting or diarrhea; bulging or flat fontanel; alert, restless, lethargic, or irritable

Older children: fever, upper respiratory or gastrointestinal illness; increasing irritability and alteration in LOC; vomiting; complaint of muscle or joint pain.

Signs of meningeal irritation: headache, photophobia, esotropia, and nuchal rigidity (resistance to neck flexion); positive Kernig or Brudzinski sign.

Symptoms can progress to include seizures, apnea, cerebral edema, photophobia, altered mental status, subdural effusion, hydrocephalus, disseminated intravascular coagulation, syndrome of inappropriate antidiuretic hormone (SIADH), and shock.

Petechiae progressing to purpura is seen in meningococcal meningitis.

Diagnostic Testing

Complete blood count, serum electrolytes and osmolality, and clotting factors.

Lumbar puncture for CSF glucose, protein, blood cells, and culture; blood culture.

CT scanning when increased ICP or brain abscess is suspected.

Clinical Therapy

IV antibiotics are administered as soon as diagnostic tests are obtained, often changed once culture and sensitivity results are known.

Corticosteroids (dexamethasone) is indicated for children older than 6 weeks of age to reduce the risk of severe neurologic sequelae such as sensorineural hearing loss. Medications to reduce ICP include antipyretics, mannitol, and high-dose barbiturates (Chávez-Bueno & McCracken, 2005).

Initial IV fluid restriction is indicated while monitoring for increased ICP and syndrome of inappropriate antidiuretic hormone. Nothing is given by mouth initially. Aggressive fluid resuscitation is indicated if child is in shock to maintain CPP.

Nursing Management
Assessment
Assess the child's physiologic status, including vital signs and LOC. Monitor for increased ICP.

Measure the infant's head circumference frequently and compare to previous measurements.

Be alert for signs of a change in the child's condition and response to treatment.

Monitor the child's ability to control secretions and to drink sufficient fluids. Monitor intake and output. Monitor the serum sodium concentration and urine specific gravity.

Assess for pain and sensory deficits.

Implementation
Use standard and droplet precaution isolation until effective treatment is under way.

Maintain hydration.

Administer medications and monitor the child's response to antibiotics. Monitor for gastrointestinal distress and blood in the stool associated with corticosteroids.

Promote comfort with reduced stimulation (dim lights, quiet room) and a side-lying position. Provide pain management.

Provide support to the family. Help the parents comfort the child and participate in daily care.

Encourage infants and children to be fully immunized to prevent potential meningitis.

Refer infants and toddlers with neurologic sequelae to an early-intervention program.

Encephalitis
Encephalitis is an acute central nervous system condition with radiographic or laboratory evidence of brain, and often meningeal, inflammation, most commonly by a viral infection (Lewis & Glaser, 2005). It often results in significant neurologic sequelae (American Academy of Pediatrics, 2006, p. 365).

Clinical Manifestations
Fever, severe headache, and vomiting are observed. Altered mental status, nuchal rigidity, photophobia, and positive Kernig and Brudzinski signs may be present.

Disorientation or confusion may progress to stupor and coma. Behavioral or personality changes may be observed. Hemiparesis, ataxia, or weakness; cranial nerve deficits; alterations in reflex response; focal or generalized seizures may develop during condition progression.

Clinical Therapy

Analysis of CSF, blood serology tests, and nasopharyngeal and stool specimens for viral pathogens is indicated. Testing for virus-specific immunoglobulin M antibodies is indicated. CT scan, MRI, and electro-encephalogram may also be performed.

Supportive care in the pediatric intensive care unit (PICU) is indicated. Condition is treated with antibiotics until bacterial pathogens have been ruled out. Acyclovir may be used for herpes viral infections. Intravenous immune globulin, corticosteroids, and other immune system modulators may be used in postinfectious encephalitis (Lewis & Glaser, 2005).

Physical therapy, occupational therapy, and speech therapy may be indicated.

Nursing Management

Monitor the child's airway, ability to handle secretions, respiratory status, vital signs, color, pulse oximetry readings, capillary refill time, arterial blood gas values, LOC, and urine output.

Anticipate and have appropriate equipment for managing seizures at bedside.

Provide skin care, position and turn appropriately, and perform passive range-of-motion exercises. Perform chest physiotherapy.

Orient child to environment as LOC improves. Offer age-appropriate toys and diversions.

Keep parents informed about the child's condition, treatment, and prognosis.

Refer parents to home care, social services, family counseling, and support groups.

HEADACHES

Headaches have both benign (migraine, inflammatory, and tension) and structural (tumors and increased ICP) causes.

Clinical Manifestations

Migraines

Triggered by stress; foods containing nitrates, glutamate, caffeine, tyramine, and salt; menses; oral contraceptives; stress; fatigue; and hunger

Aura (auditory, visual, or taste sensation) in some children

Unilateral or bilateral pulsatile throbbing pain lasting for hours or days, aggravated by routine activity, pain often in retro-orbital frontal and temporal region

Nausea and vomiting, recurrent abdominal pain

Sensitivity to light or sound

Tension Headaches

May be associated with stresses associated with school, insecurity, or conflict in the family

Dull, achy pain in band around head, in temporal or occipital areas, or in neck and shoulders that may last for days; intermittent or constant pain with fluctuations in severity.

Dizziness and fatigue may be present.

Medication-Overuse Headaches

Dull, bilateral or unilateral pain in frontal area; can vary in character, location, and severity from time to time

Usually increase in frequency and severity over time, paralleling the increase in medication use; occur at least two to four times a week or almost daily.

Headaches recur when the abortive therapy or medication wears off.

Structural (space-occupying lesion or increased ICP)

Pain increasing in frequency and severity, increases with sneezing, coughing, or straining

Awakens child or present when awakening

Vomiting is persistent or preceded by severe headache

Abnormal neurologic signs (e.g., double vision, papilledema, strabismus, weakness, ataxia)

Diagnostic Testing

Usually based on detailed history and physical examination

Radiologic studies (CT scan or MRI) when neurologic signs are present; CSF if infection or inflammatory process is suspected, such as meningitis (Gunner, & Smith, 2007).

Clinical Therapy

Migraines

Food elimination trial to identify food triggers; avoid food triggers such as caffeine, chocolate, cheese, monosodium glutamate

Noise and light avoidance during acute phase

Medications to abort migraine (e.g., sumatriptan nasal spray in adolescents); analgesic medication (ibuprofen, acetaminophen, naproxen)

Regulation of sleep and exercise

Relaxation techniques and biofeedback

Tension Headaches

Relaxation techniques and rest

Analgesic and anti-inflammatory medications

Ice pack

Medication-Overuse Headaches

Discontinuation of all medications for headaches (caffeine, acetaminophen, nonsteroidal anti-inflammatory drugs, and triptans) (Kossoff & Mankad, 2006)

Clonidine may be used to treat withdrawal symptoms.

Structural

Surgery

Analgesic medications

Nursing Management

Assess the child for potential neurologic signs associated with headaches.

Encourage the child to keep a calendar or diary of headaches, including the events and stresses occurring at the time. Analyze diary for patterns of triggers or stress. Identify and discuss strategies that may help reduce triggers or stress.

Encourage child to develop a daily routine with regular exercise, a consistent bedtime and awakening time, and regular eating schedule to avoid hunger.

If a food elimination trial is implemented, educate the child and family about foods to eat and not eat, and how to gradually add foods to identify offending food triggers.

Educate child and family that medications should be taken at first sign of headache. Teach child and parents that medications should not be used for more than 2 to 3 days a week.

NEONATAL ABSTINENCE SYNDROME

Illicit substances used during pregnancy that may cause neonatal abstinence syndrome include opiates (heroine, meperidine, methadone),

CNS stimulants (cocaine, propoxyphene, amphetamines), and CNS depressants (barbiturates, alcohol, and marijuana). Children with prenatal cocaine exposure may have difficulties with language development, attention span, memory, and motor skills (Schiller & Allen, 2005). Reduced brain volume, heart defects, strokes, cleft palate, and gastrointestinal defects have been noted in methamphetamine-exposed infants (McGuinness & Pollack, 2008).

Clinical Manifestations

Withdrawal symptoms for opiates manifest within 24 to 48 hours after birth, for barbiturates within 2 to 14 days after birth, and for cocaine or amphetamines within 7 days after birth (Stoll, 2007).

Prematurity, intrauterine growth retardation, transient tachypnea, and apnea are commonly seen with prenatal cocaine exposure. Other signs include hypertonia, tremors, and extensor leg posture; poor sucking and feeding difficulties; less time in quiet sleep; more stressed behaviors such as mouthing and clenched fists; and difficulty regulating behaviors.

Irritability, jitteriness, tremors, high-pitched cry, and excessive suck may manifest with other illicit substances (Bauer, Langer, Shankaran, et al., 2005).

Excoriated skin due to continuous movements against bed linen.

Sneezing, stuffy nose, sweating, tachycardia, and tachypnea.

Diarrhea, vomiting, and poor feeding.

Diagnostic Testing

Toxicology screening of maternal and infant urine or toxicology screening of meconium or infant hair reveals mother's drug use for the last half of the pregnancy. Chain of custody for specimens may be needed.

Diagnostic testing for human immunodeficiency virus (HIV), hepatitis B, hepatitis C, and syphilis is indicated.

Brazelton Neonatal Behavioral Assessment Scale evaluates infants on habituation, general arousal level, orientation, quality of movement and tone, autonomic stability, reflexes, and responsiveness when aroused (Olsson, 2007).

Clinical Therapy

Supportive treatment is indicated: reduced environmental stimuli and swaddling.

Medications such as phenobarbital, diazepam, methadone, clonidine, and paregoric may be prescribed to alleviate symptoms of drug withdrawal.

Breastfeeding is discouraged, as the drugs cross over into breast milk.

Nursing Management
Assessment
Observe for poor sucking, seizures, vomiting and diarrhea, dehydration, and an increased metabolic rate. Consider if the newborn could have neonatal abstinence syndrome or another condition, such as infection, bowel obstruction, electrolyte disorder, hydrocephalus, or intracranial anomaly, with similar signs.

Monitor the skin for abrasions.

Assess the strengths, safety, and competence of the mother and other potential caregivers. Determine if the infant could be going to a home with a clandestine methamphetamine lab. Determine if the mother is still using illicit drugs and identify other family supports that may help provide the care and safety needed by the newborn.

Implementation
Provide frequent, small, high-calorie feedings (24 calories per ounce formula). Be patient when feeding infants with poor coordination of sucking and swallowing. Teach parents to use a calm approach and soothing voice when feeding. Newborns may initially feed better in side-lying position while swaddled.

Administer prescribed medications if ordered for drug withdrawal and monitor the infant's response.

Use techniques to calm and soothe the newborn:
- Provide quiet environment with subdued lighting to minimize stimulation and promote sleep.
- Comfort and pacify the infant with swaddling, rocking, and a pacifier for sucking needs. Infant massage may be beneficial.
- Hold the infant with the spine flexed to decrease extensor tone.

Promote parent–infant interaction, minimizing stimulation and promoting feeding.

Refer for careful long-term follow-up (social services, physicians, and nurses) to ensure the infant's safety and to assess growth and development. Support from social services or child protective services may be needed to manage complex family situations.

NEUROFIBROMATOSIS 1 (VON RECKLINGHAUSEN DISEASE)

Neurofibromatosis 1 (NF1) is an autosomal dominant disorder in which tumors grow along nerves, leading to skin changes and bone deformities. Neurofibromas develop from cells of the nerve sheath, usually at some point along the peripheral nerves or at nerve endings. Most children and adults with mild symptoms can live a normal, productive life. Children with NF1 may be at risk for leukemia, rhabdomyosarcoma, and pheochromocytoma (Theos & Korf, 2006).

Clinical Manifestations

Six or more café au lait spots or dark macules 5 mm or larger seen at birth or by 2 years of age. In darker-skinned children, the spots are darker than surrounding skin. The spots grow to 15 mm or larger in diameter by adulthood. Freckling in the axillary or inguinal areas may be present.

Multiple neurofibromas or benign tumors begin to grow on or under the skin during puberty; plexiform neurofibromas develop, involving several nerves.

Pain is present when tumors grow around and compress a nerve or grow in the spinal cord.

Scoliosis, thinning of tibia, and fractures that do not heal well may be observed.

Vision deficits are present when tumors develop in the optic nerve (optic glioma); Lisch nodules (tan benign tumors on iris of eye).

Precocious puberty or delayed puberty with delayed menarche is present.

Diagnostic Testing

Diagnosis is based on physical examination. Prenatal diagnosis using amniocentesis or chorionic villus sampling procedures is possible. Genetic testing may be useful in some cases.

MRI of the brain and radiographs of the spine and other bones is indicated when problems are detected.

Clinical Therapy

Monitor for signs of developing problems (growth and development, hypertension, scoliosis, timing of sexual development, and neurofibromas).

Annual ophthalmic examinations are indicated to detect optic gliomas, vision deficits, and monitor Lisch nodules.

Genetic counseling may be indicated.

Surgery is indicated when neurofibromas are disfiguring, cause pain, or are life-threatening.

Nursing Management

Assess for café au lait spots, axillary and inguinal freckling, and small tumors on the body. Note growth of any mass or pain caused by a mass. Monitor for hypertension. Monitor growth and pubertal development. Perform vision and scoliosis screening on a frequent basis. Note any evidence of tibial bowing or thinning.

Monitor school performance for learning disabilities and hyper-activity.

Provide psychological support to the child and family, as tumor development causes self-image and self-esteem problems. Identify peers or refer the adolescent to support groups. Focus on the child's strengths.

SEIZURE DISORDERS

Seizures result from abnormal excessive electrical discharges in the brain, causing involuntary movement and behavior and sensory alterations. Common causes include CNS infection, hypoxia, brain injury, and a sudden rise in temperature. Other causes include electrolyte disturbance (e.g., hypoglycemia), endocrine dysfunction, toxins, and brain tumor.

Clinical Manifestations

Partial seizures—aura (sensory warning of seizure) and loss of consciousness may occur; unilateral motor movements depend on the brain region where abnormal electrical activity occurs; may progress to generalized seizure.

Generalized seizures—bilateral and symmetric movements; often begin with a tonic phase (unconsciousness, continuous muscular contraction, and sustained stiffness), followed by the clonic phase (alternating muscular contraction and relaxation as a rhythmic repetitive jerking). The postictal period follows with decreased LOC.

Febrile seizures—generalized tonic-clonic movements; eyes roll back; lasts a few seconds to 1 to 2 minutes; short postictal period; associated with a rapid temperature rise above 39°C (102°F).

Newborn seizures—subtle signs such as horizontal deviation of eye, repetitive blinking, sucking or lip smacking/tongue thrusting, rhythmic repetitive extremity movement (e.g., bicycling legs).

Status epilepticus—a generalized seizure lasting longer than 30 minutes or a series of seizures during which consciousness is not regained (Riviello, Ashwal, Hirtz, et al., 2006).

Diagnostic Testing

Testing varies with potential cause of seizures

Complete blood cell count; serum electrolytes, glucose, and blood gases may be monitored

Cultures of urine, blood, CSF

Serum drug level if the child is taking any anticonvulsants

Electroencephalogram; CT or MRI

Toxicology screening, lead level, tests for inborn errors of metabolism

Clinical Therapy

Emergency care: maintain patent airway, supplemental oxygen, benzodiazepine medication.

Anticonvulsant therapy—a single medication for seizure control is preferred; dosage adjustments are necessary as the child grows. Multivitamin with calcium is prescribed to help prevent osteoporosis.

Monitor therapeutic drug levels and perform regular blood testing to identify hematologic or liver problems (Table 23–4).

Surgery to remove a tumor, lesion, or even a portion of the brain causing the seizures when the seizures are not responsive to medication may be indicated.

A vagal nerve stimulator can minimize the severity and frequency of seizures, and reduce the number of antiepileptic medications needed (Ghatan, 2006).

A ketogenic diet is recommended for intractable seizures. The high-fat, adequate-protein, and low-carbohydrate diet produces ketosis and has anticonvulsant effects (Freeman, Kossoff, & Hartman, 2007).

Clinical Therapy for Status Epilepticus

Emergency assessment and interventions (see chapter 11) may be indicated.

Table 23–4   Commonly Used Medications for the Treatment of Seizures

Medication	Nursing Management
Diazepam IV	IV push medication is administered very slowly as close to vein as possible.
	Monitor vital signs for hypotension, tachycardia, and respiratory depression.
Phenobarbital PO, IV, IM	IV medication must be administered slowly.
	Monitor child's vital signs frequently when given intravenously.
	May crush tablets and mix with food or fluid.
Phenytoin PO, IV	Educate family to ensure adequate intake of vitamin D, folic acid, and calcium.
	Promote frequent dental care for gingival hyperplasia.
	Ginkgo may decrease anticonvulsant effectiveness.
Carbamazepine PO	Give with food to enhance absorption.
	Do not administer suspension simultaneously with another liquid medication to prevent formation of a precipitate.
	Causes photosensitivity reactions.
Valproic acid PO	Do not use carbonated beverage to dilute syrup. Do not chew tablets and capsules.
	Give with food to decrease irritation.
	Monitor platelet count and bleeding times.
	Childbearing-age females should take folic acid (Weinstein & Gaillard, 2007).
	Do not use aspirin, sedatives, and allergy medications with this drug.
Ethosuximide PO	Monitor for weight loss or anorexia.
	Give with food if gastrointestinal upset occurs.
Primidone PO	Tablet may be crushed and given with fluid; may be given with food.
	Do not combine with over-the-counter medications unless approved by healthcare provider.
	Educate family to ensure adequate intake of vitamin D, folic acid, calcium, and vitamin B_{12}.
Clonazepam PO	Monitor for signs of overdose (confusion, irritability, sleepiness, sweating, muscle cramps, diminished reflexes).
	Do not combine with over-the-counter medications unless approved by healthcare provider.

Table 23–4 Commonly Used Medications for the Treatment of Seizures (Continued)

Medication	Nursing Management
Felbamate PO	Monitor weight for gain or loss.
	Child needs regular monitoring for hematologic and liver problems.
	Careful dosing is needed when combined with other anticonvulsants.
Gabapentin PO	Vision, concentration, and coordination may be impaired by the medication.
	Do not take medication within 2 hours of an antacid.
Lamotrigine PO	Drug increases photosensitivity.
	Monitor for adverse effects if used with valproic acid.
Tiagabine PO	Give with food.
	Monitor for signs of central nervous system depression.
	Avoid using with over-the-counter medications that cause drowsiness.
Topiramate PO	Increase fluid intake to reduce risk of kidney stones.
	Psychomotor slowing as well as speech and language problems may develop with use of medication.

Note: Data from *Nurse's Drug Guide 2009*, by B. A. Wilson, M. T. Shannon, & K. M. Shields, 2009, Upper Saddle River, NJ: Pearson Prentice Hall.

Monitor electrolytes, glucose, blood gases, increasing fever, and abnormal blood pressure.

Rectal or IV benzodiazepine medications may be indicated. Monitor for respiratory depression from cumulative benzodiazepine doses. Prepare to manage the airway and to assist ventilations. Nasogastric tube insertion is indicated to reduce aspiration risk.

Nursing Management
Assessment
Assess the specific seizure activity, LOC, vital signs, and signs of hypoxia. The child's lack of responsiveness may be due to the postictal state.

Collect and analyze historical information about the seizure activity, clustering, aura, description of motor activity or changes in muscle tone, automatisms, and any changes in development or school performance.

Assess the family's adaptation. Identify how well the child copes when a seizure happens at school.

Implementation

Maintain airway patency; place nothing in child's mouth during a seizure; protect the child from self-harm during seizures.

Monitor oxygenation; supplement oxygen when SpO_2 falls below 95%.

Administer IV medications slowly for acute management of seizures to minimize risk of respiratory or circulatory collapse.

Provide emotional support to family; permit them to express fears and frustrations.

Patient and Family Education

Teach about potential causes of seizures and home management (medication administration, ketogenic diet, protecting from injury). Teach about need for medication dosage changes as the child grows.

Develop emergency care plan and individualized health plan (IHP).

Educate adolescents about potential teratogenicity of some anticonvulsants, and encourage contraception for sexually active adolescent females.

Provide child and family with safety guidelines:
- Do not leave the child alone in the bathtub. Children who bathe alone should use the shower.
- Have a buddy and lifeguard present when the child swims.
- Wear a life vest when boating.
- Use a helmet when the child has frequent seizures to protect the head during a fall.
- Keep child away from open flames or outdoor grills.
- Avoid activities where fall risks are increased (e.g., rock climbing).
- Wear medical alert identification.

STRUCTURAL DEFECTS

Hydrocephalus

Hydrocephalus is an imbalance between the production and absorption of CSF that leads to an increase in the volume of CSF. The condition may be congenital, associated with CNS malformations such as myelomeningocele, or develop as a complication of an injury, an acute illness, or intraventricular hemorrhage in the premature newborn. One or more ventricles becomes enlarged.

Communicating hydrocephalus—the CSF flows freely between normal channels and pathways, but absorption of CSF in the subarachnoid space and the arachnoid villi is impaired.

Noncommunicating hydrocephalus—the most common type; an obstruction in the channels or pathways impedes the flow of CSF and prevents it from entering the subarachnoid space.

Clinical Manifestations
Infants
Rapidly increasing head circumference; tense, full, or bulging fontanel; split sutures; Macewen's sign (cracked-pot sound); difficulty holding head up

Bossing (protrusion) of frontal area; face is disproportionate to the skull size.

Prominent, distended scalp veins, translucent scalp skin

Increased muscle tone, brisk deep tendon reflexes, Babinski sign

Irritability or lethargy, decline in LOC, poor feeding

Late signs: apnea, a shrill, high-pitched cry, sunsetting eyes (sclera visible above iris), sixth cranial nerve palsy, developmental regression, difficulty swallowing or feeding, and vomiting

Older Children with Acquired Hydrocephalus
No head enlargement

Signs of increased ICP, headache on arising with vomiting

Irritability, lethargy, altered LOC, sleepiness, confusion, apathy, poor appetite

Personality change, loss of interest in daily activities, poor judgment or verbal incoherence, worsening school performance, memory loss

Ataxia, spasticity, or other alterations in motor development

Visual defects due to pressure on second, third, and sixth cranial nerves; papilledema

Diagnostic Testing
Serial head circumference measurements

CT scanning and MRI may reveal the anatomic cause of hydrocephalus; ultrasonography or echoencephalography is indicated in infants with open fontanels.

Shunt failure is evaluated with CT scanning; MRI; lateral radiographs of the skull, neck, chest and abdomen; a radionucleotide CSF study; and a CSF culture is obtained by tapping the shunt.

Clinical Therapy

Medications (e.g., acetazolamide) are indicated to reduce the rate of CSF production until surgery is performed. Decadron is indicated to reduce cerebral edema associated with increased ICP (Chiafery, 2006).

A ventricular access device to withdraw CSF may be inserted before shunt placement.

Surgery may be indicated to remove the obstruction such as a tumor or to create a new CSF pathway (endoscopic third ventriculoscopy).

Placement of a shunt in the ventricle to divert CSF to the peritoneal cavity, atrium of the heart, or the pleural spaces may be indicated. Mechanical complications may include catheter blockage, kinking of the tubing, or valve breakdown.

For shunt infection: antibiotics, shunt removal, and placement of an external ventricular drainage system. A new shunt is inserted when the CSF cultures are sterile.

Nursing Management

Assessment

Measure the head circumference of all infants and plot on a growth curve to detect unexpected head enlargement.

After shunt placement surgery, monitor the vital signs, respiratory status, irritability, and LOC to detect increased ICP. Assess pain. Monitor intake and output.

Monitor for signs of infection; redness and swelling of the shunt tract; leakage of CSF; nuchal rigidity; neck or back pain; headache; and photophobia (Ditmyer, 2004).

Measure head circumference daily and compare to previous measurements.

Assess for shunt failure and infection at all healthcare visits. Monitor for signs of visual problems as well as cognitive, speech, and motor developmental delays.

Implementation

Postoperatively, place the child in a flat position to prevent rapid CSF drainage. Keep body in alignment with splints or towel rolls. Do not stretch or strain the neck muscles that must support the large head. Elevate the head of the bed gradually over 1 to 2 days.

Perform passive range-of-motion exercises three to four times per day as ordered.

Protect the skin, especially of the heavy head that an infant may have difficulty moving. Change position every 2 hours, inspect for areas of redness, place on pressure-reducing surface, keep skin clean and dry, and use transparent dressing over skin surfaces exposed to frequent friction.

Provide frequent, small feedings with frequent burping, as the infant is prone to vomiting.

Provide emotional support. Keep the parents informed about the child's condition and procedures to be performed. Assure parents that most children with shunts lead normal lives.

Refer to early intervention program to promote development. School children may need an IEP or individualized health plan (IHP).

Patient and Family Education

Educate about the signs and symptoms of shunt failure (signs of increased ICP) and infection (changes in LOC, irritability, personality change, malaise, headache, diplopia, nausea, loss of developmental milestones or loss of coordination and balance, and low-grade fever).

Assist with development of an emergency care plan in case of shunt failure or infection. Provide guidelines for contacting the healthcare provider.

Infants with poor head control should not be placed in forward-facing car safety seats, regardless of age, due to the risk of cervical spine injury and death in the event of a car crash.

Use a helmet for bicycle riding and skateboarding. Child should not participate in sports with high risk for head or abdominal impact.

Maintain good nutrition and promote regular bowel movements. Constipation and abdominal pressure may interfere with shunt drainage (Chiafery, 2006).

Myelodysplasia or Spina Bifida

Myelodysplasia is a malformation of the spinal cord and spinal canal or neural tube defect including the following defects:

- Anencephaly—no development of the brain above the brainstem.
- Encephalocele—protrusion of meningeal tissue or meningeal-covered brain through a defect in the skull.
- Spina bifida occulta—a vertebral defect without visible protrusion of the meninges or spinal cord tissue. An abnormal growth of hair, a dimple or sinus tract, a lipoma, or a vascular skin lesion may be present over the defect.
- Meningocele—a spinal-fluid-filled meningeal sac protruding through a vertebral defect, associated with no abnormalities of the spinal cord.
- Myelomeningocele (spina bifida)—a defect in one or more vertebrae through which a spinal-fluid-filled meningeal sac and spinal cord contents protrude.

Spina bifida is most common in the sacral and lumbar vertebrae, but can occur in any vertebrae. The cause is unknown, but genetics, maternal use of seizure or acne medications, and maternal conditions (diabetes mellitus, gestational diabetes, and folic acid deficiency) are implicated. Chiari II malformation is associated with myelomeningocele above the sacral level. Hydrocephalus causes displacement of the cerebellum, brainstem, and fourth ventricle, leading to herniation. Sudden death, respiratory difficulty, and swallowing difficulties result. Assisted ventilation and surgical decompression may be life saving (Stevenson, 2004).

Clinical Manifestations

A sac-like protrusion on the infant's back indicates meningocele or myelomeningocele. The higher the defect on the vertebral column, the greater the neurologic dysfunction:

- Thoracic or lumbar 1–2 level: paralysis of the legs, weakness and sensory loss in the trunk and lower body region
- Lumbar 3: can flex hips and extend the knees; ankles and toes paralyzed
- Lumbar 4–5 level: can flex hips and extend knees; weak or absent ankle extension, toe flexion, and hip extension
- Sacral level: mild weakness in ankles and toes; bladder and bowel function may be affected

Hip abnormalities such as hip dysplasia; clubfoot; scoliosis or kyphosis may be present.

Sensory loss occurs. Bowel and bladder sphincters may be affected, causing incontinence. Renal involvement may result from neurologic impairment and urinary retention.

Hydrocephalus and Chiari II malformation complications:
- Signs in infants: difficulty swallowing, apnea, respiratory difficulty, inspiratory stridor, weak or poor cry, sustained backward arching of the head (opisthotonus).
- Signs in older children: choking, hoarseness, vocal cord paralysis, disordered breathing during sleep, stiffness or spasticity of arms and hands, loss of feeling or sensation.

Other disabilities: mobility problems, learning disabilities, seizures, and vision impairments.

Potential complications: spinal curvatures, musculoskeletal and joint abnormalities, skin sores, urinary dysfunction, and sexual dysfunction.

Diagnostic Testing
Prenatal maternal serum tests for alpha-fetoprotein, high-resolution fetal ultrasound

Ultrasonography, radiologic imaging by CT scan, MRI, and flat films of the spinal column

Evaluation of bladder and bowel function, neurologic and motor function, and cognitive function

Clinical Therapy
Surgery to close and repair the lesion within 24 to 48 hours of birth to reduce infection

Braces to support joint position and mobility

Assistive devices such as walkers, crutches, and wheelchairs to enhance mobility

Encourage weight bearing.

A diet with adequate calcium and vitamin D to minimize risk for osteoporosis

Use nonlatex equipment and supplies; child is at risk for latex allergy because of multiple surgeries for orthopedic and urologic problems.

Surgery or an orthotic jacket to correct spinal deformities

Bowel interventions: stool softeners, glycerin or bisacodyl suppositories, added fiber in diet; surgery using appendix to create a channel between the abdominal skin and bowel for enemas (Malone antegrade continence enema)

Bladder interventions: clean intermittent catheterization, surgery to create a urine reservoir and abdominal stoma for catheterization (Mitranoff procedure)

Comprehensive healthcare planning with a team of physicians, nurses, and therapists from neurosurgery, orthopedics, urology, and physical therapy

Nursing Management
Assessment
Newborn
- Monitor for integrity of the sac and leakage of CSF. Inspect area for wound healing after surgery. Note any signs of infection.
- Assess the extremities for deformities and motor defects.
- Assess the vital signs, monitor intake and output, and assess for bladder and bowel involvement.
- Measure the head circumference daily to assess for hydrocephalus.
- Assess family's financial status, health insurance, and need for social services.

Child
- Assess the child's vital signs, growth, and head circumference. Assess the range of motion of joints and mobility status.
- Assess neurologic status for any deterioration in function that could be associated with shunt failure or problem with the spinal cord.
- After surgery to correct deformities, assess vital signs, responsiveness, and level of pain. Assess dressing sites for bleeding and draining. Monitor the distal extremities for swelling and circulation. Assess intake and output.

Implementation
Newborn before Surgery
- Cover the sac with a sterile saline dressing and protect it from pressure, infection, and trauma. Use the prone position with hips slightly flexed and legs abducted to minimize tension on the sac.
- Feed the newborn with the head turned to one side until surgery has been performed. Comfort the neonate before surgery with tactile stimulation such as touching, patting, and cuddling.

Postsurgical Care

- Observe for infection, especially meningitis. Keep the diaper away from incision site. Keep in prone position until healed, then change to supine position for sleeping.
- If a ventriculoperitoneal shunt is placed, see Hydrocephalus section for care information. Use splints to maintain extremity alignment, and gentle range of motion to promote mobility.
- Provide emotional support to parents and involve them in the care.
- Encourage use of local healthcare provider for primary care and episodic illnesses with care coordination by a multidisciplinary team of health professionals.
- Make home health nursing referral and identify a case manager until parents assume that role. Obtain special devices such as splints, wedges, and rolls for care in the home.
- Refer parents to resource groups such as the Spina Bifida Association of America.

Patient Education

General care: instruct parents how to position, handle, and feed the infant; how to perform range-of-motion exercises; and how to identify and use latex-free products. See chapter 17.

Elimination: teach the skill of intermittent catheterization. Teach bowel training to control evacuation of bowel with diet and a glycerin or bisacodyl suppository in either the morning or evening.

Nutrition: discuss nutritional needs to promote growth, reduce osteoporosis, and reduce constipation. Emphasize importance of preventing excessive weight gain.

Mobility: educate the child and families about the proper use of braces, walkers, crutches, canes, custom-designed wheelchairs, and car safety seats. Encourage independent mobility.

Skin care: inspect daily all skin areas under braces and splints, pressure areas on buttocks when in wheelchair; and provide skin care.

Emergency preparedness: teach parents the signs and symptoms of increased ICP, hydrocephalus, shunt infection or malfunction, and urinary tract infection; assist with development of emergency care plan and guidelines for contacting a healthcare professional.

Developmental issues: begin teaching children to assume responsibility for self-care as their intellectual ability and fine motor skills develop. Provide guidance on coordination of educational services, development of an IEP, and development of an individualized transition plan.

INJURIES OF THE NEUROLOGIC SYSTEM

Concussion

A concussion is a mild traumatic brain injury (TBI) that causes an alteration in mental status, but not necessarily loss of consciousness (Kirkwood, Yeates, & Wilson, 2006). Stretching, compression, or shearing of nerve fibers as the brain moves within the skull disrupts the brain chemicals responsible for brain functioning (Adirim, 2007). High-risk sports for concussion are hockey, football, and soccer.

Athletes who sustain a second concussion before complete recovery from the first may develop *second impact syndrome*. Acute brain swelling, neurologic or cognitive deficits, and sometimes death can result from the cumulative effect of these concussions.

Clinical Manifestations

Clinical manifestations are associated with severity of injury:

Grade 1—transient confusion, no loss of consciousness, mental status abnormalities last less than 15 minutes

Grade 2—transient confusion with posttraumatic amnesia, no loss of consciousness, and a duration of mental status abnormalities of 15 minutes or longer

Grade 3—Any loss of consciousness, either brief (seconds) or prolonged (minutes or longer) (Adirim, 2007)

Pediatric Concussive Syndrome

Is believed to be associated with injury to the brainstem.

Occurs in children younger than age 3 years.

Toddlers are stunned at time of injury, with no loss of consciousness.

Later become pale, clammy, lethargic, and may vomit.

Postconcussive Syndrome—Complex Concussion

Lethargy, disorientation, irritability, and behavior changes observed within 10 to 30 minutes of injury.

Postconcussive cognitive deficits do not become apparent until at least 24 hours after injury (Adirim, 2007).

Persistent recurrence of symptoms with exertion for 3 to 6 months, seizures, loss of consciousness longer than 1 minute, or prolonged cognitive impairment may be present (McCrory, Johnston, Meeuwisse, et al., 2005).

Clinical Therapy

Provide supportive treatment. Monitor over several hours for decreased LOC.

May be admitted if unconscious for more than 5 minutes or if amnesia of event.

Postconcussive syndrome: supportive treatment, prepare parents and teachers to expect child's altered behavior during weeks to months of recovery.

Removal from sports participation may be indicated according to guidelines for severity of concussion and number of concussions.

Nursing Management

See guidelines for child with a mild brain injury in Traumatic Brain Injury section on page 515.

Hypoxic–Ischemic Brain Injury (Drowning)

Drowning is the process resulting in primary respiratory impairment from submersion or immersion in a liquid medium (Meyer, Theodorou, & Berg, 2006). Children at high risk include toddlers because of inability to escape from the water, adolescent boys because of risk-taking behavior, and children with seizure disorders.

With the immersion injury the child becomes progressively more hypoxemic, impairing the cardiac muscle until it stops. Water in the airway inactivates surfactant and damages the alveoli, leading to pulmonary edema and acute respiratory distress syndrome. Pneumonia may develop. Anoxia causes cerebral edema, increased ICP, and irreversible CNS injury. Drowning may result in death, complete recovery, severe brain injury, or variable neurologic deficits.

Clinical Manifestations

Pulseless and apneic: When submerged for less than 5 to 10 minutes and resuscitated at the scene, may have few symptoms.

When submerged longer and resuscitated, decreased LOC, seizures, irregular respirations, gastric distention, cerebral edema, increased ICP, and respiratory acidosis may be present.

When submerged longer than 25 minutes, will likely die or have severe neurologic impairment (Meyer, Theodorou, & Berg, 2006).

Clinical Therapy

Upon rescue, assess for spontaneous breathing, heart rate, and responsiveness. Clear mouth of foreign matter and perform CPR. Defibrillation for ventricular fibrillation is indicated.

Cardiorespiratory monitoring equipment, arterial blood gases, chest radiograph

Oxygen (100%) by nonrebreather face mask and rewarming

Airway secured with an endotracheal tube

Mechanical ventilation to keep alveoli open, promote adequate oxygenation, and prevent hypercarbia

IV fluids are indicated if hypovolemic. Once hypovolemia is corrected, fluids are often restricted to reduce the risk of cerebral edema. Cerebral edema and increased ICP are treated (see Traumatic Brain Injury section).

Potential medications used include diuretics to reduce cerebral edema, vasopressors to maintain a normal blood pressure, and antibiotics if signs of pneumonia develop.

Nursing Management

Assessment

Monitor the child's respiratory status, oxygenation, cardiopulmonary function, neurologic status (Glasgow Coma Scale, pupil checks), and vital signs. Assess intake and output.

Monitor for signs of respiratory distress and decreasing LOC, indicating potential cerebral edema.

Assess response of family members and need for support associated with the child's life-threatening injury.

Implementation

The child with seriously compromised respiratory and neurologic status is cared for in the PICU.

Administer oxygen and positive end-expiratory pressure or mechanical ventilation if acute respiratory distress develops.

Position the child properly to promote respiratory function.

Note any change in respiratory status and blood gases, and notify the physician promptly.

Implement nursing interventions as described in the Altered States of Consciousness section.

If cerebral edema develops, implement nursing interventions described in the Traumatic Brain Injury section.

Provide emotional support to the family. Encourage parents to seek assistance from social workers, clergy, close friends, and relatives. Arrange for appropriate referrals.

If the child's prognosis is poor, an ethical consult may be offered to educate the family about options for decision making regarding sustaining or terminating life support.

When the child has significant neurologic disabilities, identify a case manager to work with the family for long-term care and rehabilitation options.

Become involved in community efforts to prevent drowning through education and enactment/enforcement of regulations such as fencing around all four sides of swimming pools.

Patient and Family Education

Teach ways to prevent drowning, such as empty buckets, fencing and controlled access around swimming pools, and close supervision of children in and near the water, including the bathtub.

Encourage parents with private pools to get CPR training and to keep a phone at poolside.

Educate adolescents about the dangers of mixing alcohol and swimming.

Traumatic Brain Injury

Traumatic brain injury (TBI) is an injury to the brain caused by blunt force or penetration that disrupts normal brain functioning such as a change in LOC. At the time of impact, scalp injuries, skull fractures, contusions, and hematomas of brain tissue may be present. The inertial injury tears nerves, fibers, and blood vessels. Secondary effects resulting from the biochemical and cellular response to the initial insult lead to hypoxia, cerebral edema, and increased ICP. TBI is the leading cause of injury mortality and disability (Jankowitz, & Adelson, 2006).

TBI is the most common injury in childhood, often caused by falls in young children. Highest risk for TBI occurs in children younger than age 5 years and during adolescence. A permanent disability such as epilepsy, cognitive impairment, learning problems, and behavioral or emotional problems may result from a moderate or severe injury.

Clinical Manifestations
Mild Brain Injury
See Concussion section for acute signs.

Glasgow Coma Scale score of 13 to 15 is observed.

Longer-term signs and symptoms: low-grade headache that will not go away; memory problems, slowness in thinking, acting, speaking, and reading; difficulty paying attention or concentrating, change in performance at school; lack of motivation or interest in favorite toys; feeling tired all the time, change in sleeping pattern; change in eating patterns; increased sensitivity to lights, sounds, distractions; easily irritated.

Moderate Brain Injury
Decreased responsiveness; Glasgow Coma Scale score of 9 to 12

Posttraumatic amnesia for 1 to 24 hours

Loss of consciousness for 5 to 10 minutes

Severe Brain Injury
Glasgow Coma Scale score of 8 or less

Posttraumatic amnesia for more than 24 hours

Coma

Increased ICP

Other Potential Clinical Manifestations
Posttraumatic seizures

Retinal hemorrhages in many children with inflicted TBI (e.g., shaken baby syndrome)

Cushing's triad, characterized by hypertension, increased systolic pressure with wide pulse pressure, bradycardia, and irregular respirations, is associated with impending brain herniation or compromised blood flow to the brainstem.

Reflexes may be hyporesponsive, hyperresponsive, or areflexic. Child may assume a decorticate, decerebrate, or flaccid posture.

Diagnostic Testing
Glasgow Coma Scale to monitor changes in responsiveness

Cranial nerve assessment

Complete blood cell count, blood chemistry, toxicology screening, and urinalysis

Radiologic testing including skull and cervical spine radiographs, CT, MRI, and positron emission tomography (PET) scanning

ICP monitoring

Clinical Therapy

Emergency care—ensure that the airway is clear and stable, intubating if necessary. Administer oxygen and assist ventilation at the child's normal respiratory rate to prevent hypoxemia and hypercarbia. Hyperventilation may be used only for initial treatment of acute significant increased ICP (Marcoux, 2005).

Maintain CPP to ensure brain has adequate oxygen and nutrients and to promote removal of accumulated neurotoxins. Treat shock aggressively with IV fluid, and inotropic medications if needed to maintain the blood pressure. Restrict fluids only after the child is hemodynamically stable.

Depressed, compound, and basilar fractures: irrigation, surgical débridement, and elevation of bone; tetanus prophylaxis; and antibiotics.

Surgical débridement of any penetrating injury tracts, evacuation of hematomas, and removal of accessible bone or bullet particles may be indicated.

Manage increased ICP. Brain swelling leads to lowered cerebral perfusion pressure, worsening cerebral ischemia, and more swelling. Hypoxia and hypercapnia can cause vasodilation and increased ICP. If unrelieved, brain shifting begins in the cranium as a precursor of herniation. Mechanical ventilation with 100% oxygen at the child's normal respiratory rate is used in the first 24 hours after injury to maintain oxygenation levels.

- Medications (mannitol and hypertonic saline) help pull fluid out of the brain and lower ICP. Sedatives and analgesics reduce pain and help prevent increases in ICP. See Table 23–5.
- Invasive procedures such as burr holes, a ventriculostomy catheter, or decompressive craniectomy may be used.
- Head of the bed elevated up to 30 degrees, head maintained at midline to promote venous drainage. Avoid hip flexion.
- Environment should be kept as quiet as possible. Body temperature should be kept within normal limits. Therapeutic hypothermia is an investigational treatment to protect the brain.

Enteral nutrition is started early using a postpyloric feeding tube to decrease risk of aspiration.

Table 23–5   Medications Used for Increased Intracranial Pressure (ICP)

Medication	Nursing Management
Analgesics and sedatives	Monitor respiratory status with pulse oximetry and blood gases to assess for respiratory depression.
	Monitor behaviors and physiologic responses to assess pain management.
	When mechanical ventilation is needed, suction airway secretions to maintain airway patency.
Mannitol	Carefully monitor ICP as well as intake and output.
	Monitor serum osmolality (should be less than 320 mOsm/L) because of potential renal toxicity.
	Monitor serum and urine electrolytes to detect syndrome of inappropriate antidiuretic hormone secretion.
Hypertonic saline (3%) infusion	Must be administered by central venous catheter due to hypertonicity (Knapp, 2005).
	Monitor serum sodium and neurologic status to detect neurologic damage associated with severe osmotic shifts.
	Serum sodium levels should be gradually returned to normal when hypertonic saline is discontinued.
Barbiturates (pentobarbital)	Use a cardiorespiratory monitor to detect dysrhythmias.
	Monitor mean arterial blood pressure, as the medication can cause decreased cardiac output and hypotension.
Anticonvulsants	Monitor the child for seizures. Immediate medications are needed to stop seizure activity.

Note: Data from "Management of Increased Intracranial Pressure in the Critically Ill Child with Acute Neurologic Injury," by K. K. Marcoux, 2005, *AACN Clinical Issues, 16*(2), 212–231; and "Severe Traumatic Brain Injury," by R. T. Mansfield, 2007, *Clinical Pediatric Emergency Medicine, 8*, 156–164.

Rehabilitation care: prevent complications from immobilization, disuse, and neurologic dysfunction. Long-term rehabilitation is indicated to promote optimal level of function.

Nursing Management
Assessment
Assess the child's ability to maintain an open airway, regulate breathing, and maintain circulation.

Assess the neurologic status frequently with the pediatric Glasgow Coma Scale (see Table 23–2), pupil size and reactivity, and cranial nerves. Note decerebrate or decorticate posturing.

Carefully inspect any area of the skull with swelling or a hematoma for a possible fracture.

Monitor vital signs closely, watching for changes indicating increased hypoxia, ICP, or Cushing's triad.

Assume that the child with increased ICP has pain. Use physiologic and behavioral signs to assess for pain.

Assess the family's coping with the child's life-threatening injury and their support systems.

Implementation

Minimize increases in ICP by maintaining oxygenation and ventilation, keeping the airway clear, suctioning the airway only when excessive secretions are present, and providing careful thermoregulation. Minimize unpleasant stimuli and pain from procedures to prevent spikes in ICP.

Administer IV fluids at the rate that maintains hydration and blood pressure to ensure adequate cerebral perfusion pressure (CPP). Monitor the effects of medications on hydration status.

Stabilize and protect the intraventricular catheter or bolt from becoming displaced.

Position the child with head at midline supine on a flat surface or side-lying with neck and head straight to prevent compression of the neck blood vessels. Turn child by logrolling. Head of bed may be elevated only when CPP is maintained.

Promote nutrition to promote wound healing; enteral feeding may be used.

Provide oral care and good skin care. Pad and cushion bony prominences and change the child's position frequently. Protect the eyes from corneal irritation with ophthalmic ointment and patching.

Prevent constipation with stool softeners and suppositories as needed.

Perform passive range-of-motion exercises to prevent contractures. Coordinate initiation of physical, occupational, and speech therapy. Use splints to position extremities in functional positions. Encourage parents to learn techniques. Promote rehabilitation.

Provide stimulation based on the child's age and ability using toys, books, music, or games. Encourage parents to bring in the child's favorite music.

When the child may die or have a new disability, provide emotional support to parents in collaboration with social services, mental health providers, or clergy members.

Following severe brain injury, coordinate rehabilitation services to help the child regain self-care skills and improve functioning. Determine what adaptations and assistive technology are needed to care for the child at home. Refer families to home health services to help care for the child and to develop case management skills.

Patient and Family Education
Following mild brain injury:
- Prepare parents for altered behavior during 6 weeks of brain healing, such as tiring easily, memory loss or forgetfulness, easy distractibility, difficulty concentrating and following directions, irritability or short temper, and needing help starting and finishing tasks.
- An educational assessment should be initiated if recovery takes longer than 6 weeks.

Following moderate to severe brain injury:
- Children often have behavior problems that include inattention, increased or decreased activity, impulsivity, irritability, lowered frustration tolerance, emotional lability, apathy, aggression, and social withdrawal.
- Children may also have long-term problems with attention, problem solving, and speed of information processing that compromise their school performance.
- Encourage neuropsychological testing to identify subtle learning disabilities, and determine appropriate educational accommodations needed.

24 ALTERATIONS IN MENTAL HEALTH AND COGNITION

DEVELOPMENTAL AND BEHAVIORAL DISORDERS

Pervasive Developmental Disorders—Autism

Description/Etiology

Pervasive developmental disorders (PDDs) begin in early childhood and are characterized by impaired social interactions and communication, with restricted interests, activities, and behaviors (Centers for Disease Control and Prevention, 2006); they are also called *autistic spectrum disorders* (ASDs).

There are five types of PDDs: autistic disorder, Asperger's syndrome, Rett disorder, child disintegrative disorder, and PDD not otherwise specified.

The etiology of autistic spectrum disorders is unclear, but they are biologically based with multiple and complex phenotypes as cause; genetic transmission, immune responses, and neuroanatomy are being investigated as causes.

Neurotransmitters such as dopamine, serotonin, and opioids are abnormal in some children and a focus of present research. Brain size and therefore head circumference may be enlarged in the young child with the disorder (DiCicco-Bloom, Lord, Zwaigenbaum et al., 2006).

Fetal alcohol syndrome, fragile X syndrome, phenylketonuria, Down syndrome, and tuberous sclerosis are all associated with a higher-than-normal incidence (Johnson et al., 2007).

Clinical Manifestations

The essential features typically become apparent by the time a child is 3 years of age and involve impairment in social interaction, communication, adaptation to new situations, attention span, and organizational responses to new situations (Volkmar, Wiesner & Westphal, 2006).

The child may be unable to converse normally, fail to initiate conversations, and have impaired observations of nonverbal behavior.

Stereotypy or rigid, obsessive, repetitive behavior may occur.

Responses to sensory stimuli are frequently abnormal and include an extreme aversion to touch, loud noises, and bright lights.

Emotional lability is common.

Communication difficulties or delays in speech and language are common and are often the first symptoms that lead to diagnosis.

Absence of babbling and other communication by 1 year, absence of two-word phrases by 2 years, and deterioration of previous language skills are characteristic; abnormal communication patterns include both verbal and nonverbal communication.

They often have rituals and become upset if normal routines are disrupted.

Autistic children may manifest disturbances in the rate or sequence of development; they are frequently cognitively impaired but can demonstrate a wide range of intellectual ability and functioning.

See further clinical manifestations of particular types in Table 24–1.

Diagnostic Tests
The first step in identification of children at risk of ASD is surveillance at each healthcare visit. Diagnosis is based on the results of the examination and the presence of specific criteria, as described in the American Psychiatric Association's *Diagnostic and Statistical Manual of Mental Disorders*, 4th edition (DSM-IV-TR).

Diagnosis includes developmental testing, neuroimaging (computed tomography scan or magnetic resonance imaging), lead screening, metabolic studies, DNA analysis, and electroencephalogram.

Clinical Therapy
Early intervention assists in maximizing the child's potential and establishing helpful support for parents (Giarelli, Souders, Pinto-Martin et al., 2005).

Treatment focuses on behavior management to teach focus and learning skills, reward appropriate behaviors, foster positive or adaptive coping skills, and facilitate effective communication.

Goals of treatment are to reduce rigidity or stereotypy (repetitive, obsessive, machinelike movements) and other maladaptive behaviors.

Some parents choose to use complementary therapies such as vitamin supplements and dimethylglycine.

Medications are used with some children to treat associated disorders but are not effective in treatment of autistic syndrome itself; they may

Table 24–1 Clinical Manifestations of Autistic Spectrum Disorders (Pervasive Developmental Disorders)

Disorder	Clinical Manifestations	Clinical Therapy
Autistic disorder	Impaired social, communicative, and behavioral development, usually noted in first year of life.	Early intervention is key to maximal performance. Interventions focus on improving behaviors and communication skills, providing physical and occupational therapy, structuring play interactions with other children, and educating parents about the child's needs.
Asperger's syndrome	Impaired social interactions with normal language development for age; pitch, tone and other speech characteristics may be abnormal. Verbal skills involving spelling and vocabulary are high, with concept formation, language flexibility, and comprehension low.	Social interactions are the focus of therapy.
Rett disorder	Early development appears normal and symptoms emerge at 6–18 mo. Ataxia, hand-wringing, intermittent hyperventilation, dementia, and growth retardation show progressive increase. Appears only in females as an X-linked dominant disorder; mutations occur in the gene MeCP2, affecting methyl-CpG-binding protein 2, which is important in brain development.	Early intervention in areas of abnormal behaviors.
Childhood disintegrative disorder	First 2–5 years of development appear normal followed by deterioration in many areas of functioning. Behaviors finally stabilize at some point without further deterioration.	Focus on areas of developmental function that show abnormality. Individualized education plans are needed in school to deal with communication, play, physical therapy, and teaching management skills to parents. Regression in toileting and other skills may occur.
Pervasive developmental disorder not otherwise specified	Severe social impairment without meeting DSM criteria for other types of autistic spectrum disorder.	Behavioral therapy focuses on building social skills.

include stimulants, selective serotonin reuptake inhibitors (SSRIs), and mood stabilizers.

Further therapy is listed in Table 24–1.

Nursing Management

Carefully evaluate the child for history of developmental milestones; perform developmental screening that considers several areas of development, including motor activity, social skills, and language. Become familiar with the "red flags" of the American Academy of Neurology and Child Neurology Society that require immediate evaluation (Johnson et al., 2007):

- No babbling or communication gestures by 12 months
- No single word by 16 months
- No spontaneous two-word combinations by 24 months
- Loss of language or social skills previously achieved

Perform hearing and vision screening if possible to rule out sensory problems.

The child needs to be oriented to new settings such as a classroom or the hospital room; ask parents about the child's usual routines and maintain these routines as much as possible.

Adjust communication techniques and teaching to the child's developmental level.

Schedule daily care and routine procedures at consistent times to maintain predictability.

Evaluate methods of communication and adapt to the child's needs.

Maintain a safe environment.

Partner with parents to promote the child's development through behavior modification and specialized educational programs.

Families of autistic children need a great deal of support to cope with the challenges of caring for the autistic child; help them to identify resources for child care, such as special toddler programs and preschools; assist them to work with schools to establish an individualized education plan.

The parent or primary caretaker often has difficulty obtaining respite care and may need assistance to find suitable resources.

Siblings of the autistic child may need help to explain the disorder to their friends or teachers.

Attention Deficit Disorder and Attention Deficit Hyperactivity Disorder

Description and Etiology

Attention deficit disorder is a variation in central nervous system (CNS) processing characterized by developmentally inappropriate behaviors involving inattention; when hyperactivity and impulsivity accompany inattention, the disorder is called *attention deficit hyperactivity disorder*.

Attention deficit hyperactivity disorder is most commonly manifested and affects from 6% to 9% of all school-age children, boys almost four times more commonly than girls (Froehlich, Lanphear, Epstein et al., 2007; Wolraich, Wibbelsman, Brown et al., 2005).

Some prenatal and environmental exposures are associated with higher incidence of the disorder; examples of known associations include exposure to high levels of lead or mercury in childhood, prenatal exposure to alcohol or tobacco smoke, preterm labor, impaired placenta functioning, and impaired oxygenation in the perinatal period; seizures and serious head injury are other potential associations.

Genetic factors may be important, as well as family dynamics and environmental characteristics.

The pathophysiology of attention deficit disorder/attention deficit hyperactivity disorder is unclear, but there may be a deficit in the catecholamines dopamine and norepinephrine in some children, lowering the threshold for stimuli input.

Clinical Manifestations

Children with attention deficit disorder and attention deficit hyperactivity disorder have problems related to decreased attention span, impulsiveness, and/or increased motor activity.

Diagnostic Tests

Obtaining an accurate diagnosis by a pediatric mental health specialist is vital; specific diagnostic criteria must be applied to all children with the potential diagnosis (see DSM criteria in American Psychiatric Association, 2000).

Behaviors both at home and school or child care must be evaluated because abnormal patterns in two settings are needed for diagnosis.

Various tests are available for use by the trained professional in establishing the diagnosis.

Diagnosis begins with a careful history of the child, including family history, birth history, growth and developmental milestones, behaviors such as sleep and eating patterns, progression and patterns in school, social and environmental conditions, and reports from parents and teachers.

A physical examination should be performed to rule out neurologic diseases and other health problems.

A mental health specialist performs testing of the child and administers questionnaires to the parent and teacher to identify the disorder and to rule out other conditions that may mimic or occur concurrently, such as depression, anxiety, learning disorder, conduct disorder, or oppositional defiant disorder.

Clinical Therapy

Treatment is established to meet the desired behavioral outcomes and includes a combination of approaches, such as environmental changes, behavior therapy, and pharmacotherapy (Brown et al., 2005).

See Table 24–2 for a listing of common pharmacologic treatments.

Nursing Management

Assess the child's development, and observe interactions and activity level.

Refer to mental health specialist for diagnosis.

When medications are used for treatment, be alert for side effects; careful periodic monitoring of weight, height, and blood pressure is necessary.

Promote the child's self-esteem by emphasizing the positive aspects of behavior and treating instances of negative behavior as learning opportunities; help the child to develop ego strengths.

Behavior modification programs can help to reduce specific impulsive behaviors.

Parents must cope simultaneously with managing the difficult needs and demands of a hard-to-handle child, obtaining appropriate evaluation and treatment, and understanding and accepting the diagnosis, even when the child exhibits different behaviors with different people; family support is essential.

Provide information on behavioral techniques, including need for daily exercise and quiet places for homework; work closely with the

Table 24–2 Medications Used to Treat Attention Deficit Hyperactivity Disorder

Medication	Action/Use	Nursing Management
Methylpheni-date	A derivative of piperidine that acts like amphetamine. May work in ADHD treatment by inhibiting reuptake of dopamine and norepinephrine, thereby enhancing catecholamine effects in the nervous system, improving attention span and task performance. Schedule II drug in Schedule of Controlled Substances.	Available in short-acting forms of 5, 10, and 20 mg as Ritalin and Methylin, and in 2.5, 5, and 10 mg forms as Focalin. Also in intermediate-acting forms of 20 mg (Ritalin SR), 10 and 20 mg (Metadate ER and Methylin ER). Available in long-acting forms of 18, 27, 36, and 54 mg (Concerta), 20 mg (Metadate CD), and 20, 30, and 40 mg (Ritalin LA). The variety of available forms makes it important to read labels carefully and inform families about proper admin-istration of the child's specific type of drug. The most common side effects are headache, insomnia, and anorexia. Periodic growth measurements are needed. Behavior and school perfor-mance are monitored.
Amphetamine salts (ampheta-mine, dextroampheta-mine, lisdix-amfetamine)	Synthetic sympa-thomimetic amine with stimulant effect on CNS. Increases release of norepi-nephrine and dopamine by blocking their reuptake. Schedule II drug in Schedule of Controlled Substances.	Available in short-acting forms (for 4–6 hours) of 5 mg (Dexedrine), 5 and 10 mg (Cextrostat) and 5 and 7.5 mg (Adderall). Intermediate-acting forms include 10, 12.5, 15, 20, and 30 mg Adderall, and 5, 10, and 15 mg Dexedrine Span-sules. A long-acting form (for 10–12 hours) is 5, 10, 15, 20, 25, or 30 mg Adderall-XR; Vynanse was approved in 2007. Read labels and instruct in proper administration. Anorexia, weight loss, insom-nia, and headache are common side effects. Monitor vital signs and growth measurements periodically.

Medication	Action/Use	Nursing Management
Atomoxetine	This is the first nonstimulant drug for treatment of ADHD. It inhibits norepinephrine reuptake. Decreases hyperactivity and impulsivity of ADHD and may assist with improving mood and decreasing anxiety.	Available as Stratterain 10, 18, 25, 40, and 60 mg capsules. Recommended starting dose for children is 0.5 mg/kg/day. Has been shown to have long-lasting effect of 1 day or longer. Side effects are uncommon and transient, with dyspepsia or vomiting, fatigue, decreased appetite, and dizziness most common. Have the child change position slowly if dizziness occurs; caution teen not to drive until effects of drug are clear. Perform periodic growth measurements. FDA has warned about uncommon side effects of hepatotoxicity and suicidal ideation.

school and healthcare provider; and provide information about medication effects, safe storage, and administration.

MOOD DISORDERS

Depression

Description and Etiology

Depression is psychological distress that can range from mild to severe.

The incidence of major depression is estimated to be approximately 0.3% in preschoolers, 2% in prepubertal children, and approximately 5% to 10% in adolescents; males and females are equally affected until adolescence, when the incidence in girls rapidly increases until they are twice as commonly afflicted (Dopheide, 2006).

Many theories have been proposed to explain the cause of depression in children and adolescents; depression may be biologic in origin (decrease in monoamines needed for neurotransmission) or a result of learned helplessness, cognitive distortion, social skills deficit, or family dysfunction; other mental health disorders commonly accompany depression.

Clinical Manifestations

Characteristic findings of major depression in children and adolescents include declining school performance, withdrawal from social activities, sleep disturbance (either too much or too little), appetite disturbance (too much or too little), multiple somatic complaints, especially headaches and stomachaches, decreased energy, difficulty concentrating and making decisions, low self-esteem, and feelings of hopelessness.

Symptoms of depression in children vary according to their developmental levels.

- Infants may fail to eat and grow.
- Toddlers can show regressive behaviors in toileting and other activities.
- Preschoolers have less symbolic and other play activities, and demonstrate self-destructive behaviors.
- School children may show a decrease in academic performance, increased or decreased activity, somatic complaints, and loss of friends; they may be irritable and manifest frequent death themes in their play.
- Adolescents can have a wide array of symptoms such as anxiety, decreased social contact, poor school performance, lack of prior involvement in activities, poor self-care, difficulty with parents and teachers, and focus on violence (Dopheide, 2006; Luby, Heffelfinger, Koenig-McNaught, et al., 2004; Pruett & Luby, 2004).

Diagnostic Tests

Initial assessment is performed by a child psychologist or child psychiatrist; a variety of scales and techniques are used, such as the following:

- Children's Depression Inventory
- Revised Children's Manifest Anxiety Scale
- Beck Depression Inventory
- Preschool Feelings Checklist
- Reynolds Child Depression Scale
- Reynolds Adolescent Depression Scale
- Center for Epidemiologic Studies Depression Scale of Children

Clinical Therapy

Treatment may include psychotherapy in combination with psychotropic medication.

Often a combination of individual, family, and group therapy provides the greatest benefits for young children and adolescents.

Involving parents and other family members in the treatment plan is essential.

Group therapy is an effective treatment measure for adolescents because of the importance of peer group relationships during the teenage years.

Cognitive behavior therapy (CBT) may be used with adolescents, and play therapy with younger children.

Antidepressant medications, most commonly the SSRIs, tricyclic antidepressants such as imipramine (Tofranil) and desipramine (Norpramin), and amitriptyline (Elavil), may be prescribed. The only antidepressant approved to treat major depressive disorders in pediatric patients is fluoxetine HCl (Prozac), but others are used by clinicians when the child does not respond to Prozac.

Nursing Management

Nursing assessment includes a thorough history, physical examination, and screening for risk factors of depression (Table 24–3).

Monitor vital signs of youth receiving antidepressant medications.

Watch for common side effects of the agent(s) used, and carefully monitor for serious side effects of tricyclic antidepressants or SSRIs. Monitor closely with face-to-face contact.

Monitor cardiovascular status, including hypertension and tachycardia; observe motor movement; and record dietary intake.

Table 24–3   Risk Factors for Child and Adolescent Depression

Child	Family	School and Social Situations
Frequent feelings of sadness, sleep problems, loss of interest in activities	Parental neglect, abuse, or loss	Academic pressures and underachievement
Increase in risk taking and impulsivity	Dysfunctional family relationships	Stressful social relationships
Previous suicide attempt	Family history of depression, suicide, substance abuse, alcoholism, other psychopathology	Declining participation in social events
Alcohol or substance abuse		
Diagnosed psychotic disorder		
Chronic illness and frequent hospitalization		

Help parents to evaluate inpatient settings if the child needs hospitalization to be certain the care provided best meets the needs of the child or adolescent.

Teach parents and school personnel to recognize signs and symptoms of worsening depression and to report these symptoms promptly.

Parents should be taught dosages and side effects of any prescribed medications.

Instruct the family to remove guns, ammunition, and other potentially harmful items from the home. Have the family immediately seek emergency care if they are concerned about the child's safety or worsening condition.

Refer the family to appropriate healthcare professionals and to support groups for family members dealing with depression.

Bipolar Disorder (Manic Depression)

Bipolar disorder is a mental illness in which extreme changes in affect and energy are manifested. Moods most often alter between mania and depression. Children often present with irritability or hyperactivity.

About 1% of children and adults suffer from bipolar illness, with a high rate of onset from 15 to 19 years (Lansford, 2005). The manic phase of bipolar illness is characterized by hyperactivity and high energy, irritability, aggression, and sometimes hallucinations.

In the depressive phase, the child is sad, has alterations in sleep and eating patterns, feels worthless, is lacking in energy, and is socially withdrawn, similar to any depressive illness. Mania may be the persistent symptom in children, or rapid cycles of mania and depression can occur throughout the day (Lansford, 2005).

Diagnosis and treatment of bipolar disorder should be performed by mental health specialists; there are not specific criteria for diagnosis of bipolar disease in children.

The treatment of bipolar disease involves a variety of drugs used to stabilize mood. Lithium, valproate, divalproex, carbamazepine, olanzapine, excarbazepine, lamotregine, quetiapine, and risperidone are examples of drugs used. Early treatment is key to preventing chronic, serious mental illness (Ferguson-Noyes, 2005; Kowatch et al., 2005). Individual and family education and therapy can be helpful.

The child with bipolar disorder needs ongoing care to ensure implementation of therapy and return to function.

The nurse administers medications in some settings and instructs parents, the child, and other family members in other settings; observe for side effects to the specific drug regimen used.

Assist parents to find resources for health care because medications and other treatments may be costly; parents and children need information about the disorder because it may recur several times during life; assist the child to find social events and groups that build a sense of self-esteem.

Anxiety and Related Disorders

Anxiety is a subjective feeling of uncertainty, worry, and helplessness, usually accompanied by CNS signs, including restlessness, trembling, perspiration, and rapid pulse.

Generalized anxiety disorder is often manifested in children by restlessness, excessive fatigue, poor concentration, irritability, muscle tension, and sleep disturbance.

Separation anxiety disorder is a particular type of anxiety characterized by an extreme state of uneasiness when in unfamiliar surroundings and often by refusal to visit friends' homes or attend school for at least 2 weeks; children with separation anxiety disorder tend to be perfectionistic, overly compliant, and eager to please; they often cling to the parent or caretaker; they may use physical complaints such as headaches, abdominal pain, nausea, and vomiting in an attempt to avoid being away from the parent, and depression frequently accompanies separation anxiety disorder.

Another type of anxiety disorder is *panic disorder*, the presence of recurrent, unexpected panic attacks; these attacks are periods of intense fear and discomfort in the absence of real danger; physical symptoms experienced are palpitations, sweating, chills, hot flashes, shaking, shortness of breath, choking, chest pain, nausea, and dizziness; the person describes feelings of danger or doom.

Another disorder is *obsessive-compulsive disorder*, in which children have recurrent ritualistic thoughts or actions that interfere with daily life. Affected children have recurrent obsessive thoughts, commonly about contamination, harm, sex, or moral concerns. These obsessions are handled through a series of compulsive behaviors that interfere with daily life; examples of behaviors and concerns are obsessions about dirt or germs, worries about harm, and sexual thoughts; common behaviors are excessive hand washing, counting objects, and hoarding substances.

School phobia (also known as social anxiety disorder) is a persistent, irrational, or excessive fear of negative evaluation or embarrassment in social situations and therefore of attending school. *Posttraumatic stress disorder* victims have experienced or witnessed a life-threatening event; the symptoms of distress continue for more than 1 month and cause impairment in functioning. The major types of manifestations cluster in three groups: (1) the person repeatedly experiences the event, such as in a nightmare or, for young children, in repetitive play about the event; (2) avoidance by purposefully avoiding places or activities that trigger the memory; and (3) arousal such as increased vigilance, and somatic complaints (Brown, 2005).

The event is persistently reexperienced through thoughts, dreams, or memories, leading to feelings of fear, terror, and helplessness; the child with posttraumatic stress disorder is often irritable and has sleep problems and inattentiveness; there is a state of hypervigilance and exaggerated startle response, such as to touch or loud noises; the child feels detached from others and alone.

The diagnosis for anxiety and related disorders is made by a mental health specialist.

Counseling by a mental health specialist is the main therapy for anxiety disorders; techniques such as play therapy and group techniques are frequently used with children. Cognitive behavior therapy (CBT) is the treatment of choice, with both the child and family members included.

Nursing Management

The nurse gathers information about family history, the events that have occurred in the child's life, behavioral descriptions and recent changes, developmental progression, and social interactions.

Nursing care for anxiety disorders focuses on behavioral and cognitive therapies to enhance coping skills—for example, mental health nurses may conduct group therapy sessions both in inpatient and community settings.

Children can learn relaxation techniques, and nurses may teach such techniques or recommend that the child consider participation in yoga or guided-imagery classes.

Parents or other significant people should be included in the treatment program; nurses often teach them basic information about the child's diagnosis and therapy, provide resources that they need to get relief from worry about the child, and help them identify financial resources to cover cost of treatment.

Nurses often administer medications to children being treated for anxiety; be alert for and promptly report side effects; ensure that the family knows how to safely administer the drugs; drugs should be kept locked securely; the child should wear a medical alert tag with the medications noted.

Have the child return for follow up as needed because some medications may take several weeks to achieve effects, and close monitoring is essential.

School personnel may need to know about the child's treatment, so partner with the families to provide needed information.

Some schools have counselors who can be instrumental in carrying out treatment plans at school and acting as a resource in that setting; school personnel may be asked to provide feedback about the child's attendance, performance, and social skills as a measure of the success of therapy, and the community or school nurse can relay this information to the mental health therapist.

SUICIDE

Suicide is the third leading cause of death in adolescents between 15 and 19 years of age and has grown in incidence in the last 5 years (Centers for Disease Control and Prevention, 2007).

The most common precursor to adolescent suicide is depression; common signs or symptoms of an underlying depression that could lead to suicide include boredom, restlessness, problems with concentration, irritability, lethargy, intentional misbehavior, preoccupation with one's own body or health, and excessive dependence on or isolation from others (especially adults or caregivers); the depression may be exacerbated by a recent psychosocial stress such as loss or perceived rejection or ridicule.

Many risk factors for suicide exist in children and adolescents, and there are also known protective factors (Table 24–4).

The child or adolescent found to be at high risk for suicide may be admitted to a psychiatric unit for care or cared for in a community mental health facility; it is important to provide crisis intervention at the time of the suicide attempt to minimize the opportunity for repeat attempts and begin a therapeutic treatment plan.

Treatment may include individual, group, or family therapy.

Negotiating a no-suicide contract is an important first step in therapy; in the contract, the child agrees not to attempt suicide during a specified

Table 24–4 Risk and Protective Factors for Suicide in Children and Adolescents

Risk Factors	Protective Factors
History of previous attempted suicide	Emotional well-being
Suicide or attempt by friend	Satisfactory school performance
School problems or changes in grades	Participation in sports or other group events
Pregnancy	Weight satisfaction
Drug use or abuse	Parent/family connectedness
Problems with a romantic relationship	Discuss issues with family frequently
Minority sexual practice	School connectedness
Loneliness, withdrawal	Safe school
Feelings of anxiety	Safe neighborhood
History of chronic family problems	Caring adult presence at school or elsewhere
Chronic illness	Availability of school counseling
Physical, emotional, or sexual abuse	School policies against fighting, bullying
History of suicide in a family member	
History of depression	
Chronic low self-esteem	
Change in behavior	
Change in weight	
Giving away special possessions	
Access to firearms and ammunition	

time period; the presence of a contract is not a guarantee of child safety, so vigilant monitoring of the youth's condition continues.

Comorbidities such as depression or substance abuse must also be addressed for treatment to be successful.

Nursing Management

The major nursing role is in prevention of suicide; all children and adolescents in health promotion visits and emergency rooms should be evaluated for risk.

During health promotion visits, be alert for children with depression, substance abuse, recent stresses, and changes in behavior.

Gather a family history of mental health disorders, suicide attempts, and stresses.

Ask about how often the youth talks with or has meals and other activities with the family.

Most suicides are committed with firearms present in the home, so ask at each healthcare visit if the family has firearms; encourage families to keep firearms unloaded, with ammunition and firearms locked in separate locations; be sure that children and adolescents do not have access to the keys for the locked firearms.

Nursing care of the child or teen hospitalized after a suicide attempt centers on taking appropriate precautions to ensure the safety of a child or adolescent at risk of suicide.

- The child and the environment of the hospital or other setting are monitored for any object that could be used for self-harm.
- All potentially harmful objects, such as shoestrings, belts, pantyhose, and hair ribbons, are removed.
- All personal care items (including toothbrush and shampoo) are kept locked at the nursing station and monitored constantly when used by the child.
- Children or adolescents who are considered at high risk for suicidal behaviors are attended by a nursing staff member at all times, including while using the bathroom and sleeping.

When the child is receiving care in the community, encourage parents to keep follow-up clinic appointments, to watch for self-destructive behaviors, and to administer any prescribed medications according to the treatment schedule; arrange home visits and other community resources for families.

Education in all school settings is appropriate to assist children in knowing about resources of help when needed and in identifying peers at risk.

- Teach students to report to teachers, nurses, or counselors about friends who have threatened suicide or seem depressed or display behaviors different than usual.
- Nurses often plan with mental health specialists to implement suicide prevention programs in schools and communities.

Provide supportive grief-counseling services to family and friends when suicide occurs.

SUBSTANCE USE

Tobacco Use

Tobacco use is the most preventable cause of adult death in the United States, Canada, and most other developed nations.

Major health problems linked to tobacco use include cardiovascular disease, cancer, chronic lung disease, increased prevalence of car crashes, low birth weight, and other maternal problems; even passive smoking or environmental tobacco smoke is linked to increased heart disease, blood pressure, and respiratory problems, and decreased youth academic performance (Collins, Wileyto, Murphy, et al., 2007; Reardon, 2007).

Cigarette use is most common; however, chewing tobacco, snuff, cigars, and bidis may also be used and also pose significant health hazards.

Characteristics that contribute to the likelihood of tobacco use include increasing age, male gender, ethnic group, ease of obtaining tobacco products, and smoking among family members; low socioeconomic group membership, access to tobacco products, low price of products, advertising, and lack of parental involvement in the youths' lives are also associated with tobacco use (U.S. Department of Health and Human Services, 2006).

Nursing Management

The roles of nurses in preventing and intervening in youth smoking are to inform youth, identify smokers, and implement programs.

Educational programs have been developed to encourage youth to avoid tobacco use, and smoking cessation programs are available to assist youth who are already regular smokers to lead to cessation or decrease in tobacco use. Use of incentives and counselor-based, individually tailored telephone interventions have been effective (Backinger, Michaels, Jefferson, et al., 2008; Liu, Pererson, Kealey, et al., 2007).

Questions about tobacco use should be inserted by nurses into all well-child visits, beginning at approximately 9 to 10 years of age; inquire about whether family members (especially parents and siblings) smoke or chew, and ask if some of the child's friends have tried smoking.

Determine the child's knowledge and beliefs about the benefits and risks of tobacco use.

Assess for associated risk behaviors such as alcohol and drug use, sexual behavior, and suicidal thoughts.

Offer information on available prevention and cessation programs to youth and families in clinics, outpatient surgery centers, community activities, and hospitals.

Use opportunities such as adolescent pregnancy and presence of illness to reinforce the hazardous effects of tobacco on the individual and on those nearby.

Speak to young athletes about the effects of tobacco on athletic performance.

Show youth the ways in which this product can interfere with their meeting of life goals.

Role-play how to tell other youth no when tobacco is offered.

Establish programs that increase the sense of self-esteem without tobacco use.

Be sure to include parents in the programs so that they see and acknowledge their role in setting an example about tobacco use and in providing guidelines for the child; influence of environmental tobacco (secondhand smoke) should be acknowledged.

Encourage positive coping techniques for youth who are engaged in cessation.

Work with the schools and school districts to help establish preventive and cessation programs.

Alcohol and Drug Use

Use of many substances—particularly marijuana, alcohol, cocaine, crack, and heroin—remains high among youth.

Substance use represents a maladaptive coping response to the stressors of childhood and adolescence.

Children in families with a history of substance use are at higher risk of using drugs and alcohol; other risk factors include rebelliousness, aggressiveness, low self-esteem, dysfunctional parental relationships, lack of adequate support systems, academic underachievement, poor judgment, and poor impulse control. A significant risk factor for initiation of alcohol use is a transition time, such as change from middle to high school, or a major family stress, such as parental separation or divorce (Loveland-Cherry, 2006). Substance use in children and adolescents is commonly overlooked and under-diagnosed by healthcare providers.

Common physical manifestations include alterations in vital signs, weight loss, chronic fatigue, chronic cough, respiratory congestion, red eyes, and general apathy and malaise; the mental status examination may reveal alterations in level of consciousness, impaired attention and concentration, impaired thought processes, delusions, and hallucinations; low self-esteem, feelings of guilt or worthlessness, and suicidal or homicidal thoughts are also common; poor school performance and changes in mood, sleep habits, appetite, dress, and social relationships are nonspecific characteristics of the substance-using child (see Table 24–5 for further information on clinical manifestations).

The primary goal of treatment is to teach the child and other family members to develop and sustain positive coping patterns and to support them during this process.

Table 24–5 Clinical Manifestations of Commonly Abused Drugs

Drug	Potential for Dependence	Clinical Manifestations
Depressants		
Alcohol, barbiturates (amobarbital, pentobarbital, secobarbital)	Physical and psychological: high; varies somewhat among drugs	Physical: decreased muscle tone and coordination, tremors Psychological: impaired speech, memory, and judgment; confusion; decreased attention span; emotional lability
Stimulants		
Amphetamines (e.g., Benzedrine), caffeine, cocaine	Physical: low to moderate Psychological: high; withdrawal from amphetamines and cocaine can lead to severe depression	Physical: dilated pupils, increased pulse and blood pressure, flushing, nausea, loss of appetite, tremors Psychological: euphoria; increased alertness, agitation, or irritability; hallucinations; insomnia
Opiates		
Codeine, heroin, meperidine (Demerol), methadone, morphine, opium, oxycodone (Percodan, OxyContin)	Physical and psychological: high; varies somewhat among drugs; withdrawal effects are uncomfortable but rarely life-threatening	Physical: analgesia, depressed respirations and muscle tone (may lead to coma or death), nausea, constricted pupils Psychological: changes in mood (usually euphoria), drowsiness, impaired attention or memory, sense of tranquility

Table 24–5 Clinical Manifestations of Commonly Abused Drugs (Continued)

Drug	Potential for Dependence	Clinical Manifestations
Hallucinogens		
Lysergic acid diethylamide (LSD), mescaline, phencyclidine (PCP)	Physical: none Psychological: unknown	Physical: lack of coordination, dilated pupils, hypertension, elevated temperature; severe PCP intoxication can result in seizures, respiratory depression, coma, and death Psychological: visual illusions and hallucinations, altered perceptions of time and space, emotional lability, psychosis
Volatile inhalants		
Glues, typing correction fluid, acrylic paints, spot removers, lighter fluid, gasoline, butane	Physical and psychological: varies with drug used	Physical: impaired coordination, liver damage (in some cases) Psychological: impaired judgment, delirium
Marijuana	Physical: low Psychological: usually low; occasionally moderate to high	Physical: tachycardia, reddened conjunctiva, dry mouth, increased appetite Psychological: initial anxiety followed by euphoria; giddiness; impaired attention, judgment, and memory

Most treatment programs offer inpatient and outpatient services, as well as aftercare programs; they usually consist of peer support focusing on the development of a lifestyle free of drugs or alcohol, healthy family relationships, and positive coping skills; family involvement is strongly encouraged.

Hospitalization is required if the physical dependence is significant and withdrawal places the child at risk for complications such as seizures, depression, or suicidal behavior.

Nursing Management

Nursing management focuses on prevention of substance use, early identification of users, and referral to treatment options.

Assessment tools provide useful information for the healthcare provider; examples are the PACES and HEEADSSS tools:

P = Parents, peers

A = Accidents, alcohol/drug use

C = Cigarettes

E = Emotional problems

S = School, sexuality
(Knight, 1997)

H = Home environment

E = Employment and education

E = Eating

A = Activities

D = Drugs (substance use)

S = Sexuality

S = Suicide/depression

S = Safety
(Goldenring & Rosen, 2004)

CHILD ABUSE

Child abuse includes physical abuse, physical neglect, emotional abuse and neglect, verbal abuse, and sexual abuse.

Abuse generally involves an act of commission—that is, actively doing something to a child physically, emotionally, or sexually, such as hitting, belittling, or molesting; neglect more often involves an act of omission, such as not providing adequate nutrition, emotional contact, or necessary physical care.

Physical abuse is the deliberate maltreatment of another individual that inflicts pain or injury and may result in permanent or temporary disfigurement or even death.

Physical neglect is the deliberate withholding of or failure to provide the necessary and available resources to the child.

Emotional abuse involves shaming, ridiculing, embarrassing, or insulting the child or the destruction of a child's personal property.

Emotional neglect is characterized by the caretaker's emotional unavailability to the child.

Child sexual abuse is the exploitation of a child for the sexual gratification of an adult.

The most common abuser is the child's parent or guardian or the male friend of the child's mother.

Risk factors associated with abusive behavior in adults include the following:
- Psychopathology, such as drug addiction or alcoholism, low self-esteem, poor impulse control, and other personality disorders
- Poor parenting experiences, such as abuse in the abuser's own childhood, rejection by the abuser's own parent(s), lack of knowledge of alternative methods of discipline, strong belief in or family tradition of harsh discipline, and lack of parental affection
- Marital stressors and problems with partners, such as hostile-dependent, abusive, or nonsupportive relationships and one-sided decision making
- Environmental stressors, such as legal, financial, medical, or housing problems
- Social isolation, such as few friends and limited use of sitters, family, or other resources
- Inappropriate expectations for the developmental level of the child

See Tables 24–6 and 24–7 for some common clinical manifestations of abuse.

Table 24–6   Clinical Manifestations of Child Abuse

Multiple bruises in various stages of healing

Scald burns with clear lines of demarcation and in a glove or stocking distribution

Rope, belt, or cord marks, usually seen on the mouth, buttocks, back, legs, and arms

Burn scars in various stages of healing

Multiple fractures in various stages of healing; spiral fractures not explained by accident

Shortness of breath and distress on being moved, indicating chest contusions and possible rib fractures

Cranial or abdominal injuries

Sedation from overmedication

Change in behavior or school performance

Fear and avoidance of certain people or situations

Anger and violent play

Exacerbation of chronic illness (such as diabetes or asthma) because of withholding of medication evaluation

Table 24–7 Clinical Manifestations of Sexual Abuse in Children and Adolescents

Vaginal discharge

Blood-stained underpants or diaper

Genital redness, pain, itching, or bruising

Difficulty walking or sitting

Urinary tract infection

Sexually transmitted disease

Somatic complaints, such as headaches or stomachaches

New or excessive sexual curiosity or play

Child or adolescent works as a prostitute

Sleeping problems, such as nightmares or night terrors

Bedwetting

Unwillingness to go to babysitter, family member, neighbor, or other person

Fear of strangers

New or excessive sexual curiosity or play

Constant masturbation

Curling into fetal position

Phobias about particular places, people, or things

Abrupt changes in school performance and attendance

Changes in eating habits

Abrupt changes in behavior (especially withdrawal)

Child or adolescent female acts like a wife or mother

Diagnosis of abuse is made on the basis of a careful history and thorough physical examination; radiologic, computed tomography, and magnetic resonance imaging studies may be ordered to identify signs of recurrent abuse such as healed fractures and other damaged tissues; laboratory studies may involve urine culture for signs of infection or screening for sexually transmitted diseases; genitourinary examination may be performed if sexual abuse is suspected.

Neglect, which is more difficult to define and identify, frequently requires hospitalization with a comprehensive medical, social, and psychiatric evaluation.

Initial therapy focuses on providing safety; physical injuries are treated, and the child is removed from the abusive situation.

Children who have been physically, emotionally, or sexually abused are at risk for major mental health problems, such as depression and posttraumatic stress disorder; they require skilled care by mental health professionals who are specially trained in this area.

Initially, the treatment goals include prevention of self-destructive or other dangerous acts.

Children are encouraged to express their fears and feelings in a safe and supportive environment.

The child is assisted to build coping skills and self-esteem.

The child must be reassured and convinced that he or she is in no way responsible or to blame for what happened.

Nursing Management

Nursing assessment in instances of suspected child abuse or neglect requires a comprehensive history and physical examination, with documentation of findings.

Be alert for discrepancies between the history and physical assessment data.

Work with social services and community agencies to assess the child's home environment, individuals living in the home, and the actions surrounding the abuse.

Assist in removing the child from the home to temporary custody of the court or foster care of another relative, if indicated.

Counsel family members about abuse and refer for appropriate therapy.

Protect and treat the child's injuries.

Work within schools to inform all children about where they may turn in abusive situations, and help establish information sessions for teens about date rape and safety precautions.

FEEDING AND EATING DISORDERS

Feeding Disorder of Infancy and Early Childhood (Failure to Thrive)

Feeding disorder of infancy and early childhood, or failure to thrive (FTT), describes a syndrome in which infants or young children fail to eat enough food to be adequately nourished.

The cause of FTT can be organic, as in congenital acquired immun-odeficiency syndrome, inborn errors of metabolism, neurologic disease, and esophageal reflux; however, most cases of FTT are nonorganic in origin; FTT resulting from nonorganic causes is called *feeding disorder of infancy or early childhood.*

Infants and children whose parents or caretakers experience poverty, depression, substance abuse, mental retardation, or psychosis are at risk for this disorder; parents may be socially and emotionally isolated or may lack knowledge of infant nutritional and nurturing needs. Preterm and small-for-gestational-age babies more commonly have eating disorders (Block, Krebs, and Committee on Children Abuse and Neglect, 2005).

A reciprocal interaction pattern may exist whereby the parent does not offer enough food or is not responsive to the infant's hunger cues, and the infant is irritable, not soothed, and does not give clear cues about hunger.

The characteristics of this feeding disorder are persistent failure to eat adequately with no weight gain or with weight loss in a child 6 years of age or younger that is not associated with other medical conditions or mental disorders and is not caused by lack of or unavailability of food. Weight is generally < the 5th percentile, and weight-for-length is < 80% of ideal weight (Block et al., 2005; Olsen, 2006). Infants with feeding disorders refuse food, may have erratic sleep patterns, are irritable and difficult to soothe, and are often developmentally delayed.

A thorough history and physical examination are needed to rule out any chronic physical illness; the infant or child may be hospitalized so that healthcare providers can establish a routine for feeding and sleeping.

The goals of treatment are to provide adequate caloric and nutritional intake, promote normal growth and development, and assist parents in developing feeding routines and responding to the infant's cues of physical and psychological hunger.

Nursing Management

Nurses perform accurate measurement of weight and height each time any child is seen for health care to provide a record of growth patterns over time.

The child's activity level, developmental milestones, and interaction patterns provide important information.

When feeding the child, the nurse observes how the child indicates hunger or satiety, the ability of the child to be soothed, and general interaction patterns such as eye contact, touch, and cuddliness.

Nursing care centers on performing a thorough history and physical assessment, observing parent–child interactions during feeding times, and providing necessary teaching to enable parents to respond appropriately to their child's needs.

Observations of feeding and continued careful physical assessments are needed; the child's intake is carefully recorded at each meal or feeding.

Parents are taught how to understand and respond to the child's cues of hunger and satiety; they are taught to hold, rock, and touch the infant during feedings and to establish eye contact with infants and children during feeding situations.

Refer the family to an agency that can continue monitoring of the home situation; this provides an opportunity to observe feeding during a home visit and evaluate stresses and behavior patterns among family members.

Frequent growth measurement and development must be ensured so the child is adequately nourished.

Parents may need referral to community resources to help them manage stressful situations in their lives and to enhance their parenting skills.

Finding a nurturing relationship for the parent may provide the support needed to enhance parenting.

Anorexia Nervosa

Anorexia nervosa is a potentially life-threatening eating disorder that occurs primarily in teenage girls and young women, but also can be seen in males.

Adolescents with anorexia are characterized by extreme weight loss accompanied by a preoccupation with weight and food, excessive compulsive exercising, peculiar patterns of eating and handling food, and distorted body image.

Cultural overemphasis on thinness may contribute to the overconcern with dieting, body image, and fear of becoming fat that is experienced by many adolescents; chemical changes have been found in the brain and blood of anorectic patients, leading to theories about a biologic cause; often a significant life stress, loss, or change precedes the onset of anorexia. Stress hormones are commonly elevated, and immune system function may be disturbed (Gluck, 2006).

The adolescent may engage in lengthy and vigorous exercise (up to 4 hours daily) to prevent weight gain; laxatives or diuretics may be used to induce weight loss.

Leukopenia, electrolyte imbalance, and hypoglycemia develop as a result of protein–energy malnutrition; once the body mass decreases below a critical level, menstruation ceases.

Accompanying signs and symptoms of depression, crying spells, feelings of isolation and loneliness, and suicidal thoughts and feelings are common; the disorder is often associated with mental illness such as obsessive-compulsive disorder, anxiety disorders, and history of abuse (American Dietetic Association, 2006).

Physical findings include cold intolerance, dizziness, constipation, abdominal discomfort, bloating, irregular menses, and malnutrition; hypothalamic suppression can lead to disturbances of gynecologic function, osteoporosis, decreased bone density, and fractures; lanugo (fine, downy body hair) may be present.

Fluid and electrolyte imbalances, especially potassium imbalances, are common; extreme weight loss often leads to cardiac arrhythmias (bradycardia).

Diagnosis is based on a comprehensive history, physical examination revealing characteristic clinical manifestations, and the DSM-IV criteria.

Diagnostic tests commonly include hematocrit and hemoglobin, serum electrolytes, and serum vitamins and vitamin precursors; bone density studies may be warranted.

The goal of treatment is to address the physiologic problems associated with malnutrition, as well as the behavioral and cognitive components of the disorder.

A firm focus is placed on reaching a targeted weight, with a gradual weight gain of 0.1–0.2 kg/day (0.25–0.5 lb/day); enteral feedings or total parenteral nutrition may be necessary to replace lost fluid, protein, and nutrients.

Individual treatment and family therapy are used to address any individual and family patterns that may contribute to the disorder.

Nursing Management

Nursing care centers on meeting nutritional and fluid needs, preventing complications, administering medications, and providing referral to appropriate resources.

Monitor nutritional and fluid intake, encourage consumption of food, and observe eating behaviors at mealtime; elimination patterns may be altered as a result of increased intake during hospitalization, so monitor for abdominal distention, constipation, or diarrhea. Daily monitoring of serum electrolytes is necessary during acute hospitalizations with electrolyte imbalance.

If total parenteral nutrition is administered, watch for complications such as circulatory overload, hyperglycemia, or hypoglycemia; use strict aseptic technique when changing tubing or dressings.

Monitor vital signs if the adolescent is receiving antidepressants; watch for signs of hypertension and tachycardia, as well as changes in mood and behavior.

Refer parents and other family members to the American Anorexia and Bulimia Association, National Anorectic Aid Society, and National Association of Anorexia Nervosa and Associated Disorders for further information about the disorder and a list of support groups in their area.

Bulimia Nervosa

Bulimia nervosa is an eating disorder characterized by binge eating (a compulsion to consume large quantities of food in a short period of time); usually the episodes of bingeing are followed by various methods of weight control (purging), such as self-induced vomiting, large doses of laxatives or diuretics, or a combination of methods.

Causes of bulimia nervosa are similar to those of anorexia nervosa: sensitivity to social pressure for thinness, body image difficulties, and long-standing dysfunctional family patterns; depression is commonly associated with the disorder.

Adolescents with bulimia are preoccupied with body shape, size, and weight; they may appear overweight or thin and usually report a wide range of average body weight over the years.

Physical findings depend on the degree of purging, starvation, dehydration, and electrolyte disturbance; erosion of tooth enamel, increased dental caries, and gum recession, which result from vomiting of gastric acids, are common findings; the back of a hand can have calluses from inducing vomiting; abdominal distention is often seen; esophageal tears and esophagitis may also occur. Lowered potassium levels are related to repetitive vomiting, since gastric contents have a high potassium level (American Psychiatric Association, 2006).

Treatment includes management of physiologic problems, behavior modification, and psychotherapy.

Nursing Management

During hospitalization, the patient should keep a food diary.

Be alert to the adolescent who hides, gives away, or discards food from the tray or who exits to use the bathroom after meals; the adolescent should be monitored for at least 30 minutes after meals by remaining in a central area in the company of the nurse or other responsible individuals.

Withdrawal from laxatives and diuretics is managed with careful observation for alterations in fluid and electrolyte status.

Cardiac monitoring may be necessary if potassium levels are seriously altered.

Esophageal tearing or esophagitis is treated to promote mucosal healing.

Medications such as antidepressants may be administered.

Encourage continuation of group and other therapy sessions.

COGNITIVE DISORDERS

Learning Disabilities

Learning disabilities affect approximately 5% of school children.

The brain is unable to receive or process information in the normal manner.

Common types of learning disorders are listed in Table 24–8.

Children may have difficulty in processing visual information, which may be manifested in reading, writing, and mathematics performance; others may have more difficulty with oral information, leading to problems in language development and reading (Kelly & Aylward, 2005; National Center for Learning Disabilities, 2004).

Table 24–8   Clinical Manifestations of Various Learning Disabilities

Disorder	Clinical Manifestations
Dyslexia	Difficulty with writing, reading, and spelling
Dyscalculia	Mathematics and computation problems
Dysgraphia	Difficulty with writing, spelling, and composition
Dyspraxia	Problems with manual dexterity and coordination

The causes of learning disorders are complex. Sometimes they are related to low birth weight or problems during the perinatal period; there may be a genetic component because their occurrence is more common when other family members are affected.

Treatments involve learning how to compensate for the difficulties by using capabilities that are intact.

Children with learning disabilities should have individualized education plans established with realistic goals for school performance.

Nurses play a major role in identification of children with learning disabilities; assess the child for the following developmental milestones that can indicate learning disability:

- Lack of ability to phrase sentences together by 2.5 years
- Inability to use speech that is understandable at least 50% of the time by 3 years
- Inability to tie shoes, button, hop, or cut by kindergarten
- Inability to sit for a short story by 3 to 5 years (Kelly & Aylward, 2005)

When a child may have a learning disability, refer the family to the school or other testing resource.

Partner with the family to plan for the child's learning needs.

Help the family to work closely with the child, provide a setting at home to maximize potential for learning, and build healthy self-esteem in the child.

Assist the family to work with the school to establish annual goals for the child.

Mental Retardation
Description and Etiology

Mental retardation is defined as significant limitation in intellectual functioning and adaptive behavior. It is manifested in differences in conceptual, social, and practical life skills and begins before the age of 18 years (American Association of Mental Retardation, 2004).

Intellectual functioning is generally characterized by an IQ below 70–75, and there are significant impairments in adaptive functioning (the ability of an individual to meet the standards expected for his or her cultural group); the child with mental retardation has adaptive deficits in at least two areas, such as communication, self-care, home living, social/interpersonal skills, use of community resources, self-direction, functional academic skills, work, leisure, health, or safety.

The causes of mental retardation can be grouped into three general categories: prenatal errors in the development of the CNS, prenatal or postnatal changes in the biologic environment of the person, and external forces leading to CNS damage; in each instance, the precipitating factor causes a change in the form, function, and adaptation of the CNS (Table 24–9).

Three common conditions associated with mental retardation from prenatal conditions are Down syndrome, fragile X syndrome, and fetal alcohol syndrome; see Table 24–10 for physical characteristics of children with each of these conditions.

In the United States, approximately 1 in 800 to 1,000 infants, or 5,500 infants each year, are born with Down syndrome (Centers for Disease Control and Prevention, 2006a; Van Riper, 2007); the condition is caused by an extra chromosome, so the child has 47 rather than 46 chromosomes.

Fragile X syndrome is caused by a single recessive gene abnormality on the X chromosome.

Fetal alcohol syndrome is caused by the effect of ethyl alcohol on the developing fetus; alcohol ingestion by the pregnant woman can influence development of many body organs and effects can range from mild to severe. The term *fetal alcohol spectrum disorder* (FASD) describes the wide range of effects from the condition, which can range from FAS to a milder condition called fetal alcohol effects (FAE) (Caley, Shipkey, Winkelman, et al., 2006).

Table 24–9 Common Conditions Associated with Mental Retardation

Prenatal Conditions	Biologic Environment	External Forces
Down syndrome	Inborn errors of metabolism (e.g., phenylketonuria, hypothyroidism)	Traumatic brain injury (e.g., accident)
Fragile X syndrome		Poison ingestion (acute or chronic)
Fetal alcohol syndrome		Hypoxia/anoxic insult
Maternal infection (e.g., rubella, cytomegalovirus)		Infection (e.g., meningitis)
		Environmental deprivation

Table 24–10 Characteristics of Three Common Conditions Associated with Mental Retardation

Down Syndrome	Fragile X Syndrome	Fetal Alcohol Syndrome
Small head (microcephaly)	Long face	Flat midface
	Prominent jaw	Low nasal bridge
Flattened forehead	Large ears	Long philtrum with narrow upper lip
Wide, short neck	Frequent otitis media	
Epicanthal eye folds	Large testicles	Short, upturned nose
White spots on eye iris (Brushfield spots)	Epicanthal eye folds	Poor coordination
	Strabismus	Failure to thrive
Congenital cataracts	High-arched palate	Skeletal and joint abnormalities
Flat nose	Scoliosis	
Small, low-set ears	Pliable joints	Hearing loss
Protruding tongue		
Short, broad hands		
Simian line on palm		
Wide space between first and second toes		
Hearing loss		
Increased incidence of diabetes, congenital heart defect, and leukemia		
Hypotonia		

Clinical Manifestations

Children who are mentally retarded manifest delays in all areas of development, including motor movement, language, and adaptive behavior.

Children achieve developmental milestones more slowly than the average child.

Mental retardation is sometimes accompanied by sensory impairment, speech problems, motor and orthopedic disabilities, and seizure disorders.

Diagnostic Tests

Mental retardation is diagnosed and initial treatment is planned in a multistep process and by involving a multidisciplinary team; members of the team are commonly a developmental specialist, physician, geneticist, nurse, teacher, language therapist, occupational therapist, and physical rehabilitation specialist.

A comprehensive history and evaluation of the child's physical characteristics, developmental level, and intellectual and adaptive functioning are carried out.

Laboratory tests such as chromosome analysis, blood enzyme levels, and lead levels and cranial imaging provide valuable information in some circumstances.

Tests of intellectual and adaptive functioning are performed when mental retardation is suspected.

A neurologic examination may indicate asymmetry of movement or strength, irritability or lethargy, or abnormal pitch to an infant's cry.

Because mental retardation may be accompanied by physical abnormalities, it is important to observe the child for facial symmetry, distance between the eyes, level of the ears, hair growth, and palmar creases.

Clinical Therapy
Based on the results of the evaluation, a multidisciplinary team plans the support needed to maximize the child's potential for development.

Management focuses on early intervention to improve the degree of adaptive functioning.

Simultaneous treatment of associated physical, emotional, and behavioral problems is provided.

Depending on the child's condition, special education programs and physical or occupational therapy may be necessary.

Nursing Management
Assessment
Nurses can help to identify children with mental retardation through history taking, observation, and developmental screening during early childhood.

The history should provide information about the mental and adaptive functioning of birth parents and other family members, as mental retardation may cluster in some families and conditions such as fragile X syndrome are genetic in origin.

The pregnancy and birth history can provide important information relating to alcohol and drug use by the mother during pregnancy; be alert for a history of difficult pregnancy and problems.

During home visits, during clinic appointments, in childcare centers, and during hospitalization, be alert for signs of developmental delays, multiple (more than three) physical anomalies associated with a specific condition, or neurologic alterations.

Developmental assessment should be part of each health promotion/ health maintenance visit to aid in early identification.

Once the diagnosis of mental retardation has been made, assess the adaptive functioning of the child and family.

A functional assessment of the child should be performed, including toileting, dressing, and feeding skills.

Assess the child's language, sensory, and psychomotor functioning.

Assess the home and community for safety hazards.

Observe how the family is managing with the child.

To determine the impact of the child with mental retardation on the family, ask parents to describe (1) family activities that include the child; (2) strategies that parents and siblings use to deal with community attitudes about the child; and (3) the case of a child with other disabilities, methods of managing the child's care and planning for future care needs.

Assess the availability of services such as support groups for parents and special education opportunities for children.

Intervention
Family members need empathy and support both at the time of diagnosis and in the ensuing years.

Parents and other family members may be in an acute or chronic state of grief over the loss of the perfect child.

Encourage the family members to verbalize their feelings.

Introduce the parents to parents of other mentally retarded children to provide assistance and support as they learn how to manage the child's needs.

Discuss the availability of respite care to provide parents with a break from caretaking.

Parents need honest information and answers to their questions about the child's condition.

Reinforce information provided by genetic counselors and other healthcare professionals.

Inform parents about community resources designed to assist children with mental retardation, including the Zero to Three Project, special education preschools and schools, county health services, and respite care.

Assist with plans for education and services such as physical or speech therapy; children need an individualized education plan designed to meet their specific learning needs.

Children with mental retardation require close supervision because they may lack an understanding of common hazards; ensure safety in the hospital environment, and assist parents to provide safety at home and school and to teach their child necessary skills such as pedestrian safety; consider both physical and emotional safety because the child with mental retardation may be trusting of others and sometimes is at risk for physical or sexual abuse.

Encourage parents' efforts to maximize the child's areas of strength and identify needs related to adaptive behaviors.

Assist parents as necessary to acquire the skills required to coordinate the child's plan of care.

Continue to evaluate the child's needs regularly, and assist parents with the treatment plan revision as necessary.

25 ALTERATIONS IN MUSCULOSKELETAL FUNCTION

DISORDERS OF FEET AND LEGS

Metatarsus Adductus

Most common congenital foot deformity

Characterized by an inward turning of the forefoot at the tarsometatarsal joints

Caused by both intrauterine positioning and genetic factors

Foot radiographs and physical assessment performed for diagnosis

Clinical Therapy

Simple exercises may correct the problem by approximately 3 months of age.

Serial casting is the treatment of choice for curvature angles of more than 15 degrees, or in cases that do not improve.

Braces and orthopedic shoes may also be used to maintain correction after casting.

Nursing Management

Reassure parents that the child's condition can be corrected.

Teach parents simple stretching exercises that can be performed at each diaper change:
- Hold the infant's foot securely by the heel. Maintain the heel in this position.
- Move the forefoot outward away from the body with the other hand.
- Hold the foot in this position for 5 seconds.
- Repeat five times during each diaper change.

If casting is necessary, provide cast care, and teach parents how to care for the child in a cast at home.

Clubfoot

Clinical Manifestations

Occurs in approximately 1 to 2 in 1,000 births, affects boys nearly twice as often as girls, and is bilateral in approximately half of affected infants (Hart et al., 2005).

Involves three areas of deformity: The midfoot is directed downward (equinus), the hindfoot turns inward (varus), and the forefoot curls toward the heel (adduction) and turns upward in partial supination.

Muscles, tendons, and bones are all involved in the abnormality, and clubfoot cannot be corrected by exercise.

The foot is small, with a shortened Achilles tendon; muscles in the lower leg are atrophied, but leg lengths are generally normal.

Diagnostic Tests

Visual inspection, examination, and radiographs confirm the diagnosis and extent of involvement.

Clinical Therapy

Serial casting beginning as soon as possible after birth is the first therapy; the foot is manipulated to achieve maximum correction first of the varus deformity and then of the equinus deformity.

A long leg cast is applied to hold the foot in the desired position and is changed every 1 to 2 weeks; the regimen of manipulation and casting continues for approximately 8 to 12 weeks until maximum correction is achieved.

If the deformity has been corrected, the child may then wear a splint with a crossbar between shoes (most commonly called a *Denis Browne splint*) or reverse last corrective shoes (shoes with the toes pointing outward rather than inward) to maintain the correction (Morcuende, Dolan, Dietz, et al., 2004).

If the deformity has not been corrected, surgical intervention using posteromedial release is required at approximately 3 to 12 months of age.

Surgery is followed by casting for 6 to 12 weeks, followed by a physical rehabilitation program and, commonly, use of a brace and corrective shoes.

Nursing Management

The goals of nursing care for the child with a clubfoot are to provide necessary information to parents and ensure safety and adequate healing during the treatment process.

Assessment

Perform a physical examination, including position and appearance of the foot.

Assess the child's motor development.

Evaluate the family's coping mechanisms and access to transportation to healthcare agency for serial casting visits.

Intervention

Explain the treatment to parents and involve them in the child's care.

Provide cast care to ensure skin and neurovascular integrity (see Box 25–1).

| Box 25–1 | Nursing Care of the Child in a Cast |

- A plaster cast takes anywhere from 24 to 48 hours to dry. When handling the cast, be gentle and use the palms of your hands, as fingertips can indent plaster and create pressure areas.
- After the cast is applied, elevate the extremity on a pillow above the level of the heart. Elevation helps to reduce swelling and increases venous return.
- If the cast is applied after surgery, there may be drainage or bleeding through the cast material. Circle the stain, and note the date and time on the cast to provide a means of assessing the amount of fluid lost. Once a cast is dry, a "window," or opening, is sometimes cut so that a wound can be viewed or to allow the stomach to expand more comfortably.
- Assess the distal pulses, and check the fingers and toes for color, warmth, capillary refill, and edema. Assess sensation as well as movement. Any deviation from normal may indicate nerve damage or decreased blood supply.
- During the first 24 hours, the casted extremity should be checked every 15 to 30 minutes for 2 hours, then every 1 to 2 hours thereafter. The skin should be warm. It should blanch when slight pressure is applied and then return to its normal color within 3 seconds. For the next 2 days, the casted extremity should be assessed at least every 4 hours.
- Check the edges of the cast for roughness or crumbling. If necessary, pull the inner stockinette over the edge of the cast and tape.
- The rough edges of the cast may also be alleviated by "petaling." This is done by securing tape or padding to the inside of the cast and pulling it over the edge, covering the jagged or broken pieces of plaster, and securing it to the outer surface of the cast. Moleskin may be used on the cast as well. Petal the opening around a window in the cast if one is present.
- Keep the cast as clean and dry as possible. Cover the cast with a plastic bag or plastic wrap when the child bathes or showers.
- The skin under the cast may itch; however, do not use powders or lotions near the edges or under the cast, as they can cause skin irritation.
- Be sure that children do not put small objects between the casts and their extremities; these actions can cause skin irritation as well as neurovascular compromise.

Routine postoperative care after surgical correction includes neurovascular status checks every 2 hours for the first 24 hours and observing for any swelling around the cast edges, application of ice bags to the foot, and keeping the ankle and foot elevated on a pillow for 24 hours to promote healing and help with venous return.

Keep new casts open to air to facilitate drying; monitor, record, and report drainage or bleeding.

Administer pain medication routinely for 24 to 48 hours after surgery; popliteal or epidural blocks may be placed during surgery and used in the immediate postsurgical period for pain control; monitor these blocks for effectiveness and any undesired effects.

Patient and Family Education
Parents should be given written instructions for care of the child with a cast.

Skin care:
- Check the skin around the cast edges for irritation, rubbing, or blistering. The skin should be clean and dry.
- Cleanse the skin just under the cast edges and between the toes or fingers with a cotton-tipped applicator and rubbing alcohol. Avoid using lotions, oils, and powders near the cast, as they may cause caking.
- Avoid poking sharp objects down inside the cast, as this may result in sores.

Cast care:
- Keep the cast dry. Protect plaster with a cast shoe, thick sock, or sling.
- Allow a new, wet cast to air dry for 24 hours.
- Begin walking on a leg cast only when the physician gives permission.

Be alert for possible complications:
- Toes or fingers should be pink, not blue or white.
- Skin should be warm and the tips of the toes should blanch when pinched.
- Raise the casted arm or leg above heart level, and rest it on pillows to prevent or reduce any swelling.

Notify the healthcare provider if any of the following occur:
- Unusual odor beneath the cast
- Tingling
- Burning or numbness in the casted arm or leg
- Drainage through the cast
- Swelling or inability to move the fingers or toes
- Slippage of the cast

- Cast cracked, soft, or loose
- Sudden, unexplained fever
- Unusual fussiness or irritability in an infant or child
- Fingers or toes that are blue or white
- Pain that is not relieved by any comfort measures (e.g., repositioning or pain medication)

General care:
- Demonstrate the use of a sponge bath to protect the cast from water breakdown.
- Discuss several options for clothing that accommodate a cast, for example, one-piece snap suits or sweatpants.
- Discuss potential safety hazards that may result from awkward positioning. Be sure the child is properly situated in a car safety seat for the trip home.
- Suggest that parents make an effort to place toys within the child's reach because movements of a child in a cast may be slowed.
- Have parents avoid use of "umbrella" strollers and infant swings because they do not provide adequate support for the casted leg.

Adapted from and courtesy of Shriners Hospital for Children-Spokane (Washington).

Parents should be given written instructions for care of the child with a brace:
- Braces should be as comfortable as possible and the child should have adequate mobility while wearing the brace.
- Begin wearing the brace for periods of 1 to 2 hours and then progress to 2 to 4 hours.
- Check the skin at 1- to 2-hour intervals initially, then lengthen to every 4 hours once skin has been clear for several days. If redness is apparent, leave the brace off and allow the skin to clear. If breakdown has occurred, the brace cannot be replaced until healing is complete.
- Always have the child wear a clean white sock, T-shirt, or other thin white liner beneath the brace. Be sure the liner is wrinkle-free under the brace. Avoid using powders or lotions that can cause skin to break down. Toughen any sensitive areas using alcohol wipes.
- Reapply the brace when the skin returns to its normal color.
- Return to the physician or orthotic specialist if discomfort or red areas persist or if the brace needs adjustment or repair or is outgrown.
- Check the brace daily for rough edges.

Genu Varum and Genu Valgum

Genu varum is a deformity in which the knees are widely separated while the ankles are close together and the lower legs are turned inward (varus).

In genu valgum (knock-knees), the knees are close together while the ankles are widely spaced so that the lower legs are directed outward (valgus).

At certain stages of a child's development, the appearance of bowlegs or knock-knees is normal. Until 2 to 3 years, the knees are normally bowed, showing varus alignment, and by 4 to 5 years, some knock-knee or valgus alignment commonly emerges.

Blount's disease and rickets are two pathologic causes of bowlegs and should be ruled out if the condition is severe or has not improved by 2 years of age.

Excessive or continued knock-knees should also be evaluated by an orthopedist, although unlike genu varum, the condition has no pathologic causes.

Physical measurements, radiographic studies, arthrography (joint radiograph), magnetic resonance imaging (MRI), and computed tomography imaging may be used for accurate diagnosis of varus and valgus conditions.

Treatment may include braces, supplementation with calcium and vitamin D if rickets is a cause, and occasional surgery.

Nursing care centers on instruction on brace wear or dietary supplementation as needed, along with postsurgical care for that intervention.

DISORDERS OF THE HIP

Developmental Dysplasia of the Hip

Developmental dysplasia of the hip (DDH) refers to a variety of conditions in which the femoral head and the acetabulum are improperly aligned with an unstable connection. These conditions include hip instability, dislocation (displacement of the bone from its normal articulation with the joint), subluxation (in this instance, a partial dislocation), and acetabular dysplasia (abnormal cellular or structural development leading to instability; Shipman, Helfand, Nygren, et al., 2006).

Clinical Manifestations

Limited abduction of the affected hip.

Asymmetry of the gluteal and thigh fat folds.

Telescoping or pistoning of the thigh.

The older child with untreated developmental dysplasia of the hip walks with a significant limp.

Diagnostic Tests

Physical examination, including Allis' sign (one knee lower than the other when the knees are flexed) and positive Ortolani-Barlow maneuver.

Sonogram may be used until 4 months of age and radiographs after that time.

Clinical Therapy

Pavlik harness, a dynamic splint that allows movement but ensures hip flexion and abduction while not allowing hip extension or adduction.

Surgery and application of spica cast may be needed.

Nursing Management

Encourage families to make regular healthcare visits so assessment of hips can occur throughout the infancy period.

Provide care for the child in traction or who has surgery and has spica cast application (see Box 25–1). If permitted by physician's orders, release the child from traction for meals and daily care. The time out of traction should not exceed 1 hour per day. Encourage parents to hold and cuddle the child at this time to promote comfort and bonding.

Special care after surgery for developmental dysplasia of the hip includes the following:
- Use adequate padding and skin wrapping to avoid placing pressure on the popliteal space. Such pressure could lead to nerve damage.
- Change the casted child's position every 2 to 3 hours while awake to help avoid areas of pressure and promote increased circulation. The child can be placed either prone or supine or positioned on the floor and supported with pillows.
- Help prevent skin irritation and breakdown in the child with a cast. Use moleskin to provide protection from rough edges. Place tape around the perineal opening of the cast to prevent soiling.
- Increase fluids and fiber in the child's diet, as a change in bowel or bladder status is commonly associated with immobility.
- Assess respiratory system carefully, and plan games to encourage deep breathing by the young child.

Patient and Family Education

Instruct families on proper use of the Pavlik harness when it is prescribed:
- Position the chest halter at nipple line and fasten with Velcro.
- Position the legs and feet in the stirrups, being sure the hips are flexed and abducted. Fasten with Velcro.

- Connect the chest halter and leg straps in front.
- Connect the chest halter and leg straps in back.
- All the straps are marked at the first fitting with indelible ink so they can be reattached easily after the harness is rinsed and dried.

Instruct parents on care of the child in a spica cast, including safe transport home in a car (see Box 25–1).

Emphasize importance of neurovascular checks and reporting promptly any signs of circulatory impairment.

Consider safety because the child cannot move away from dangers such as heat and may easily fall from high places.

Instruct about ways to encourage normal growth and development while the child is immobilized in a cast.

Legg-Calvé-Perthes Disease (Perthes' Disease)

This is a self-limiting condition in which there is avascular necrosis of the femoral head.

Clinical Manifestations

Usually occurs between the ages of 2 and 12 years, with an average age of 7 years at onset, and is about four times more common in males (Hosalkar, Horn, Friedman, et al., 2007).

Child may complain of hip pain and/or manifest a limp.

The disease progresses in several stages over a time of approximately 2 years:

Prenecrosis	An insult or coagulation disorder causes loss of blood supply to the femoral head.
I Necrosis	Avascular stage (3–6 months); the child is asymptomatic, bone radiographs are normal, and the head of the femur is structurally intact but avascular.
II Revascularization	Period of 1–4 years characterized by pain and limitation of movement. Bone radiographs show new bone deposition and dead bone resorption. Fracture and deformity of the head of the femur can occur.
III Bone healing	Reossification takes place; pain decreases.
IV Remodeling	The disease process is over, pain is absent, and improvement in joint function occurs.

Diagnostic Tests

Diagnosis is made using standard anteroposterior and frog-leg radiographs.

Bone scans and MRI may show the disease process earlier than radiographs.

Laboratory studies of the blood, such as white blood cell count, help to rule out inflammatory synovitis of the hip.

Clinical Therapy

The femoral head must be contained within the hip socket by abduction until reossification is complete to promote healing and prevent deformity.

At the beginning of treatment, traction can be used to maintain the hips in an abducted and internally rotated position.

Once abduction is accomplished, treatment consists of Petrie (leg abduction) casting, or surgical soft tissue releases such as adductor tenotomy, followed by application of Toronto or Scottish Rite braces.

Nursing Management

Teach the parents and child about the course of the disease and expected treatment, emphasizing the importance of keeping the hip non-weight-bearing.

Offer suggestions for activities that redirect energy and promote normal development; these may include horseback riding, which promotes hip abduction; swimming to increase mobility; handcrafts to promote fine motor skills; and reading or computer activities to stimulate cognitive development.

Assist the family to work with the school to plan for the child's mobility to classes.

Teach cast or brace care as required by the child's treatment.

Slipped Capital Femoral Epiphysis

Occurs when the femoral head is displaced from the femoral neck.

Most common during the adolescent growth spurt, between the ages of 12 to 15 years in boys and 10 to 13 years in girls.

Boys are more often affected than girls; blacks are affected more often than other ethnic groups, as are children who are overweight, with sports injuries or other trauma, with a history of radiation therapy, or with endocrine disease (Manoff, Banffy, & Winell, 2005).

Symptoms include limp, pain in knee, thigh, groin or hip, and decreased mobility of hip.

Acute slipped capital femoral epiphysis has a sudden onset of less than 3 weeks' duration. The child with an acute slip has sudden, severe pain and cannot bear weight. This may be associated with traumatic injury.

Chronic slipped capital femoral epiphysis has a duration of longer than 3 weeks. It presents with persistent hip pain, which is generally aching or mild and can be referred to the thigh, knee, or both. A limp and decreased range of motion may also occur.

Acute-on-chronic is an additional slippage in a child with a chronic condition. The child with a chronic slip sustains a traumatic incident that causes further slippage of the femoral head, causing sudden, severe pain.

Radiographs are used to confirm the diagnosis. A bone scan, ultrasound, computed tomography, and MRI are sometimes performed to verify the extent of injury.

Surgical treatment is usually necessary; this involves fixation of the epiphysis with screws or pins.

Medical treatment, which is occasionally used, includes a regimen of no weight bearing, bed rest, a spica cast, and Buck or Russell traction.

Nursing care involves encouraging recommended weight among children and adolescents and recognizing and referring those with symptoms of the disorder.

Care during traction and after surgical correction is an important nursing intervention (Tables 25–1 and 25–2).

DISORDERS OF THE SPINE

Scoliosis

Scoliosis is a lateral S- or C-shaped curvature of the spine that is often associated with a rotational deformity of the spine and ribs; spinal curvatures of more than 10 degrees are abnormal.

Clinical Manifestations

Idiopathic scoliosis is the most common type and frequently occurs in girls, especially during the growth spurt between the ages of 10 and 13 years.

Scoliosis can also occur in congenital diseases involving the spinal structure and in the musculoskeletal changes seen in conditions such

Table 25–1   Types of Traction

Skin traction

Pull is applied to the skin surface, which puts traction directly on the bones and muscles. Traction is attached to the skin with adhesive materials or straps, or foam boots, belts, or halters.

Dunlop traction (can be either skeletal or skin)

Used for fracture of the humerus. The arm, which is flexed, is suspended horizontally with straps placed on both the upper and lower portions for pull from both sides.

Bryant's traction

Used specifically for the child 3 years of age or younger and weighing less than 17.5 kg (35 lb) who has developmental dysplasia of the hip or a fractured femur. This bilateral traction is applied to the child's legs and kept in place by wrapping the legs from foot to thigh with elastic bandages. The hips are flexed at a 90-degree angle, with knees extended. This position is maintained by attaching the traction appliance to weights and pulleys, which are suspended above the crib. The buttocks do not rest on the mattress, but are slightly elevated off the bed.

Buck traction

Used for knee immobilization; to correct contractures or deformities or for short-term immobilization of a fracture. It keeps the leg in an extended position, without hip flexion. Traction is applied to the extremity in one direction (straight line) with a single pulley system.

Russell traction

Used for fractures of the femur and lower leg. Traction is placed on the lower leg while the knee is suspended in a padded sling. The hips and knees, which are slightly flexed, are immobilized. One force is applied by a double pulley to the foot, and another force is applied upward using a sling under the knee and an overhead pulley.

Skeletal traction

Pull is directly applied to the bone by pins, wires, tongs, or other apparatus that have been surgically placed through the distal end of the bone.

Skeletal cervical traction

Used for cervical spine injuries to reduce fractures and dislocations. Crutchfield, Gardner-Wells, or Vinke tongs are placed in the skull with burr holes. Weights are attached to the apparatus with a rope and pulley system to the hyperextended head.

Halo traction

Used to immobilize the head and neck after cervical injury or dislocation. Also used for positioning and immobilization after cervical injury.

90–90 traction

Used for fractures of the femur or tibia. A skeletal pin or wire is surgically placed through the distal part of the femur; the lower part of the extremity is in a boot cast. Traction ropes and pulleys are applied at the pin site and on the boot cast to maintain the flexion of both the hip and knee at 90 degrees. This traction can also be used for treatment of an upper extremity fracture.

Table 25–1 Types of Traction (Continued)

External fixators

These devices can be used in the treatment of simple fractures, both open and closed; complex fractures with extensive soft tissue involvement; correction of bony or soft tissue deformities; pseudoarthroses; and limb length discrepancy. They are attached to the extremity by percutaneous transfixing of pins or wires to the bone.

Table 25–2 Nursing Care of the Child with Traction

1. Assess the child in traction by first checking the equipment. Make sure that the equipment is in the proper position. Observe both the body appliance and the attached weights and pulleys. Make certain that the child's body is in proper alignment.
2. Assess the skin under the straps and pin insertion sites for any signs of redness, edema, or skin breakdown.
3. Assess the extremity by checking neurovascular status frequently (check warmth, color, distal pulses, capillary refill time, movement, sensation).
4. Provide pin care when ordered using sterile technique. Clean the area surrounding the pin with cotton-tipped applicators saturated with normal saline or half-strength hydrogen peroxide. Clean the area again with sterile water or more saline. Apply an antibacterial ointment, if ordered, using another cotton-tipped applicator.
5. With skin tractions, perform skin care every 4 hours when the traction device is removed.
6. Place a sheepskin pad under the child's extremity if prescriptions permit.

as myelomeningocele, cerebral palsy, or muscular dystrophy; it can also be acquired after injury to the spinal cord.

Truncal asymmetry, uneven shoulder and hip height, a one-sided rib hump, and a prominent scapula occur; compensatory problems may develop for curvatures of more than 40 degrees, such as hip and back pain and lung compromise leading to fatigue or dyspnea with exertion.

Diagnostic Tests

Observation and radiographic examination are used to diagnose scoliosis.

MRI, computed tomography scan, and bone scan may be used to assess the degree of curvature.

Clinical Therapy

Treatment of children with mild scoliosis (curvatures of 10–20 degrees) consists of exercises to improve posture and muscle tone and to maintain, or possibly increase, flexibility of the spine.

Moderate scoliosis (curvatures of 20–40 degrees) includes bracing, commonly with a Boston brace, worn for 23 hours daily.

Electrical stimulation is used occasionally as an alternative treatment.

Children with severe scoliosis (curvatures of 40 degrees or more) require surgery, which involves spinal fusion and instrumentation.

Nursing Management

Nursing management focuses on screening and early detection, teaching about brace wear, caring for the adolescent having surgery for scoliosis, and partnering with the adolescent and family to provide support during all treatments.

Assessment

Assess all children for scoliosis, particularly those entering puberty:
- Visual observation from the front:
- Is the head midline?
- Are the shoulders at the same height?
- Is there the same amount of space between arms and body on each side?

From the back:
- Is the head midline?
- Are the shoulders at the same height?
- Are the scapula equally prominent and at the same height?
- Is the spine straight?
- Is there the same amount of space between arms and body on each side?
- Are the hips at the same height?

With the adolescent holding hands together and bent over slightly:
- Are the scapula humps even?

With the adolescent holding hands together and bent over toward floor:
- Are the flank humps even?
- Is the spine straight?
- Is there a marked roundness when viewed from the side? (evidence of kyphosis)

Assess skin condition and hours of daily wear for the adolescent who wears a brace.

For the child who requires spinal fusion, postoperative care requires intensive assessment of all systems, including respiratory, neurologic, musculoskeletal, integumentary, fluid and electrolytes, and pain control.

Intervention

Emphasize importance of continued care to monitor for continuation of curvature.

Provide information for families about the treatment that is prescribed for the child/adolescent.

Prepare the family and child when surgical intervention is planned.

Provide care for the child with spinal fusion, to include the following:

- Monitor respiratory status and use pulse oximeter; administer oxygen if needed; have the teen deep breathe and use incentive spirometer.
- Reposition at least every 2 hours.
- Perform neurovascular checks of each extremity, including color, circulation, capillary refill, warmth, sensation, and motion, every 2 hours for first 24 hours and then every 4 hours.
- Monitor presence of pedal and distal tibial pulses.
- Apply antiembolism stockings until the teen is ambulatory.
- Monitor for pain, swelling, or positive Homans' sign in legs.
- Evaluate for edema.
- Perform range-of-motion exercises when ordered.
- Assess level of pain, and initiate pain management strategies.
- Administer pain medication around the clock, especially in the first 48 hours.
- As the teen becomes ambulatory, instruct in brace or cast care as needed; provide instructions about activities that are allowed and those to avoid.

DISORDERS OF BONE

Osteoporosis and Osteopenia

Osteoporosis is a metabolic bone disease in which bone mineral density is more than 2.5 standard deviations below the norm; osteopenia is low bone mass between 1.0 and 2.5 standard deviations below norm (Bowman & Russell, 2006).

Conditions associated with these disorders include osteopenia of prematurity, low mechanical loading due to inability to ambulate or treatment of a condition by immobilization, inadequate nutritional intake, Turner syndrome, growth hormone deficiency, osteogenesis imperfecta, juvenile rheumatoid arthritis, and diabetes.

The disorders are silent diseases and may go undetected for years until a fracture occurs. Bone mineral content and density are measured by single photon absorptiometry (SPA), dual photon absorptiometry

(DPA), or dual-energy x-ray absorptiometry (DEXA). Serum studies such as bone-specific alkaline phosphatase, phosphorus, and type I collagen can be used to measure osteoblastic and osteoclastic activity. Premature newborns at risk of osteopenia of prematurity need collaborative management by neonatologists, neonatal nutritionists, and neonatal nurses.

For children at risk of developing osteoporosis, calcium and vitamin D intake is encouraged, and oral supplements may be given.

Standing therapy for those who are nonambulatory can provide mechanical weight and enhance bone density. Extremity range of motion for very-low-birth-weight newborns may decrease bone loss in the period after birth (Litmanovitz, Dolfin, Arnon, et al., 2007).

When a cast or other immobilizing device is removed from a child, a gradually increasing program of exercise in collaboration with physical rehabilitation professionals promotes bone strengthening and lowered risk for fractures or related sequelae.

Nurses perform dietary analysis of children at risk.

Refer children at risk to nutritionists and physicians for further education and diagnosis.

Administer nutritional supplements when prescribed, and teach families how to give these medications.

Partner with families to provide therapy for nonambulatory children that stimulates weight bearing.

Teach parents how to recognize fractures in children who may not have normal sensation and are unable to report them. Swelling, unusual shape of a limb, fussiness of the child, and falls should be reported promptly.

Osteomyelitis

An infection of the bone, most often one of the long bones of the lower extremity.

Clinical Manifestations

Common causes of osteomyelitis include *Staphylococcus aureus*, *Escherichia coli*, group B streptococci, *Streptococcus aureus*, *Streptococcus pyogenes*, *Pseudomonas aeruginosa*, and *Haemophilus influenzae*.

Symptoms include constant bone pain, edema, decreased mobility of the infected joint, and fever.

Redness may be present over the area of infection.

The child may refuse to walk or may limp.

The onset of acute osteomyelitis is generally rapid and is therefore sometimes misdiagnosed as a sports injury (Kaplan, 2005; Kocher et al., 2006).

Diagnostic Tests

A history suggestive of osteomyelitis includes an upper respiratory infection or blunt trauma followed by pain at the area of a growth plate.

Laboratory evaluation shows leukocytosis and an elevated erythrocyte sedimentation rate and C-reactive protein (Gutierrez, 2005); the degree of erythrocyte sedimentation rate elevation is directly related to the severity of the infection.

Radiographs and bone scans may identify the area of involvement.

A needle aspiration of the site or a blood culture can confirm the diagnosis and provide a culture of the causative organism.

Clinical Therapy

Medical management of infection begins with the intravenous administration of a broad-spectrum antibiotic, even before culture results are available.

When an adequate response to antibiotic is not obtained within 2 to 3 days, the area may be aspirated again, or surgical drainage may be performed.

Intravenous fluids may be administered to ensure adequate hydration.

Nursing Management

Assess the onset of symptoms and a history of recent infections or trauma; include questions about immunization status, especially tetanus.

Evaluate the affected area for signs of redness, swelling, pain, and decreased range of motion.

Measure vital signs; increased temperature and pulse may provide clues about worsening infection.

Blood cultures and other cultures of the body must be performed before the first dose of antibiotic when osteomyelitis is suspected.

Obtain continuing blood samples as needed to monitor erythrocyte sedimentation rate and C-reactive protein.

Administer intravenous fluids as ordered, and offer oral fluids frequently to maintain hydration status of the child.

Administer intravenous and oral antibiotics as ordered.

Monitor the intravenous site and provide care for the central or other lines.

Administer analgesics, and use other comfort measure to relieve bone pain and joint tenderness.

Strict aseptic technique and transmission-based precautions should be used during all nursing care; instruct the family in these techniques.

Osteogenesis Imperfecta
Clinical Manifestations

Osteogenesis imperfecta is a connective tissue disorder characterized by a biochemical defect in the production of collagen.

It is genetically transmitted, generally in an autosomal-dominant inheritance pattern.

Clinical manifestations include multiple and frequent fractures; blue sclerae; thin, soft skin; increased joint flexibility; enlargement of the anterior fontanel; weak muscles; soft, pliable, brittle bones; and short stature; conductive hearing loss can occur by adolescence or young adulthood (Devogelaer & Coppin, 2006); most children with osteogenesis imperfecta are short in height and may have decreased range of motion in several joints.

The disease is classified into four types:

- Type I: Most common form; children have fragile bones, blue sclerae, weakened tooth dentin, and hearing loss that manifests in adolescence.
- Type II: Ribs and skeleton are extensively involved; most children with this form of the disease die *in utero* or shortly after birth.
- Type III: The newborn or infant sustains numerous fractures and manifests blue sclerae; severe bone fragility and kyphoscoliosis are observed; most children with type III disease die in childhood as a result of cardiorespiratory failure.
- Type IV: Characterized by fractures without other symptoms of the disease; bowing of the legs and other structural deformities can occur; however, the incidence of fractures decreases beginning in puberty.

Diagnostic Tests

Because the disease is genetic in origin, ultrasound or collagen analysis of chorionic villus cells can be used for diagnosis before birth in babies at known risk.

Diagnosis may be made only when the child has a delay in walking or sustains a fracture. Radiographic evaluation may detect both old and new fractures.

Tests such as dual energy x-ray absorptiometry can be used to measure bone density.

Serum alkaline phosphatase level may be elevated; other measures of bone metabolism such as serum osteocalcin, procollagen 1 C-terminal peptide, collagen 1 teleopeptide, and urine deoxypyridinoline may be performed occasionally to measure effects of experimental medication.

Clinical Therapy

There is no cure for osteogenesis imperfecta; clinical therapy consists primarily of fracture care and prevention of deformities.

Treatment includes physical therapy; casting, bracing, or splinting; surgical stabilization; nutritional management with high vitamin D and calcium intake; and bisphosphonate medication such as pamidronate.

Surgery to insert telescoping rods in long bones may be helpful to stabilize bones. Hematologic stem cell transplant has been used successfully in some children with severe osteogenesis imperfecta and is under further research (Lee & Hui, 2006).

Nursing Management

Assessment

Assess the child carefully and frequently for signs of fractures.

Ask about favorite activities of the child because they need to be integrated into plans for physical activity and developmental progression.

Perform careful growth measures and developmental screening.

Intervention

Handle the child gently: The trunk and extremities should be supported when the child is moved; perform tasks such as bathing and diapering carefully; use a blanket or pillow under the child for additional support when lifting and moving; do not pull the infant's legs upward when changing a diaper, as this can cause a fracture, but slip a hand under the hips to raise them, slide the diaper carefully in, and then bring it up as the legs are slightly abducted.

Partner with families to provide safe activities for the child. Discourage contact sports and other activities that are likely to lead to fractures.

Encourage a well-balanced diet with additional vitamin C, vitamin D, and calcium to encourage healing and bone growth; calories should be limited to maintain weight at recommended levels because immobility can lead to overweight and the child is generally short for age.

Provide preparatory teaching for the child who requires surgical intervention for management of fractures.

Parents may feel guilt, anger, and worry over the child; support them and refer to organizations such as the Osteogenesis Imperfecta Foundation.

Evaluate the child's developmental progress periodically, and make suggestions for interventions that parents can use to foster cognitive, social, and physical milestones.

DISORDERS OF MUSCLES

Muscular Dystrophy

The muscular dystrophies are a group of inherited diseases characterized by muscle fiber degeneration and muscle wasting; the disorders can begin early or late in life, and onset can be at birth or gradual during childhood.

Clinical Manifestations

With Duchenne muscular dystrophy, muscle weakness begins in the lower extremities in early childhood; parents may notice the child tripping, toe walking, and displaying enlargement of the calf muscles (in fact, the calf is not enlarged but muscle is replaced by fat). By the middle teen years, the child's condition has usually progressed so that walking is not possible. The disease progresses up the body, potentially causing conditions such as scoliosis, other musculoskeletal conditions, cardiomyopathy, and respiratory distress. Fractures may occur when the child falls due to weakness. Becker's dystrophy is similar but emerges later and more slowly.

The dystrophies of infancy are manifested by generalized weakness and hypotonia. The baby may have difficulty with sucking and swallowing. Ocular problems may be present.

Diagnostic Tests

Diagnosis and classification are most often based on clinical signs and the pattern of muscle involvement.

Biochemical examinations such as serum enzyme assay, muscle biopsy, and electromyography confirm the diagnosis.

Serum creatine kinase level is elevated early in the disease.

Dystrophin, the muscle protein that is deficient in muscular dystrophy, can be measured by muscle biopsy.

Genetic testing establishes the specific abnormality and type of disease present.

Clinical Therapy

There is no effective treatment for childhood muscular dystrophy; research is being directed at several techniques to repair mutations by gene therapy and stem cell therapy (Kuehn, 2007; Lee & Hui, 2006).

The steroids prednisone and deflazacort may preserve muscle function, preserving walking for a longer period.

Surgery may be used to correct scoliosis, a commonly accompanying disorder, to facilitate lung expansion.

Respiratory infections are vigorously treated with deep breathing, coughing, nebulizer treatments, and antibiotics when indicated.

Nursing Management

Assessment

Monitor all vital signs as well as cardiac and respiratory functioning.

Comprehensive and regular cardiac evaluations are recommended (American Academy of Pediatrics, Section on Cardiology and Cardiac Surgery, 2005).

Assess urinary function and frequency of bowel movements.

Periodically measure strength and range of motion.

Assess mobility via ambulation or assisted device.

Perform periodic developmental assessments.

Evaluate the family's risk and protective factors for dealing with this chronic and fatal disorder.

Intervention

Nurses often provide home healthcare services to such children, work with them in school nursing positions, and partner with parents in clinics and other facilities to provide health promotion and maintenance as the child grows.

Administer oxygen or respiratory therapy as ordered.

Ensure that regular cardiac and respiratory evaluations are performed by specialists in those fields.

Soft foods or enteral tube feedings may be needed to promote nutrition; the infant with a rare dystrophy in infancy may need gavage feedings.

Maintain bowel function with fluids, high-fiber foods, and medications as needed.

Monitor and ensure adequate fluid output.

Be alert for signs of infection.

Perform range of motion and provide for physical activity to level of ability.

Physical therapy helps the child ambulate and prevents joint contractures; provide good back support and posture by keeping the child's body in alignment when confined to a wheelchair; splints may be needed to maintain extremities in proper position.

Perform periodic developmental assessments, and provide parents with suggestions for encouraging the child's development.

Meet with teachers to evaluate the child's learning needs and functioning in the classroom; an individualized education plan should be established.

Partner with the school to provide tutors or home computers if needed.

Young children should be enrolled in early intervention programs before they are old enough for school.

Encourage the child to be independent for as long as possible, concentrating on what the child can accomplish.

Exercise as tolerated contributes to muscle strength and a general sense of well-being.

The family is challenged to manage the child's care, provide a nurturing environment for other children and family members, and obtain necessary financial resources over many years.

Refer the family to respite care, assist them in finding resources, and be certain that either a family member or health professional acts as case manager to coordinate various services needed; refer family members to resource and support groups such as the Muscular Dystrophy Association; refer for genetic counseling.

Parents need bereavement counseling and end-of-life care as the child becomes weaker and the disease progresses.

INJURIES TO THE MUSCULOSKELETAL SYSTEM

Fractures

A fracture is a break in a bone that occurs when more stress is placed on the bone than the bone can withstand.

Clinical Manifestations

Fractures, which may occur at any age, occur frequently in children because their bones are less dense and more porous than those of adults.

Due to their porous nature, the bones of children may bow, leading to more common greenstick or spiral fractures in children.

Childhood fractures most often involve the clavicle, tibia, ulna, and femur, with distal forearm fractures the most common type (Carson, Woolridge, Colletti, et al., 2006). Fractures to the pelvis are often associated with motor vehicle crashes. Epiphyseal (growth plate) injuries are dangerous in children, as they can interfere with future growth at the site. Fractures are generally characterized by pain, abnormal positioning, edema, immobility or decreased range of motion, ecchymosis, guarding, and crepitus.

Types of fractures are described using the Salter-Harris classification system (Table 25–3).

Diagnostic Tests

Radiographs are used to diagnose fractures and to determine the exact location and type of fracture.

Clinical Therapy

Immobilization is essential for the bone healing process to take place.

A closed reduction aligns the bone by manual manipulation or traction.

An open reduction requires surgical alignment of the bone, often using pins, plates, wires, or screws.

For open fractures, surgery must also be performed for débridement to remove dead tissue and clean the wound.

Casting is the most common external method of immobilization.

Nursing Management

Assess the diets of all youth who might be at risk for fractures and insert dietary teaching in health promotion visits.

Table 25–3   Salter-Harris Fracture Classification System

Type I
  Common
  Fracture between bone and growth plate
  Growth plate undisturbed
  Growth disturbances rare

Type II
  Most common
  Fracture through bone above growth plate
  Growth disturbances rare

Type III
  Less common
  Fracture through growth plate
  Serious threat to growth and joint

Type IV
  Fracture through growth plate and bone
  Serious threat to growth

Type V
  Rare
  Crush injury causes cell death in growth plate, resulting in arrested growth
  and limited bone length
  If growth plate is partially destroyed, angular deformities may result

When dealing with an injured child, be alert to the signs and symptoms of fractures before moving the child; when in doubt about the nature of an injury, apply a splint.

Evaluate pain, swelling, and any abnormal positioning of the injured area.

When a child is admitted to the emergency department or hospital, nursing assessment includes the extent of the injury, the degree of pain, and the child's vital signs (respiratory status, pulse, blood pressure).

Nursing care focuses on care of the child before and after fracture reduction, encouraging mobility as ordered, maintaining skin integrity, preventing infection, and teaching the parents and child how to care for the fracture.

If conscious sedation or pain blocks are used, nursing care for these procedures is needed. When caring for a child who has undergone fracture reduction, it is important to be aware of the signs of complications; notify the physician immediately if these signs occur.

Document assessments and report changes and abnormal results immediately. The major serious complication is compartment syndrome, or a condition of increased pressure in a limited space such as the soft tissue of an extremity that is casted, which compromises circulation and nervous innervation (Altizer, 2004); manifestations of the syndrome begin approximately 30 minutes after tissue ischemia starts and include the following:

- Paresthesia (tingling, burning, loss of two-point discrimination)
- Pain (unrelieved by medication, characterized by crying in the young child)
- Pressure (skin is tense, cast appears tight)
- Pallor (pale, gray, or white skin tone)[1]
- Paralysis (weakness or inability to move extremity)[1]
- Pulselessness (weak or absent pulse)[1]

Check extremities every 15 minutes until stable and then every 1 to 2 hours for the following:

- Color
- Temperature
- Capillary refill
- Peripheral pulses
- Edema
- Sensation
- Motor ability
- Pain

(Altizer, 2004; Grottkau, Epps, & Di Scala, 2005) See Box 25–1 for further details on cast care.

Teach the parents and child cast care, activity restrictions, and how to identify problems that should be reported.

Help parents to identify any modifications that may be needed at home and school; the child who has to manage steps at home or school may need special training with crutches or a temporary ramp.

Refer parents to home health nurses or home teaching services if indicated.

Provide pertinent teaching to prevent future injuries.

Sports Injuries

Sports injuries are the most common type of injury in youth from 13 to 19 years of age.

---

[1]Indicates a late sign

Football, wrestling, soccer, and gymnastics are the sports most commonly associated with injury.

Fractures, described previously, are common sports injuries of young athletes.

See Table 25–4 for common sports injuries.

Children and adolescents should receive instruction in correct techniques from a person qualified to coach and supervise children.

Have parents inquire about the coach's experience and also verify that the coaching staff is prepared in emergency care.

Encourage youth to gradually increase time and intensity at a sport rather than immediately playing a new sport for long periods of time.

Ask about sports participation for all youth, but especially when there are complaints of sore muscles, edema of body parts, and bruises.

Perform neurovascular assessment of extremities, including color, temperature, capillary refill time, edema, pulses, sensation, and pain.

Teach youth to warm up for 10 to 15 minutes before participation and to cool down for a corresponding period at the end of activity; they should not ignore pain.

Table 25–4 Common Sports Injuries

Sport	Types of Injuries
Baseball/Basketball	Hand and finger fractures and sprains
	Contusions and sprains of upper or lower extremities; wrists, elbows, knees, and ankles are common sites
	Injury to body parts when hit by a ball—e.g., broken teeth; face, head, eye, and chest injuries
Football	Head and neck injury such as skull or cervical vertebrae fracture
	Pulled muscles or dislocations in shoulders and legs
Gymnastics	Wrist and elbow fractures and strains
	Tendonitis in elbows and ankles/legs
Hockey (ice and inline)	Dental injuries
	Leg fractures
	Head and neck injuries
Soccer	Head and neck injuries
	Strains and fractures of legs
Wrestling	Fractures and dislocations of upper and lower extremities

Ensure that youth wear recommended gear for their sports, including equipment such as well-fitted protective helmet, face masks, eye protection, mouth guards, elbow and wrist guards, gloves, and knee and shin pads.

Injuries such as muscle strains should be treated promptly with the following:

- Resting the injury for 24 to 48 hours; applying ice for 20 minutes four times daily; compression with an elastic wrap to provide comfort and decrease edema; elevating the part affected above heart level
- Gradually increasing motion to the part
- Adding flexibility and resistance or strengthening exercises
- Returning gradually to the sport, usually 2 to 3 weeks after injury

26 ALTERATIONS IN INTEGUMENTARY FUNCTION

SKIN LESIONS

Skin lesions vary in size, shape, color, and texture characteristics. Primary lesions arise from previously healthy skin (Table 26–1). Secondary lesions result from changes in primary lesions (Table 26–2).

ACUTE INFLAMMATORY SKIN CONDITIONS

Contact Dermatitis

Contact dermatitis is an inflammation of the skin that occurs in response to direct contact with an allergen or irritant. Sweating and friction enhance the absorption of the substance.

An irritant (soaps, detergents, fabric softeners, bleaches, lotions, urine, or stool) in contact with skin in adequate duration and concentration causes an inflammatory reaction. No memory T-cell function or antigen-specific immunoglobulins are activated.

Allergic contact dermatitis is a delayed hypersensitivity reaction. Common allergens include nickel, poison ivy, poison oak, lanolin, neomycin, rubber, potassium dichromate (a leather tanning agent), fragrances, and latex.

Table 26–1   Primary Skin Lesions

Lesion Name	Description	Example
Macule	Flat, nonpalpable, diameter <1 cm (0.5 in.)	Freckle, rubella, petechiae
Papule	Elevated, firm, diameter <1 cm (0.5 in.)	Warts, pigmented nevi
Patch	Macule diameter >1 cm (0.5 in.)	Vitiligo, mongolian spot
Nodule	Elevated, firm, deeper in dermis than papule, diameter 1–2 cm (0.5 –1 in.)	Erythema nodosum
Tumor	Elevated, solid, diameter >2 cm (1 in.)	Neoplasm, hemangioma
Vesicle	Elevated, filled with fluid, diameter <1 cm (0.5 in.)	Early chickenpox, herpes simplex
Pustule	Vesicle filled with purulent fluid	Impetigo, acne
Bulla	Vesicle diameter >1 cm (0.5 in.)	Burn blister
Wheal	Irregular elevated solid area of edematous skin	Urticaria, bee sting

Table 26–2   Common Secondary Skin Lesions

Lesion Name	Description	Example
Crust	Dried residue of serum, pus, or blood	Impetigo
Scale	Thin flake of exfoliated epidermis	Dandruff, psoriasis
Lichenification	Thickening of skin with increased visibility of normal skin furrows	Eczema (atopic dermatitis)
Scar	Replacement of destroyed tissue with fibrous tissue	Healed surgical incision
Keloid	Overdevelopment or hypertrophy of scar, extends beyond wound edges and above skin line	Healed skin area after traumatic injury
Excoriation	Abrasion or scratch mark	Scratched insect bite
Fissure	Linear crack in skin	Tinea pedis (athlete's foot)
Erosion	Loss of superficial epidermis; moist but does not bleed	Ruptured chickenpox vesicle
Ulcer	Deeper loss of skin surface; bleeding or scarring may ensue	Chancre
Comedone	A plug of sebaceous and keratin material in a hair follicle opening	Acne
Burrow	A narrow, raised irregular channel caused by a parasite	Scabies
Telangiectasia	Dilated, superficial blood vessels	

Clinical Manifestations

Irritant—A discrete area of redness matching the exposure location is followed by a rash that develops within a few hours of contact, peaks within 24 hours, and quickly resolves with removal of the irritant. Reactions to some irritants may include edema, vesiculation, dryness of the skin, scaling, fissuring, and necrosis.

Allergic—erythema, edema, pruritus, and vesicles or bullae that rupture, ooze, and crust characterize the rash of allergic contact dermatitis that develops within hours to 3 days after exposure, when the immunologic response has been activated. The rash is usually limited to the area of contact and may take 2 to 4 weeks to resolve without treatment (Amer & Fischer, 2006).

Clinical Therapy

The distribution of the lesions provides clues about the source and identity of the allergen or irritant.

Remove the offending agent (e.g., clothes, plant, soap).

Skin care may involve calamine lotion, cool compresses with aluminum acetate (Burow's solution) to promote drying, and wet dressings or colloidal oatmeal soaks to relieve itching.

Antihistamines may be given to reduce itching or for a sedative effect when the child is too irritable to sleep.

Topical medium-potency corticosteroids may be used for 2 to 3 weeks for allergic contact dermatitis when less than 10% of the body surface area (BSA) is affected, but they should not be applied on open lesions.

Oral corticosteroids are used for 7 to 10 days when more than 10% of the BSA is affected, followed by tapering doses over the next 7 to 10 days.

Nursing Management

Assess the skin, and identify the potential source of inflammation. Identify the family's knowledge of potential allergens and irritants.

Teach parents proper application of topical corticosteroids and to continue their use for 2 to 3 weeks, even when the skin shows signs of healing, to prevent rebound dermatitis. Teach proper administration of oral corticosteroids if prescribed.

Educate parents to use Burow's solution or aluminum acetate (Domeboro solution) for blistered or oozing lesions for 20 minutes daily to help dry lesions (Allen, 2004).

Familiarize parents with the symptoms of infection and need for follow-up care.

Patient and Family Education

Wash all clothes before the first wearing. Rinse clothes an extra time to remove all soap. Use mild soap to clean the skin.

Place a barrier between the allergen and the skin (e.g., cover all metal snaps on clothing with cloth, wear socks to avoid exposure to shoe leather), or seek clothing or shoes made without allergens.

Avoid use of nickel jewelry and belt buckles if a nickel allergy exists.

Remove clothing worn after outside activities and shower if exposure to poison ivy is possible, and then put on clean clothes.

Diaper Dermatitis

Diaper dermatitis is the most common irritant contact dermatitis in infants from 4 to 12 months of age and is caused when urine and feces interact with the skin. *Candida albicans* is a secondary infection complication, but may also occur after antibiotic therapy for another condition.

Clinical Manifestations

Primary irritant rash—glazed red plaques over the skin in direct contact with the diaper area; the skin folds are spared; in severe cases, a fiery-red, raised, and confluent rash or pustules with tenderness may be seen.

Candida albicans infection—bright-red scaly plaques with sharp margins; small papules and pustules may be seen, along with satellite lesions; skin folds are involved.

Clinical Therapy

Diagnosis is usually based on appearance. When *Candida albicans* is suspected, a skin scraping is examined with potassium hydroxide (KOH) under a microscope.

Irritant rash—with each diaper change for 5 to 7 days, apply a water-permeable barrier or protective sealant, such as zinc-oxide paste, Aquaphor, Desitin, or Balmex. A combination product, containing a diaper ointment or cream plus a protective powder (e.g., karaya powder, Stomahesive Protective Powder), may be used.

Candida albicans—antifungal creams (clotrimazole or nystatin) are applied to the affected areas at each diaper change and covered with the barrier or protective sealant until 3 days after the rash has cleared (Nield, & Kamat, 2006). An oral antifungal agent may be given to clear the candidiasis from the intestines.

Nursing Management

Change the diaper as soon as it is wet, or at least every 2 hours during the day and once during the night. Use superabsorbent disposable diapers. Expose the diaper area to air.

Wash the perianal area with warm water and a mild soap or a nonwater cleanser (Aquanil HC lotion or Cetaphil) only after a bowel movement. Use soft paper towels with warm tap water or baby wipes without alcohol.

Avoid use of powders until the skin has healed.

Apply the barrier ointment to protect the skin from urine and stool.

Observe for signs of infection. Encourage parents to return if significant improvement is not seen within a week.

INFECTIOUS DISORDERS

Cellulitis

Cellulitis is an acute inflammation of the dermis and underlying connective tissue that usually occurs on the face and extremities after injury to the skin barrier, an abscess, or sinusitis. Common causative organisms are *Staphylococcus aureus, Streptococcus pyogenes,* and *Streptococcus pneumoniae.*

Clinical Manifestations

Rapid onset of erythema, edema of the face or infected limb, warmth, and tenderness in an ill-appearing child.

Fever, chills, malaise, and enlargement and tenderness of regional lymph nodes may be present, as well as erythematous streaks extending in a proximal direction from the infection.

Diagnostic Tests

A complete blood count with differential may show an increase in white blood cells.

Culture of the site is indicated; blood cultures and a lumbar puncture are indicated if the child has a toxic appearance.

Clinical Therapy

Intravenous antibiotics are indicated if the face or a large surface area is involved to prevent complications and sepsis; oral antibiotics are indicated when other sites are involved. The child may be hospitalized. Analgesics are given for pain. See chapter 14 for periorbital cellulitis.

Nursing Management

Administer prescribed oral or intravenous antibiotics and analgesics as scheduled.

Apply warm compresses to the affected area four times daily.

Elevate head or affected limb, and keep child on bed rest.

Monitor for complications such as abscess formation, spread of the infected area in the 24- to 48-hour period after the start of treatment, increased lethargy, and fever.

Impetigo

Impetigo is a highly contagious, superficial infection of minor skin abrasions, lacerations, insect bites, burns, or dermatitis caused by streptococci, staphylococci, or both.

Clinical Manifestations

The lesion begins as a papule and then a vesicle surrounded by edema and redness at an injured site. The vesicle ruptures, leaving a honey-colored crust covering an ulcerated base. Multiple lesions may develop through self-inoculation. Pruritus and regional lymphadenopathy may be present.

Clinical Therapy

Impetigo is diagnosed by appearance. A Gram stain and bacterial culture may be used.

Crusts are soaked in warm water and gently scrubbed off with an antiseptic soap.

Topical bactericidal ointment (mupirocin) is applied three times a day for 5 to 7 days. Retapamulin 1% ointment (Altabax) applied twice a day for 5 days has recently been approved for treatment of impetigo in children 9 months of age and older (Bell, 2007). If there is no response, a culture and a systemic oral antibiotic may be needed.

Nursing Management

Educate parents to cleanse the lesions and apply topical medications. Emphasize the need to use the topical or oral antibiotic for the full number of days prescribed.

The infection is communicable for 48 hours after antibiotic ointment treatment is begun. Inform parents how to reduce the spread of infection to others. Inform the childcare center about the child's infection, so that toys and surfaces can be sanitized.

Ringworm (Dermatophytoses)

Dermatophytoses are fungal infections that affect the skin, hair, or nails that may be acquired from contact with infected human, cat, dog, or horse (Monroe, 2005). Dermatophytes produce enzymes to penetrate keratinized tissues and invade the hair shaft, leading to an immune reaction to fungal antigens (Shy, 2007). Tinea capitis involves the hair of the scalp. Tinea corporis involves the skin of the body but not the scalp, beard, groin, hands, or feet.

Clinical Manifestations
Tinea Capitis

Circumscribed hair loss, erythema, or a lesion lighter than skin color; broken hairs, dotted stubbed appearance where weakened hair has broken off; diffuse fine scaling, may appear as seborrhea, with yellow, greasy scales; mild itching

May have large, purulent, tender boggy mass on scalp with drainage (kerion); papules, pustules, and crusting on scalp; enlarged suboccipital or posterior cervical nodes

Tinea Corporis
Pink, scaly circular patch with an expanding border, may be scaly or erythematous throughout; slightly raised borders with a clearing center. Multiple lesions on the face, neck, and arms may be present.

Diagnostic Tests
Microscopic examination of the hair and scale scrapings using a potassium hydroxide wet mount or a fungal culture

Clinical Therapy
Tinea Capitis
Griseofulvin orally for 6 to 8 weeks or 2 weeks after symptoms disappear or Terbinafine orally once a day for 6 weeks in children older than 4 years; fluconazole and itraconazole for children 12 years and older; selenium sulfide shampoo two to three times weekly, leave on for 10 minutes before rinsing to help eliminate scalp spores.

Children being treated may develop a hypersensitivity reaction to the fungal antigen, an extensive, itchy rash on the trunk, extremities, and face similar to atopic eczema. This *id* reaction is not a medication reaction. Mild topical corticosteroids and a systemic antihistamine are used to treat it. Continuing the antifungal agent is critical to resolving the fungal infection (Shy, 2007).

Tinea Corporis
Topical antifungal cream (e.g., clotrimazole, miconazole, ketoconazole, naftifine, terbinafine) twice a day for 4 weeks; wash body with selenium sulfide shampoo two to three times a week.

An oral antifungal agent may be needed when lesions are extensive, involve hair follicles, or there is no response to topical therapy.

Nursing Management
Emphasize the need to take the oral antifungal medication for at least 6 weeks. Medication absorption is enhanced if given with a high-fat food such as whole milk or peanut butter. Inform parents about the potential *id* reaction.

Assess all family members and household pets for fungal lesions.

Educate the child and family to avoid personal contact with hair and sharing of hair accessories, brushes, and hats. Encourage all family members to bathe with selenium sulfide shampoo two to three times a week.

Inform parents and children with tinea capitis that hair regrowth is slow and may take 6 to 12 months.

INFESTATIONS

Pediculosis Capitis (Lice)

Pediculosis capitis is an infestation of the hair and scalp. Head lice live and reproduce only on humans and are transmitted by direct hair-to-hair contact or indirect contact by sharing hair accessories, brushes, hats, towels, and bedding.

Clinical Manifestations

Intense pruritus, sesame-sized bugs or nits (eggs) in the hair, open sores from scratching are present.

Nits look like silvery white, yellow, or darker 1-mm teardrops adhering to one side of the hair shaft, commonly behind the ears and at base of the head.

Posterior cervical nodes may be palpable.

Clinical Therapy

Lice are diagnosed by their presence in the hair.

A pediculicide shampoo, such as pyrethrin with an enzymatic lice egg remover, or an ovicidal rinse, such as permethrin (Nix), is used and left on the hair for 10 minutes. Second-line therapy includes malathion (Ovide) or lindane; however, toxicity, flammability, odor, and higher cost are a concern. Products without pesticides include Lice B Gone, Lice Away Enzyme Shampoo, and Hair Clean 1-2-3.

The hair is towel dried, and the nits are removed with a fine-toothed comb. A second treatment is needed in 7 days because the neurotoxin is ineffective on nits.

Cetaphil cleanser may alternatively also be applied to a wet scalp and dried with a hair dryer to shrink-wrap and suffocate the lice (Pearlman, 2004).

Nursing Management

Assessment

Use a bright light and magnifying glass to see the lice and nits along the hair shaft, close to the scalp. Distinguish lice and nits from dandruff flakes. Examine all family members and contacts for lice.

Implementation

Educate parents to use the pediculicide for the time specified on the directions. If the child has very long hair, use a second bottle of pediculocide. The pediculocide does not kill the nits.

Remove the nits with a fine-toothed comb, tweezers, and a basin filled with water or isopropyl alcohol to dip and clean the comb and tweezers. Nits adhere to the hair shaft and must be manually pulled down it. If the nit cannot be removed, cut the hair shaft below the level of the nit. Make sure the parents know that it may take hours for all the lice and nits to be removed because they are firmly cemented to the hair shaft.

Check the hair every 2 to 3 days, and remove any lice or nits seen. Repeat treatment 1 week later, as lice may hatch in 8 to 10 days. The child may return to child care or school after the first pediculicide treatment (Sciscione & Krause-Parello, 2007).

Teach the child not to share clothing, headwear, or combs. Bedding and clothing used by the child should be changed daily, laundered in hot water with detergent, and dried in a hot dryer for 20 minutes. Seal toys and other personal items that cannot be washed or dry cleaned in a plastic bag for 2 weeks.

Scabies

Scabies is a highly contagious infestation caused by the mite *Sarcoptes scabei* and spread by skin-to-skin contact, often within a household. The female mite burrows into the outer layer of the epidermis to lay her eggs, leaving a trail of debris and feces. The larvae hatch in approximately 2 to 4 days and proceed toward the surface of the skin. The cycle is repeated 14 to 17 days later. A delayed type IV hypersensitivity reaction to the mites, debris, and feces occurs within 2 to 4 weeks of the infestation (Sladden & Johnston, 2005).

Clinical Manifestations

Rash with various lesions (papules, vesicles, pustules, and nodules), severe pruritus that worsens at night, and restlessness

Lesions located in the webs of fingers and skin folds, on the palms and wrists of hands and feet

Linear, threadlike, grayish burrows 1 to 10 cm in length

Secondary infection from scratching may obscure burrow lesions.

Diagnostic Tests

Microscopic view of burrow scrapings often reveals actively moving mites, fecal pellets, and eggs or nits.

Clinical Therapy

A scabicide, such as 5% permethrin lotion, is applied over the entire body, including the scalp, ears, and forehead, after a bath when the skin is cool and dry. Apply the lotion to the child's face if lesions are present. Do not apply to an infant's face. Leave the lotion on for 8 to 12 hours before washing it off. The treatment is repeated 1 week later. Topical and oral invermectin has FDA approval for children weighing more than 15 kg for use when other treatments are unsuccessful. Treat all family members and childcare givers at the same time, even if not symptomatic. An oral antihistamine may be prescribed for itching.

Nursing Management

Advise parents that scabies is highly contagious and transmitted by close contact. All family members should be treated simultaneously. Uninfested individuals should wash hands well if touching the child before first treatment is completed.

Change all clothing, bedding, and pillowcases used by the child daily, wash with hot water, and iron before reuse. Seal nonwashable toys and other items in plastic bags for 5 to 7 days.

VASCULAR TUMORS (HEMANGIOMAS)

Vascular tumors, or *hemangiomas*, are neoplasms of endothelial cells and increased numbers of small blood vessels that undergo rapid growth and proliferation during the first 6 to 10 months during infancy. This phase is followed by involution, a slow decrease in size, that is completed in adolescence (Cohen, 2004). Complications may be caused by the rapid growth and pressure against or obstruction of vital structures.

Clinical Manifestations

Superficial hemangiomas—bright-red vascular cutaneous plaques that resemble strawberries.

Deep hemangiomas—bluish tumors covered with normal-appearing epidermis.

Mixed hemangiomas have features of both superficial and deep tumors.

Lesions are minimally compressible and have no bruit or thrill. Ulceration of the vascular tumor may occur during the period of rapid growth. Tissue atrophy, wrinkles, telangectasias, and hypopigmentation may be seen with involution.

Diagnostic Tests

Initial diagnosis is by physical examination and monitoring the growth of the vascular tumor. Ultrasound, computed tomography scanning, or magnetic resonance imaging may also be used for potential pressure or obstruction of a vital organ.

Clinical Therapy

Oral corticosteroids are used during the proliferation phase for infants with extensive facial hemangiomas. Injections of corticosteroids into small, localized hemangiomas are sometimes performed.

Pulsed dye laser treatments at 2- to 3-week intervals are used for superficial hemangiomas during the proliferative phase. The hemangioma darkens for 1 to 2 weeks, fades to red, and then lightens (Jones, 2007).

Surgical removal of an ulcerated hemangioma is considered if the scarring outcome would be acceptable (Christinson-Lagay & Fishman, 2006).

Nursing Management

Assessment

Assess the distribution of the hemangioma and the potential complications during the rapid growth stage. Monitor for ulceration of the hemangioma.

Monitor the infant's growth, because corticosteroid treatment may slow growth.

Assess the parents' response to the infant's appearance.

Implementation

Educate parents about the type of vascular lesion, administration of corticosteroids, and potential medication side effects (gastrointestinal upset, sleep disturbance, temporary growth retardation, decreased appetite, and transient facial edema).

Inform parents about possible ulceration as the hemangioma grows rapidly and signs to expect. Tell them to cover and protect the skin from infection until seen by the physician.

Help parents see positive characteristics in the infant (e.g., responsiveness to interaction and smiling). Show parents photographs of other children who have completed therapy to show that gradual improvements are possible. Take photos of the child at intervals during treatment to show parents when improvements have occurred.

Prepare parents for changes to the child's appearance with pulsed dye laser therapy. Protect treated skin from sun exposure, and use sunscreen in the future.

CHRONIC SKIN CONDITIONS

Acne

Acne is a chronic inflammatory disorder of the pilosebaceous hair follicles located on the face and trunk. Abnormal shedding of keratinocytes within the pilosebaceous hair follicles and increased production of sebum by the sebaceous glands obstruct the follicular canal, causing *comedones* (whiteheads and blackheads). The sebum behind the comedone is an ideal environment for the anaerobic *Propionibacterium acnes,* and an inflammatory reaction results (Zaenglein & Thiboutot, 2006).

Clinical Manifestations

The three main types of acne are
1. Comedonal (characterized by open and closed comedones)
2. Papulopustular (characterized by red papules and pustules)
3. Cystic (characterized by nodules involving multiple hair follicles and cysts)

Scars form when the surrounding dermis is damaged and may be pitted, atrophic, or hypertropic (keloid). Lesions occur most often on the face, upper chest, shoulders, and back.

Inflammatory acne in adolescents with darker skin color is associated with a hyperpigmented macule that can last for 4 months or longer. Hyperpigmented areas may fade over time if inflammation is controlled (Keri, 2006).

Clinical Therapy

Diagnosis is based on examination of the skin. Treatment is customized to the predominant type of lesion present and severity of the lesions. Options include long-term use of keratolytics, retinoids, and oral antibiotics to suppress lesions and reduce scarring (Table 26–3). Oral contraceptives may be prescribed because they suppress gonadotropin secretion and reduce ovarian androgen production.

Isotretinoin (Accutane) is reserved for the most serious cases of acne that do not respond to other therapies, but it is a strong fetal teratogen (Lipper, 2007).

- Adolescent females need two negative pregnancy tests before starting treatment; a monthly pregnancy test before each prescription refill; and to use two forms of contraception (strict abstinence can count as one form) 1 month before, during, and 1 month after treatment.
- Monthly laboratory monitoring of liver function, cholesterol, and triglycerides is required. A 1-month supply of isotretinoin is provided to promote compliance.
- An Internet registry system exists for the physician to report the negative pregnancy test that the pharmacist must review prior to filling the prescription.

Table 26–3 Medications for Acne Treatment

Medication	Nursing Management
Tretinoin (Retin-A) 0.025% cream daily Salicylic acid, adapalene, tazarotene For mild and moderate comedonal and papulopustular acne	Use a lower concentration initially as skin irritation is common. Divide and spread a pea-sized amount over the entire face. Do not use as spot therapy. Apply only at night, its stability is affected by light.
2.5% benzoyl peroxide gel For mild or moderate papulopustular acne	A lower strength may be used initially if skin irritation occurs. Apply in the morning.
Topical antibiotics (clindamycin, erythromycin, tetracycline) Topical for mild inflammatory acne Oral for moderate to severe inflammatory acne	Combined with topical retinoid and benzoyl peroxide to reduce antibiotic resistance. Takes 6 to 8 weeks to see improvement, antibiotic is changed if no response. Discontinued once inflammatory lesions are under good control.
Isotretinoin (Accutane)	Requires informed consent. Females must use contraception due to teratogenic effects of the medication and have monthly pregnancy tests. Given twice a day for 15–20 weeks. A second course of treatment may be prescribed. Take medication with food to increase oral absorption.
Oral contraceptives For persistent inflammatory papules and nodules	Teach adolescent the correct administration schedule.

Nursing Management
Assessment

Assess the distribution, predominant type, and severity of acne lesions.

Assess knowledge about the cause and treatment of acne and the home therapies used.

Explore the amount of emotional distress the acne is causing the adolescent.

Implementation

Encourage good nutrition to help the skin heal.

Teach correct procedures for taking prescribed drugs such as tetracycline and isotretinoin, and discuss possible side effects. Emphasize the importance of return visits to the adolescent's healthcare provider to monitor side effects of medications.

Provide psychological support to adolescents.

Patient and Family Education

Avoid picking and squeezing pimples. Wash your hands often, and avoid touching your face to reduce the transfer of oils and bacteria to the face.

Use gentle skin cleansers without an oil base to wash the face twice a day. Do not use abrasive sponges or cloths. Wait 20 minutes until the skin is thoroughly dry before applying a topical retinoid.

For topical medications, use a pea-sized dose of topical medications to spread in a thin film over the skin. Avoid getting the topical medications near the eyes, lips, and mucous membranes.

Avoid the use of astringents and aftershaves that contain alcohol. They may further dry the skin and make it difficult to tolerate the prescribed topical medications.

Avoid hats or gear that can cause friction and occlusion of the skin.

Greasy foods may leave a residual oil on the face and hands that can be occlusive. Wash your hands after handling greasy foods.

Limit the use of pomades or petrolatum-based hair products. Keep hair spray and mousse away from the face.

Use noncomedonic (for acne-prone skin) moisturizers to reduce irritation. Use oil-free or water-based makeup. Avoid waterproof makeup.

Use noncomedonic sunscreen and protective clothing even on cloudy days, as the medications make the skin more sensitive to sun exposure.

Protect the face from cold, windy weather. Sweating, heat and humidity, and emotional stress may exacerbate acne.

Do not get discouraged with daily treatments, as it will take 6 to 12 weeks before improvement is seen. Continue daily topical therapies when acne has improved significantly so that acne does not return.

ATOPIC ECZEMA (ATOPIC DERMATITIS)

Atopic eczema is a chronic, superficial inflammatory skin disorder with intense pruritus. It affects 17% of infants, children, and adolescents (Tofte, 2007). While the etiology is unknown, a complex interaction of genetic predisposition, environmental exposure, infectious agents, defects in skin barrier function, and immunologic responses is involved (Akdis, Akdis, Bieber, et al., 2006).

The child's generally dry skin is more likely to crack and fissure. The impaired lipid barrier gives irritants a greater chance to penetrate. The child is more susceptible to infection from organisms such as staphylococcus, herpes simplex, and molluscum contagiosum.

Clinical Manifestations

Acute atopic eczema is characterized by pruritus and erythematous patches with vesicles, exudate, and crusts. Subacute cases are characterized by scaling with erythema and excoriation. Erythema and warmth may indicate a secondary bacterial skin infection.

Infantile form—pruritic exudative, crusty, papulovesicular, and erythematous lesions on cheeks, scalp, forehead, neck, trunk, and extensor surfaces of extremities; diaper area spared; some patches weep or have exudate; secondary infection; lichenification

Childhood form—pruritic, erythematous, dry scaly or weeping, well-circumscribed, papular lesions; buttocks become excoriated once toilet trained; thickened and lichenified lesions on antecubital, popliteal, flexor, and extensor surfaces of extremities, neck, and behind ears

Adolescent form—similar to childhood eczema in distribution and lesions, but less acute; other affected areas may include the eyelids, where the earlobe touches the face, fingertips, toes, nipples, and the vulvar area

Clinical Therapy

No laboratory tests are diagnostic. Skin prick tests or radioallergosorbent tests (RAST) may be used to identify food allergies. Skin cultures are used for a suspected secondary infection.

The goals of treatment are to hydrate and lubricate the skin, reduce pruritus, minimize inflammatory changes, and identify flare-up triggers. Therapy includes the following:

- Apply occlusive topical ointment after bathing to trap moisture and prevent drying of the skin. Apply moisturizing ointments and creams three to four times a day and when skin feels dry (Table 26–4).

Table 26–4   Medications Used for Atopic Eczema

Medications	Nursing Management
Emollients Eucerin cream Aquaphor ointment Vanicream Cetaphil cream SBR-lipocream White petrolatum	Use only fragrance-free or bland emollients, as fragrances and preservatives in products may cause irritation. Apply before skin is dry after bathing to trap in moisture. Apply whenever skin is dry.
Oral antihistamines	Give an hour before naptime or bedtime. If used during the day sleepiness could interfere with school.
Antibiotics Topical Oral	Monitor for a hypersensitivity reaction.
Corticosteroids Topical Oral	Avoid use around the eyes as it can induce glaucoma or cataract formation. Use lowest potency that has beneficial effect and avoid use on healthy skin to prevent skin atrophy.
Immunomodulators Tacrolimus ointment Pimecrolimus (Elidel, SDZ ASM 981)	Prepare family for the sensation of burning, redness, and itching for the first few days of therapy. Educate about the need for sunscreens because of the potential increased risk for skin cancer. Approved for children older than 2 years.

- Apply topical corticosteroids twice daily before the skin moisturizer is used. Corticosteroids are used for 2 weeks only on inflamed skin and then tapered in frequency of use or potency before discontinuing to reduce the risk of steroid side effects. Use lower-potency nonfluorinated ointments for infants and for thinner skin areas (face, diaper area, and skin folds). A higher-potency ointment is used for flare-ups.
- Oral corticosteroids may be used for a severe acute exacerbation, but a rebound effect occurs.
- Immunomodulator ointments inhibit T-lymphocyte activation and the release of cytokines and inflammatory mediators from anti-IgE-activated skin mast cells and basophils. They may be the treatment of choice for some children not responsive to or intolerant of conventional therapy.

- Topical antibiotics are used to treat excoriated, open lesions that appear infected.
- Antihistamines do not help itching, but the sedative effect may help promote sleep. Humidification in the winter and air conditioning in the summer may help reduce pruritus.
- Avoidance of highly allergenic foods, such as eggs, wheat, milk, and peanuts, in the diets of infants and lactating mothers may improve the skin condition of some children.
- Supplementation with a probiotic may be beneficial in young children with moderate to severe atopic eczema (Weston, Halbert, Richmond, et al., 2005).

Nursing Management

Assessment

Take a thorough history, including any family history of allergy, environmental or dietary factors, and past exacerbations.

Attempt to identify a trigger for the child's skin flare, such as house mites, animal dander, pollens, food allergies, irritants (detergents, chemicals, and abrasive clothing), hormonal changes, and emotional stress.

Note the distribution and type of lesions, as well as presence of weeping lesions or signs of infection.

Determine whether the sleep of the child or other family members is disturbed.

Identify whether the child's self-esteem is disturbed.

Intervention

If an oral antihistamine is ordered to promote sleep, make sure the parents understand the best time to give the medication for that purpose.

Help parents and children of all ages deal with the frustration of the acute flare-ups. Encourage good home care to improve the child's skin. Reassure parents that the condition usually improves with age and generally does not leave scars.

Identify activities that the child can participate in to improve self-esteem.

Help identify potential food allergens. Increased itching within hours of eating a certain food may be associated with atopic eczema flares. Provide alternative foods to fulfill daily nutritional requirements when allergens are identified. Refer the family to the Food Allergy and Anaphylaxis Network.

Patient and Family Education

Avoid wool clothing and clothing washed in harsh laundry detergents to decrease skin irritation and pruritus. Wear loose cotton clothing.

Bathe and let the child soak in tepid water for 5 to 15 minutes once or twice a day. Salt or baking soda can be added to the water if it causes stinging. Use mild unscented soap, such as Dove or Cetaphil liquid cleanser, only on dirty skin. Rinse well. Apply emollients to wet skin.

Immediately apply a thin layer of medication (corticosteroid, topical antibiotic, or immunomodulator) to the inflamed area and rub in completely. Then apply the ointment or cream emollient on top of the medication and over the entire body. Avoid the use of lotions that have less oil.

Consider the cost of ointments and creams, as large quantities are needed to cover the body at least twice a day. Petrolatum or Vaseline is inexpensive, safe, and easily applied.

In areas where the humidity is low, more frequent application of lubricants to the skin is needed.

Help assure that parents use enough corticosteroids for effective treatment. It takes 5 to 8 g to cover the entire body of a child who weighs 10 kg, so a 15-g tube of corticosteroid ointment is enough for only *1* day. It takes 45 g to cover the entire body of an adolescent once (Hansen, 2003). The steroid is only used where there is inflammation. Apply corticosteroids no more than twice a day.

For immunomodulators, a pea size amount should cover a 2-in. circle.

INJURIES TO THE INTEGUMENTARY SYSTEM

Animal Bites

Children are at a higher risk for animal bites, and most cases involve dogs. Bites are commonly associated with inappropriate behavior by the child, such as teasing, playing, or interfering with feeding or with care of puppies.

Clinical Manifestations

Dog bites tend to be crushing, rather than clean, sharp lacerations. Cat bites tend to be puncture wounds.

Clinical Therapy

Puncture wounds and damage to nerves, muscles, tendons, and vascular structures are identified by physical examination. Bites to the head and neck require radiographic examination to rule out any associated injury, such as airway trauma or a depressed skull fracture.

Initial treatment includes irrigation of the wound, removal of devitalized tissue, and a clean dressing. Sedation and pain management are often needed. Many wounds are closed with adhesive bandages. Wounds over joints are immobilized and elevated. Some wounds require surgical closure or reconstruction. Puncture wounds are not irrigated or sutured because of infection risk. Antibiotics may be prescribed.

Report the animal bite to the police and arrange to have the animal observed for 10 days for signs of rabies. Human rabies immune globulin or human diploid cell rabies vaccine should be given to all children bitten by a wild animal, any animal proven to be rabid, or in which rabies cannot be excluded. Cats less commonly get the rabies vaccine.

Nursing Management
Observe and document the extent of the injury, circumstances surrounding the attack, present location of the animal, and attempts to assess the animal's health.

Irrigate the wound with large quantities of sterile saline or lactated Ringer's solution. Apply a clean pressure dressing, and elevate the affected part to reduce bleeding.

Determine whether a tetanus booster is needed.

Teach parents how to care for the wound and how to identify signs of infection.

Patient and Family Education to Prevent Animal Bites
General guidelines for pets in the home:
- Never leave a young child alone with an animal.
- Do not buy a pet unless you are confident of your child's ability to respect it.
- Spay or neuter the pet to reduce aggression.

Teach children the following rules:
- Avoid unfamiliar animals, and report them to a parent.
- Avoid contact with all wild animals. If an animal (wild or unknown) is sick or acting strangely, notify the health department.
- Do not touch an animal when it is eating, sleeping, or nursing.
- Never overexcite an animal. Do not roughhouse or play games that stimulate aggressive behavior.
- Never tease or throw objects at an animal.

- Never put your face close to an animal. Seek permission before hugging or petting an animal.
- If approached by a dog, stay calm, stand still, talk softly, and back away slowly until the dog loses interest; do not run.
- If attacked, pretend to be a tree or a log, and protect the face.

Burns

Burns result from different mechanisms.
- Thermal burns, the most common burns in children, may occur through exposure to flames, scalds, or contact with a hot object.
- Chemical burns occur when children touch or ingest caustic agents.
- Electrical burns occur from exposure to direct or alternating current in electrical wires, appliances, or high-voltage wires, as well as lightning strikes.
- Radiation burns result from exposure to radioactive substances or sunlight.

A full-thickness burn can occur in an infant or young child after immersion for only 5 seconds in water with a temperature of 60°C (140°F). Coffee and other hot beverages are often served at temperatures between 71° to 82°C (160° to 180°F), (Grant, 2004).

After the burn, intense vasoconstriction results in ischemia that may increase the depth of the burn injury. Vasoactive hormone release increases capillary permeability, resulting in edema and decreased circulating blood volume as fluid and plasma shift into the interstitial spaces. Water and heat is lost through the injured skin. The child's metabolic rate and need for calories increase as the child tries to maintain body temperature and begin healing.

Clinical Manifestations

Burns are classified by depth:
- Superficial partial-thickness burns (first-degree burns) are red and painful.
- Partial-thickness burns (second-degree burns) have blisters, bullae, erythema, blanching on pressure, pain, and sensitivity to cold air.
- Full-thickness burns (third-degree burns) are those in which the injured tissue cannot regenerate, appear black, brown, white to gray, waxy, or deep cherry red, and are not painful.

Diagnostic Tests

Burn severity is determined by the depth of the burn injury, percentage of body surface area (BSA) affected, and involvement of specific body parts. BSA is calculated using a Lund-Browder chart. Specialized burn center care is needed for the following burns:

- A partial-thickness burn greater than 10% BSA in a child under 10 years; greater than 20% in an older child; full-thickness burns greater than 5%
- Burns involving the hands, face, feet, genitalia, perineum, and major joints
- Electrical burns, lightning injury, or an inhalation injury

Other major burns include those that are circumferential (injury completely surrounding the thorax or an extremity) or anterior chest burns.

Clinical Therapy

Initial care involves ensuring that the child has an airway, is breathing, and has a pulse. Use moist soaks or ice over small areas to stop the burning process and to relieve pain. Treatment focuses on decreasing burn fluid losses, preventing infection, controlling pain, promoting nutrition, and salvaging all viable burned tissue. Intravenous fluid replacement with lactated Ringer's or normal saline is given to prevent hypovolemic shock in cases of significant burn injury using the Parkland or Galveston formula for calculation. The child's temperature is maintained.

Continuous enteral feedings are often initiated within 6 hours of the burn injury to support the child's nutritional requirements. The child needs increased calories and additional protein, vitamins, and minerals for the increased metabolic rate and stress response to the burn injury (Klein & Herndon, 2004).

Débridement (removal of dead tissue to speed the healing process) is performed using sedation and anesthesiology support for pain management. Hydrotherapy may be used to help clean the wound before débridement. Traditional burn care involves antibacterial topical creams (sulfadiazine, mafenide acetate [Sulfamylon], or bacitracin) covered with a dressing, with dressing changes once or twice daily. Silver-based antimicrobial dressings (e.g., Aquacel, Acticoat) absorb exudate from the wound, and dressings are changed every 2 to 3 days (Duffy, McLaughlin, & Eichelberger, 2006). Superficial second-degree burns re-epithelialize within 3 weeks.

Skin grafting is used for deep second- or third-degree burns. A temporary skin substitute (e.g., Integra or Biobrane) or an allograft may be applied to debrided skin to form a protective barrier over the wound. An autograft, skin from the child's body, is a permanent graft.

Physical therapy and occupational therapy are important in promoting joint and muscle function. Splints may help prevent contractures and reduce scarring. Jobst or pressure garments reduce the development of hypertrophic scarring.

Nursing Management

Assessment

Perform an initial emergency assessment of airway, breathing, and circulation. Assess for signs of smoke inhalation, burns to the face and neck, or other injuries if the child fell or was involved in an explosion.

Inspect the location, extent, and shape of the burn injury. Consider the potential for child abuse when burns have a glove or stocking distribution, spare flexor surfaces, or have the shape of a hot iron, grate, or cigarette.

Frequently monitor vital signs, circulatory and respiratory status, pain management, intake and output, and daily weight measurement. Be alert to signs of infection.

Assess the child's and family's concerns over appearance and the stress of hospitalization. Identify how well the family is coping with the child's injury and other family stressors.

Implementation

Provide nursing care that includes fluid and nutrition management, pain management, and play therapy. Increase the child's fluid intake to compensate for fluid loss through damaged skin. Encourage a high-calorie, high-protein diet to meet the increased nutritional requirements of healing.

Provide wound care according to guidelines and physician orders, including dressing changes, hydrotherapy, and antibiotic therapy.

Prevent complications, such as infections, pneumonia, renal failure, and irreversible loss of function. Perform range-of-motion exercises.

Encourage the child and parents to voice concerns, and show understanding and support.

Children with minor burns are cared for at home after the initial emergency department visit to débride any open blisters and apply a topical antibiotic and dressing. Educate parents to provide pain medication before dressing changes. Parents should soak the dressing with saline to remove it, clean off old antibiotic and drainage, and reapply antibiotic and the dressing. Educate the parents to observe for signs of infection.

Insect Bites and Stings

Insect and spider bites, as well as stings in some cases, are venomous or produce an allergic reaction.

Clinical Manifestations

Bee or Wasp Sting

Venoms contain enzymes that affect vascular tone and permeability. Local reaction includes mild, local pain, erythema, and edema. Systemic reaction includes generalized urticaria, flushing, angioedema, pruritus, and wheezing. Anaphylaxis is rare.

Fire Ants

Venom is hemolytic and neurotoxic, causing a histaminelike response. Local reaction includes a black center at the bite or a trail of lesions across the skin; initial wheal becomes a vesicle within a few hours, and, in 24 hours, the fluid is cloudy and a red halo surrounds the vesicle; pruritus; and erythema, edema, and induration. Systemic and anaphylactic reactions can occur.

Black Widow Spider

Venom is neurotoxic. Local reaction includes stinging at the time of bite, localized edema and erythema, two fang marks, and petechiae branching from site. A systemic reaction occurs in 1 to 3 hours, with muscle rigidity of torso and abdomen, priapism, and muscle cramps near the bite; malaise, sweating, nausea, vomiting, dizziness, hypertension, and arrhythmias; oliguria; and restlessness and insomnia. Symptoms peak in 3 to 12 hours and diminish within 72 hours.

Brown Recluse Spider

Venom contains proteolytic enzymes and a cytotoxic factor. Reaction includes erythema and edema evolving to a purple bull's-eye lesion with an outer white zone of induration; progression to severe necrosis with scab that hardens and falls off in 7 to 14 days; and an ulcerated depression that heals in 6 to 8 weeks with scarring. Severe systemic reactions may occur in 12 to 72 hours, including fever, chills, restlessness, malaise, joint pain, and nausea and vomiting.

Clinical Therapy

Ice, cool compresses; elevate the extremity; antihistamine medication; remove bee stinger.

The child with a severe allergic reaction to insects should wear medical alert identification and carry an epinephrine injector kit (epipen).

Desensitization injections may be given to children with an anaphylactic reaction or severe systemic reaction to bees, wasps, and fire ants.

Antivenom, diazepam, and opioids may be given for black widow spider bites.

Excision and skin grafting may be performed in cases of severe necrosis due to brown recluse spider bites.

Nursing Management

Assess the child and identify the child in need for emergency care. Teach the child, parents, and school personnel how to use the epipen. If an epipen is used, call 911 as the epinephrine effect lasts 20 minutes.

Encourage parents and children to become familiar with insects and spiders in the geographic area. Teach children to avoid spiders and other biting or stinging insects.

Use an insect repellent. Avoid the use of perfumed shampoos, powders, soaps, lotions, or bright-colored or floral-print clothing when outdoors. Avoid eating sweet foods and beverages outdoors, as these attract bees and wasps.

Teach children to stay calm when a bee or wasp approaches and to slowly walk away without swatting.

Pressure Ulcers

Tissue ischemia due to pressure deprives cells of oxygen and nutrients, leading to a soft tissue injury. Without intervention, the injury rapidly progresses and a pressure ulcer forms. Children at greatest risk are those with paralysis, limited mobility or low activity, sensory deficits, or the inability to change positions and chronic fecal or urinary soiling.

Sites and potential causes of pressure ulcers include:
- Occipital region of scalp—inability to lift head
- Sacrum and buttocks—confinement to bed or wheelchair
- Legs and feet—orthotics, leg braces, casts
- Spine and neck—scoliosis brace
- Knees and elbows—rubbing against bed sheet

Clinical Manifestations

Stage 1—an area of redness that remains 30 minutes after removing the pressure or skin irritant. Children with dark skin may have persistent red, blue, or purple discoloration.

Stage 2—an area that looks rubbed or raw like an abrasion or blister

Stage 3—an ulcer forms as skin damage extends through the epidermis and dermis

Stage 4—the injury deepens to underlying tissue, muscles, bone, or connective tissue

Clinical Therapy

Diagnosis is based on appearance of the skin.

Remove pressure from the affected site until the skin has healed. Frequent repositioning or removing a brace is necessary.

A transparent film may be applied to affected red skin to minimize friction.

Pressure ulcers are treated with various dressings, such as hydrocolloids, gels or hydrogels, and calcium alginates, that create a moist environment and promote healing.

Nursing Management

Assessment

Identify factors that place the child at risk for pressure ulcers. Inspect the skin of all children at risk during healthcare visits.

Inspect the dependent skin surfaces of all infants and children confined to bed at least three times a day. Identify the size (diameter and depth) and character of the skin lesion. Note any signs of infection, the appearance of wound edges, and the type of tissue at the wound base. Describe any drainage.

Implementation

Develop protocols for pressure ulcer prevention for children at high risk.

- Increase ambulation, post a turning schedule or encourage frequent position changes, and encourage use of pressure-reducing surfaces and use of moisture barriers.
- Ensure adequate intake of fluids, proteins, and vitamins.
- Provide wound care and dressing changes according to agency guidelines.
- Avoid the use of tape to hold dressings in place unless a protective skin barrier is used.

Teach children with impaired mobility and diminished pain sensation and their parents to inspect the skin under the braces daily for signs of irritation (redness or blisters). Check the edges of braces for roughness that can pinch or scrape the skin. Brace should not be worn if any redness does not diminish within 30 minutes. Have the child wear cotton socks under the braces to prevent rubbing of bare skin.

Sunburn

Sunburn is a burn injury caused by excess ultraviolet light exposure or sun exposure after taking phototoxic drugs (acne medication, sulfonamides, tetracycline, nonsteroidal antiinflammatory drugs, and birth control pills (Boe & Tillotson, 2006). Sunburn occurs more often in children with red or blond hair, light-colored eyes, and fair skin that freckles easily. The risk for melanoma and basal cell carcinoma is strongly related to a history of one or more severe blistering sunburns during childhood or adolescence.

Clinical Manifestations

Erythema and skin tenderness develop within 4 hours after sunlight exposure. Prolonged exposure can result in edema, vesiculation, bullae, or ulceration. A melanoma in childhood may be manifested by a nodular, raised, and pink lesion (Ferrari, Bono, Collini, et al., 2006).

Clinical Therapy

Increase oral fluids. Relieve pain with cool compresses followed by the application of a low-potency topical corticosteroid (on unblistered skin) to relieve discomfort. Nonsteroidal anti-inflammatory drugs may be used for pain relief and to reduce inflammation.

Nursing Management

Teach adolescents how to monitor for changes in moles (asymmetric, have an irregular border, have color variations, and have a diameter larger than 0.6 cm) that could signal the development of skin cancer and to seek care immediately.

Patient and Family Education: Preventing Sunburn

Keep children out of direct sunlight as much as possible. Avoid scheduling outdoor activities during the hours of maximum exposure (10 AM to 4 PM).

When outdoors, minimize exposure by wearing hats and long-sleeve, closely woven cotton clothing and pants; wear T-shirts while swimming. Special sun-protection clothing can be purchased.

Water, concrete, and sand reflect up to 85% of ultraviolet rays and increase exposure.

Use sunscreen (of at least 15 skin protection factor). For optimal protection, apply as thickly as directed to all exposed areas 30 to 45 minutes before sun exposure. Reapply every 2 hours as needed, or sooner if swimming, toweling off, or perspiring heavily. Use a waterproof sunscreen when swimming, as it provides protection in water for approximately 60 to 80 minutes. Then reapply.

Call the poison control center immediately if sunscreen gets in the eyes, as it causes a chemical burn.

Avoid using sunscreens in infants younger than 6 months; they may absorb the chemicals through the skin.

A child can be burned on a cloudy day, as 80% of ultraviolet rays can penetrate the cloud cover.

If the child is prescribed a medication that causes hypersensitivity to sunlight, take extra care to avoid sun exposure.

REFERENCES

Abelson, M. B., & Granet, D. (2006). Ocular allergy in pediatric practice. *Current Allergy and Asthma Reports, 6,* 306–311.

Adelson, P. D., Bratton, S. L., Carney, N. A., Chestnut, R. A., duCoudray, H. E. M., Goldstein, B., et.al. (2003). Threshhold for treatment of intracranial hypotension: Guidelines for management of severe traumatic brain injury. *Pediatric Critical Care Medicine, 4*(3 Supp), S25–S27.

Adirim, T. A. (2007). Concussions in sports and recreation. *Clinical Pediatric Emergency Medicine, 8,* 2–6.

Aehlert, B. (2005). *PALS: Pediatric Advanced Life Support Study Guide.* St. Louis: Elsevier Mosby.

Agency for Toxic Substances & Disease Registry. (2006). *Lead toxicity clinical evaluation.* Atlanta: Author.

Aiken, J. J., & Oldham, K. T. (2005). Malrotation. In K. W. Ashcraft, G. W. Holcomb, & J. P. Murphy (Eds.), *Pediatric surgery* (4th ed., pp. 435–447). Philadelphia: Saunders.

Aitken, M. E., Graham, C. J., Killingsworth, J. B., Mullins, S. H., Parnell, D. N., & Dick, R. M. (2004). All-terrain vehicle injury in children: strategies for prevention. *British Medical Journal, 10*(5), 303–307.

A-Kader, H. A., & W. F. Balistreri. (2007). Cholestasis. In R. M. Kliegman, R. E. Behrman, H. B. Jenson, & B. F. Stanton (Eds.), *Nelson textbook of pediatrics* (18th ed., pp. 1168–1675). Philadelphia: Saunders Elsevier.

Akdis, C. A., Akdis, M., Bieber, T., Bindslev-Jensen, C., Bogunlewicz, M., et al. (2006). Diagnosis and treatment of atopic dermatitis in children and adults: European Academy of Allergology and Clinical Immunology/American Academy of Allergy, Asthma and Immunology/PRACTALL consensus report. *Journal of Allergy and Clinical Immunology, 118*(1), 152–169.

Alavi, S., Arzanian, M. T., Abbasian, M. R., & Ashena, Z. (2006). Tumor lysis syndrome in children with non-Hodgkin lymphoma. *Pediatric Hematology and Oncology, 23,* 65–70.

Alemzadeh, R., & Wyatt, D. T. (2007). Diabetes mellitus in children. In R. M. Kliegman, R. E. Behrman, H. B. Jenson, & B. F. Stanton, *Nelson textbook of pediatrics* (18th ed., pp. 2402–2431). Philadelphia: Saunders Elsevier.

Allen, P. L. J. (2004). Guidelines for the diagnosis and treatment of celiac disease in children. *Pediatric Nursing, 30*(6), 473–476.

Altizer, L. (2004). Compartment syndrome. *Orthopedic Nursing, 23,* 391–396.

Alvarez, A. M., & Rathore, M. H. (2007). Hot topics in pediatric HIV/AIDS. *Pediatric Annals, 36*(7), 423–432.

Amer, A., & Fischer, H. (2006). Linear rash leaves your patient itching. *Contemporary Pediatrics, 23*(10), 20, 23.

Amer, K. S. (2005). Advances in assessment, diagnosis, and treatment of hyperthyroidism in children. *Journal of Pediatric Nursing, 20*(2), 119–126.

American Academy of Pediatrics. (2004a). Hospital stay for healthy term newborns. *Pediatrics, 113*(5), 1434–1436.

American Academy of Pediatrics. (2004b). Management of hyperbilirubinemia in the newborn infant 35 or more weeks of gestation. *Pediatrics, 114,* 297–316.

American Academy of Pediatrics. (2004c). Managing acute gastroenteritis among children: Oral rehydration, maintenance, and nutritional therapy. *Pediatrics, 114,* 507.

American Academy of Pediatrics. (2005a). Policy statement: Breastfeeding and the use of human milk. *Pediatrics, 115*(2), 496–506.

American Academy of Pediatrics. (2005b). The changing concept of sudden infant death syndrome: Diagnostic coding shifts, controversies regarding the sleeping environment, and new variables to consider in reducing risk. *Pediatrics, 116*(5), 1245–1255.

American Academy of Pediatrics. (2006). *Red book: 2006 Report of the Committee on Infectious Diseases* (27th ed.). Elk Grove Village, IL: Author.

American Academy of Pediatrics. (2007). Car safety seats: A guide for families 2007. Retrieved June 11, 2007 from http://www.aap.org/family/carseatguide.htm

American Academy of Pediatrics, Committee on Practice and Ambulatory Medicine and Section of Ophthalmology. (2003). Eye examination in infants, children, and young adults by pediatricians. *Pediatrics, 111*(4), 902–907.

American Academy of Pediatrics, Section on Cardiology and Cardiac Surgery. (2005). Cardiac health supervision for individuals affected with Duchenne or Becker muscular dystrophy. *Pediatrics, 116,* 1569–1573.

American Academy of Pediatrics, Section on Ophthalmology. (2006). Screening examination of premature infants for retinopathy of prematurity. *Pediatrics, 117,* 572–576.

American Academy of Pediatrics, Subcommittee on Diagnosis and Management of Bronchiolitis. (2006). Diagnosis and management of bronchiolitis. *Pediatrics, 118*(4), 1774–1793.

American Academy of Pediatrics, Subcommittee on Management of Acute Otitis Media. (2004). Diagnosis and management of acute otitis media. *Pediatrics, 113,* 1451–1465.

American Association of Mental Retardation. (2004). Definition of mental retardation. Retrieved August 15, 2008, from http://www.aamr.org/Policies/faq_mental_retardation.shtml

American Diabetes Association. (2008). Diagnosis and classification of diabetes mellitus. *Diabetes Care*, 31(Supp 1), S45–S60.

American Dietetic Association. (2006). Nutrition intervention in the treatment of anorexia nervosa, bulimia nervosa, and eating disorders not otherwise specified (EDNOS). Retrieved August 3, 2006 from http://www.eatright.org/cps/rde/xchg/ada/hs.xls/advocacy_adapo701_ENU_HTML

American Heart Association. (2005). Pediatric advanced life support. *Circulation, 112* (Suppl IV), 167–187.

American Psychiatric Association. (2000). *Diagnostic* and *statistical manual of mental disorders* (4th ed., text revision). Washington, DC: American Psychiatric Association.

American Psychiatric Association, Working Group on Eating Disorders. (2006). Practice guideline for the treatment of patients with eating disorders (3rd ed.) Retrieved on May 20, 2007, from http://www.psych_pract/treatg/pg/Eating Disorder3ePG_04-28-06.pdf

The American Sickle Cell Anemia Association. (2005). How common is sickle cell anemia? Retrieved September 1, 2007, from http://www.ascaa.org/comm.htm.

American Speech-Language-Hearing Association. (2008). Type, degree, and configuration of hearing loss. Retrieved April 23, 2008, from http://www.asha.org/public/hearing/disorders/types.htm

Anderson, S. E., & Must, A. (2005). Interpreting the continued decline in the average age at menarche: Results from two nationally representative surveys of U.S. girls studied 10 years apart. *Journal of Pediatrics, 147,* 753–760.

Antoon, A. Y., & Donovan, M. K. (2007). Burn injuries. In R. M. Kliegman, R. E. Behrman, H. B. Jenson, & B. F. Stanton (Eds.), *Nelson textbook of pediatrics* (18th ed., pp. 450–458). Philadelphia, PA: Saunders Elsevier.

Arguin, A. L., & Swartz, M. K. (2004). Gastro-esophageal reflux in infants: A primary care perspective. *Pediatric Nursing, 30,* 45–52.

Arndt, C. A. S. (2007). Malignant tumors of bone. In R. M. Kliegman, R. E. Behrman, H. B. Jenson, & B. F. Stanton (Eds.), *Nelson textbook of pediatrics* (18th ed., pp. 2146–2149). Philadelphia: Saunders Elsevier.

Ater, J. A. (2007). Neuroblastoma. In R. M. Kliegman, R. E. Behrman, H. B. Jenson, & B. F. Stanton (Eds.), *Nelson textbook of pediatrics* (18th ed., pp. 2137–2139). Philadelphia: Saunders Elsevier.

Aungst, H. (2008, December 15). Asthma medications: What you need to know. Retrieved January 19, 2009 from http://contemporarypediatrics.modernmedicine.com/contpeds/article/articleDetail.jsp?id=572484

Backinger, C. L., Michaels, C. M., Jefferson, A. M., Fagan, P., Hurd, A. L., & Grana, R. (2008). Factors associated with recruitment and retention of youth into smoking cessation intervention studies: A review of the literature. *Health Education Research, 23,* 359–368.

Bagolan, P., Casaccia, G., Crescenzi, F., Nahom, A., Trucchi, A., & Giorlandino, C. (2004). Impact of a current treatment protocol on outcome of high-risk congenital diaphragmatic hernia. *Journal of Pediatric Surgery, 39,* 313–318.

Baker, C. J. (2007). *Red Book atlas of pediatric infectious diseases.* Elk Grove Village, IL: American Academy of Pediatrics.

Balaji, S. (2004). Medical therapy for sudden death. *Pediatric Clinics of North America, 51,* 1379–1387.

Banasiak, N. C. (2007). Childhood asthma: Part two: Management update. *Journal of Pediatric Health Care, 21,* 184–191.

Baron, M., & Blaber, M. E. (2005). Short-bowel syndrome in children. *American Journal of Nursing, 105*(9), 72C–72H.

Bauer, C. R., Langer, J. C., Shankaran, S., Bada, H. S., Lester, B., Wright, L. L., et al. (2005). Acute neonatal effects of cocaine exposure during pregnancy. *Archives of Pediatric and Adolescent Medicine, 159,* 824–834.

Belay, B., Belamarich, P., & Racine, A. D. (2004). Pediatric precursors of adult atherosclerosis. *Pediatrics in Review, 25*(1), 4–13.

Bell, E. (2006). Pulmonary pharmacotherapy options changing for cystic fibrosis patients. *Infectious Diseases in Children, 19*(10), 12–13.

Bell, E. A. (2007). New topical offers a choice in impetigo treatment. *Infectious Diseases in Children, 20*(10), 12.

Benfield, M. R. (2003). Current status of kidney transplant: Update 2003. *Pediatric Clinics of North America, 50,* 1301–1334.

Bernius, M., & Perlin, D. (2006). Pediatric ear, nose, and throat emergencies. *Pediatric Clinics of North America, 53,* 195–214.

Bernstein, D. (2007). Congenital heart disease. In R. M. Kleigman, R. E. Behrman, H. B. Jenson, & B. F. Stanton (Eds.), *Nelson textbook of pediatrics* (18th ed., pp. 1878–1942). Philadelphia: Saunders Elsevier.

Berry, D., Urban, A., & Grey, M. (2006). Management of type 2 diabetes in youth (Part 2). *Journal of Pediatric Health Care, 20*(2), 88–97.

Bezerra, J. A. (2005). Potential etiologies of biliary atresia. *Pediatric Transplantation, 9,* 646–651.

Biggs, W. S., & Dery W. H. (2006). Evaluation and treatment of constipation in infants and children. *American Family Physician, 73*(3), 469–477.

Bindler, R. C., & Ball, J. W. (2007). *Clinical skills manual for pediatric nursing: Caring for children* (4th ed.). Upper Saddle River, NJ: Pearson Prentice Hall.

Bindler, R. M., & Howry, L. B. (2005). *Pediatric drug guide.* Upper Saddle River, NJ: Prentice Hall Health.

Bismuth, E., & Laffel, L. (2007). Can we prevent diabetes ketoacidosis in children? *Pediatric Diabetes, 8*(6), 24–33.

Black, T. L. (2005). Congenital megacolon. In M. R. Dambro & J. A. Griffith (Eds.), *Griffith's 5-minute clinical consult* (13th ed., p. 260). Philadelphia: Lippincott, Williams, & Wilkins.

Blackwell, J. T. (2003). Management of hyperbilirubinemia in the healthy term newborn. *Journal of the American Academy of Nurse Practitioners, 15*(5), 194–198.

Block, R.W., Krebs, N. F., & Committee on Child Abuse and Neglect and Committee on Nutrition. (2005). Failure to thrive as a manifestation of child neglect. *Pediatrics, 116,* 1234–1237.

Boamah, L., & Balistreri, W. F. (2007). Manifestations of liver disease. In R. M. Kliegman, R. E. Behrman, H. B. Jenson, & B. F. Stanton (Eds.), *Nelson textbook of pediatrics,* (18th ed., pp. 1661–1668). Philadelphia: Saunders Elsevier.

Bodamer, O. A., & Lee, B. (2006). Maple syrup urine disease. *Emedicine.* Retrieved December 15, 2007, from http://www.emedicine.com/ped/topic1368.htm

Boe, K., & Tillotson, E. A. (2006). Encouraging sun safety for children and adolescents. *Journal of School Nursing, 22,* 136–141.

Boger, M. S., & Perrier, N. D. (2004). Advantages and disadvantages of surgical therapy and optimal extent of thyroidectomy for the treatment of hyperthyroidism. *Surgical Clinics of North America, 84,* 849–874.

Boland, E. A., & Grey, M. (2004). Diabetes mellitus (Types 1 and 2). In P. L. Jackson & J. A. Vessey (Eds.), *Primary care of the child with a chronic condition* (4th ed., pp. 426–444). St Louis: Mosby.

Bowman, B. A., & Russell, R. M. (Eds.). (2006). *Present knowledge of nutrition* (9th ed.). Washington, DC: International Life Sciences Institute.

Brand, D. A., Altman, R. L., Purtill, K., & Edwards, K. S. (2005). Yield of diagnostic testing in infants who have an apparent life-threatening event. *Pediatrics, 115*, 885–893.

Brandenberg, M. A. (2004). All-terrain vehicle injuries: A growing epidemic. *Annals of Emergency Medicine, 43*(4), 536–537.

Branson, B. M. (2006). Revised recommendations for HIV testing in health care settings in the United States. Available online at http://www.cdc.gov/hiv/topics/testing/resources/slidesets/pdf/testing_healthcare.pdf

Brashers, V. L. (2006). Alterations in pulmonary function. In K. L. McCance & S. E. Huether (Eds.), *Pathophysiology: The biologic basis for disease in adults and children* (5th ed., pp. 1205–1248). St. Louis: Elsevier Mosby.

Braverman, P. K. (2006). Body art: Piercing, tattooing, and scarification. *Adolescent Medicine, 17*, 505–519.

Brown, E. J. (2005). Clinical characteristics and efficacious treatment of post-traumatic stress disorder in children and adolescents. *Pediatric Annals, 34*, 139–146.

Brown, P. (2006). Answers to key questions about childhood leukemias. *Contemporary Pediatrics, 23*(3), 81–84, 87, 90.

Brown, R. T., Amler, R. W., Freeman, W. S., Perrin, J. M., Stein, M. T., Feldman, H. M., Pierce, L., Wolraich, M. L., & Committee an Quality Improvement Subcommittee on Attention–Deficit/Hyperactivity Disorder. (2005). Treatment of hyperactivity disorder: Overview of the evidence. *Pediatrics, 115*, e749–e757.

Buchanan, G. R. (2005). Thrombocytopenia during childhood: What the pediatrician needs to know. *Pediatrics in Review, 26*, 401–409.

Buka, R. L., & Cunningham, B. B. (2005). Connective tissue disease in children. *Pediatric Annals, 34*(3), 225–238.

Burger, C. M. (2004a). Hyperkalemia. *American Journal of Nursing, 104*(10), 66–70.

Burger, C. M. (2004b). Hypokalemia. *American Journal of Nursing, 104*(11), 61–65.

Burstein, G. R., & Murray, P. J. (2003). Diagnosis and management of sexually transmitted disease pathogens among adolescents. *Pediatrics in Review, 24*(3), 75–81.

Butowski, N. A., Sneed, P. K., & Chang, S. M. (2006). Diagnosis and treatment of recurrent high-grade astrocytoma. *Journal of Clinical Oncology, 10*, 1273–1280.

Caley, L. M., Shipkey, N., Winkelman, T., Dunlap, C., & Rivera, S. (2006). Evidence-based review of nursing interventions to prevent secondary disabilities in fetal alcohol spectrum disorder. *Pediatric Nursing, 32*, 155–162.

Capper-Michel, B. (2004). Bronchopulmonary dysplasia. In P. J. Allen & J. A. Vessey (Eds.), *Primary care of the child with a chronic condition* (4th ed., pp. 282–298). St. Louis: Mosby.

Carinci, F., Scapoli, L., Palmieri, A., Zollino, I., & Pezzetti, F. (2007). Human genetic factors in nonsyndromic cleft lip and palate: An update. *International Journal of Pediatric Otorhinolaryngology, 71,* 1509–1519.

Carley, A. (2003). Anemia: When is it iron deficiency? *Pediatric Nursing, 29*(2), 128–133.

Carson, S., Woolridge, D. P., Colletti, J., & Kilgore, D. (2006). Pediatric upper extremity injuries. *Pediatric Clinics of North America, 53,* 41–67.

Cassidy, J. T., & Petty, R. E. (2005). Chronic arthritis in childhood. In J. T. Cassidy, R. E. Petty, R. M. Laxer, & C. B. Lindsley (Eds.), *Textbook of pediatric rheumatology* (5th ed., pp. 206–260). Philadelphia: Elsevier Saunders.

Centers for Disease Control and Prevention. (2004a). *Guide to contraindictions and vaccinations guide.* Retrieved July 3, 2008, from http://www.cdc.gov/vaccines/recs/vac-admin/contraindications.htm

Centers for Disease Control and Prevention. (2004b). Vision impairment. Retrieved August 30, 2006, from http://www.cdc.gov/ncbddd/dd/vision3.htm

Centers for Disease Control and Prevention. (2005a). Hepatitis E fact sheet. Retrieved October 21, 2007, from http://www.cdc.gov/hepatitis

Centers for Disease Control and Prevention. (2005b). Hepatitis C fact sheet. Retrieved October 21, 2007, from http://www.cdc.gov/hepatitis.

Centers for Disease Control and Prevention. (2005c). SEARCH for Diabetes in youth. Retrieved June 8, 2008, from http://www.cdc.gov/diabetes/pubs/factsheets/search.htm

Centers for Disease Control and Prevention. (2006a) Hepatitis D fact sheet. Retrieved October 21, 2007, from http://www.cdc.gov/hepatitis

Centers for Disease, Control and Prevention. (2006b). HPV and HPV vaccine information for health care providers. Retrieved May 2007 from http://www.cdc.gov/std/HPV/hpv-vacc-hcp-3-pages.pdf

Centers for Disease Control and Prevention. (2006c). Improved national prevalence estimates for 18 selected major birth defects—United States, 1999–2001. *Morbidity and Mortality Weekly Report, 54,* 1301–1305.

Centers for Disease Control and Prevention. (2006d). Outbreaks of *Escherichia coli* 0157:H7 Associated with petting zoos—North Carolina, Florida, and Arizona, 2004 and 2005. *Journal of American Medical Association, 295*(4), 378–380.

Centers for Disease Control and Prevention. (2006e). Revised recommendations for HIV testing of adults, adolescents, and pregnant women in health-care settings. *Morbidity and Mortality Weekly Report, 55*(No. RR-14), 1–24.

Centers for Disease Control and Prevention. (2006f). Sexually transmitted diseases treatment guidelines, 2006. *Morbidity and Mortality Weekly Report,* 55(RR-11), 1–94.

Centers for Disease Control and Prevention. (2007a). Hepatitis A fact sheet. Retrieved October 21, 2007, from http://www.cdc.gov/hepatitis

Centers for Disease Control and Prevention. (2007b). Hepatitis B fact sheet. Retrieved October 21, 2007, from http://www.cdc.gov/hepatitis

Centers for Disease Control and Prevention. (2007c). Suicide trends among youths and young adults aged 10–24 years—United States, 1990–2004. *Morbidity and Mortality Weekly Report, 56*, 905–908.

Centers for Disease Control and Prevention. (2007d). Update to CDC's *Sexually Transmitted Diseases Treatment Guidelines, 2006*: Fluoroquinolones no longer recommended for treatment of gonococcal infections. *Morbidity and Mortality Weekly Report, 56*, 332–336.

Centers for Disease Control and Prevention. (2007e). Updated recommended treatment regimens for gonococcal infections and associated conditions— United States, April 2007. Retrieved June 3, 2008, from http://www.cdc .gov/std/treatment/2006/updated-regimens.htm

Centers for Disease Control and Prevention. (2009). Immunization schedules. Retrieved January 15, 2009, from http://www.cdc.gov/vaccines/recs/schedules/default.htm

Chávez-Bueno, S., & McCracken, G. H. (2005). Bacterial meningitis in children. *Pediatric Clinics of North America, 52*, 795–810.

Chehade, M. (2007). IgE and Non-IgE-mediated food allergy: Treatment in 2007. *Current Opinion in Allergy and Clinical Immunology, 7*(3), 264–268.

Chen, M-J., Change, W-H., Chu, C-H., Wang, T-E., Lin, S-C., & Shih, S-C. (2007). Rapid response of Henoch-Schönlein purpura to corticosteroids: Correlation between skin and gastric mucosal lesions. *Digestive Diseases and Sciences, 52*, 1706–1708.

Chiafery, M. (2006). Care and management of the child with shunted hydrocephalus. *Pediatric Nursing, 32*(3), 222–225.

Child restraints for newborn infants: A health care provider's guide. (2006). Edmonds, WA: Safe Ride News Publications.

Christinson-Lagay, E. R., & Fishman, S. J. (2006). Vascular anomalies. *Surgical Clinics of North America, 86*, 393–425.

Cibulka, N. J. (2006). Mother-to-child transmission of HIV in the United States. *American Journal of Nursing, 10*(7), 56–63.

Cleary, A. M., Insel, R. A., & Lewis, D. B. (2005). Disorders of lymphocyte function. In R. Hoffman, E. J. Benz, S. J. Shattil, B. Furie, H. J. Cohen, L. E. Silberstein, & P. McGlave (Eds.), *Hematology: Basic principles and practice* (4th ed., pp. 831–855). St. Louis: Elsevier.

Clement, A., Tamalet, A., Leroux, E., Ravilly, S., Fauroux, B., & Jais, J. P. (2006). Long term effects of azithromycin in patients with cystic fibrosis: A double blind, placebo controlled trial. *Thorax, 61*(10), 895–902.

Cohen, B. A. (2004). Another baby and another cutaneous lesion—and more on efficient recognition and management. *Contemporary Pediatrics, 21*(10), 39–57.

Cohen, S. M. (2006). Jaundice in the full-term newborn. *Pediatric Nursing, 32*(3), 202–208.

Colletti, J. E. (2004). Pyloric stenosis. *Canadian Journal of Emergency Medicine, 6*, 444–445.

Collins, B. N., Wileyto, E. P., Murphy, J. F., & Munafo, M. R. (2007). Adolescent environmental tobacco smoke exposure predicts academic achievement test failure. *Journal of Adolescent Health, 41*, 363–370.

Committee on Drugs and Committee on Hospital Care. (2003, 2007, Policy Reaffirmed May 1, 2007). Prevention of medication errors in the pediatric inpatient setting. *Pediatrics, 112*, 431–436.

Cook, E. H., & Higgins, S. S. (2004). Congenital heart disease. In P. Jackson Allen & J. A. Vessey (Eds.), *Primary care of the child with a chronic condition* (4th ed., 382–403). St. Louis: Mosby.

Corbeel, L. (2005). Immune-mediated aplastic anemia. *European Journal of Pediatrics, 164*, 698–699.

Corneli, H. M., Zorc, J. J., Mahajan, P., Shaw, K., Holubkov, R., et al. (2007). A multicenter, randomized controlled trial of dexamethasone for bronchiolitis. *New England Journal of Medicine, 357*(4), 331–339.

Coyer, S. M. (2005). Anemia: Diagnosis and management. *Journal of Pediatric Health Care, 19*(6), 380–385.

Cromwell, P. F., Munn, N., & Zolkowski-Wynne, J. (2005). Evaluation and management of hypertension in children and adolescents (Part Two): Evaluation and management. *Journal of Pediatric Health Care, 19*(5), 309–313.

Curry, H. (2004). Bleeding disorder basics. *Pediatric Nursing, 30*, 402–429.

Cystic Fibrosis Foundation. (2007). *About cystic fibrosis: What you need to know*. Retrieved September 4, 2007, from http://www.cff.org/AboutCF/

Davies, S. M. (2005). Hematopoietic stem cell transplantation for immunodeficiencies and genetic diseases. In R. Hoffman, E. J. Benz, S. J. Shattil, B. Furie, H. J. Cohen, L. E. Silberstein, & P. McGlave (Eds.), *Hematology: Basic principles and practice* (4th ed., pp. 1703–1712). St. Louis: Elsevier.

Davis, I. D., & Avner, E. D. (2007). Conditions particularly associated with hematuria. In R. M. Kliegman, R. E. Behrman, H. B. Jenson, & B. F. Stanton (Eds.), *Nelson textbook of pediatrics* (18th ed. pp. 2168–2188). Philadelphia: Saunders Elsevier.

Davis, K. F., Parker, K. P., & Montgomery, G. L. (2004). Sleep in infants and young children: Part one: Normal sleep. *Journal of Pediatric Health Care, 18*, 65–71.

De Andrade, A. F., da Hora Barbosa, R., Vargas, F. R., Ferman, S., Eisenberg, A. L., Fernandes, L., & Bonvicino, C. R. (2006). A molecular study of first and second RB1 mutational hits in retinoblastoma patients. *Cancer Genetics and Cytogenetics, 167*, 43–46.

DeBaun, M. R., & Vichinsky, E. (2007). Hemoglobinopathies. In R. M. Kliegman, R. E. Behrman, H. B. Jenson, & B. F. Stanton (Eds.), *Nelson textbook of pediatrics* (18th ed., pp. 2025–2038). Philadelphia: Saunders Elsevier.

Delaney, C. (2005). Antenatal hydronephrosis: Trends and management. *Urologic Nursing, 25*(3), 173–183.

Devogelaer, J. B., & Coppin, C. (2006). Osteogenesis imperfecta: Current treatment options and future prospects. *Treatments in Endocrinology, 5*, 229–242.

Diana-Zerpa, J. A., & Shapiro-Stolar, T. J. (2007). Malrotation and volvulus. In N. T. Browne, L. M. Flanigan, C. A. McComiskey, & P. Pieper (Eds.),

Nursing care of the pediatric surgical patient (2nd ed., pp. 333–342). Boston: Jones & Bartlett Publishers.

DiCicco-Bloom, E., Lord, C., Zwaigenbaum, L., Courchesne, E., Dager, S. R., Schmitz, C., Scholtz, R. T., Crawley, J., & Young, L. J. (2006). The developmental neurobiology of autism spectrum disorder. *Journal of Neuroscience, 26,* 6897–6906.

Ditmyer, S. (2004). Hydrocephalus. In P. J. Allen & J. A. Vessey (Eds.), *Primary care of the child with a chronic condition* (4th ed., pp. 543–560). St. Louis: Mosby.

Dome, J. S., Perlman, E. J., Ritchey, M. L., Coppes, M. J., Kalapurakal, J., & Grundy, P. E. (2006). Renal tumors. In P. A. Pizzo & D. G. Poplack (Eds.), *Principles and practice of pediatric oncology* (5th ed., pp. 905–932). Philadelphia: Lippincott Williams & Wilkins.

Donahue, S. P. (2007). Pediatric strabismus. *New England Journal of Medicine, 356,* 1040–1047.

Doniger, S. J., & Shariefff, G. Q. (2006). Pediatric dysrhythmias. *Pediatric Clinics of North America, 53,* 85–105.

Dopheide, J. A. (2006). Recognizing and treating depression in children and adolescents. *American Journal of Health-Systems Pharmacy, 63,* 233–243.

Doshi, N. R., & Rodriguez, L. F. (2007). Amblyopia. *American Family Physician, 75,* 361–368.

Doughty, D. (2004). Structure and function of the gastrointestinal tract in infants and children. *Journal of Wound, Ostomy and Continence Nursing, 31,* 207–212.

Doyle, D. A., & DiGeorge, A. M. (2007). Disorders of the parathyroid. In R. M. Kliegman, R. E. Behrman, H. B. Jenson, & B. F. Stanton (Eds.), *Nelson textbook of pediatrics* (18th ed., pp. 2340–2348). Philadelphia: Saunders Elsevier.

Duffy, B. J., McLaughlin, P. M., & Eichelberger, M. R. (2006). Assessment, triage, and early management of burns in children. *Clinical Pediatric Emergency Medicine, 7,* 82–93.

Dulczak, S., & Kirk, J. (2005). Overview of the evaluation, diagnosis, and management of urinary tract infections in infants and children. *Urologic Nursing, 25*(3), 185–191.

Dykes, J. (2005). Managing children with croup in emergency departments. *Emergency Nurse, 13*(6), 14–19.

Eaton, S. H., Cendron, M. A., Estrada, C. R., Bauer, S. B., Borer, J. G., Cilento, B. G., Diamond, D. A., Retik, A. B., Peters, C. A. (2005). Intermittent testicular torsion: Diagnostic features and management outcomes. *The Journal of Urology, 174*(4, Part 2), 1532–1535.

Eckert, K. (2005). Penetrating and blunt abdominal trauma. *Critical Care Nursing Quarterly, 28,* 41–59.

Ecklund, M. M., & Ecklund, C. R. (2007). How to recognize and respond to hypovolemic shock. *American Nurse Today, 2*(4), 28–31.

Edelman, C. L., & Mandle, C. L. (2006). *Health promotion throughout the life span* (6th ed.). St. Louis: Mosby, Inc.

Ehrenkranz, R. A., Walsh, M. C., Vohr, B. R., Jobe, A. H., Wright, L. L., et al., (2005). Validation of the National Institutes of Health consensus definition of bronchopulmonary dysplasia. *Pediatrics, 116*(6), 1353–1360.

Elder, J. S. (2007). Urologic disorders in infants and children. In R. M. Kliegman, R. E. Behrman, H. B. Jenson, & B. F. Stanton (Eds.), *Nelson textbook of pediatrics* (18th ed., pp. 2221–2271). Philadelphia: Saunders Elsevier.

Elkins, M. R., Robinson, M., Rose, B. R., Harbour, C., Moriarty, C. P., et al. (2006). A controlled trial of long-term inhaled hypertonic saline in patients with cystic fibrosis. *New England Journal of Medicine, 354*(3), 229–240.

Emery, H. (2004). Pediatric rheumatology: What does the future hold? *Archives of Physical Medicine and Rehabilitation, 85*, 1382–1384.

Erickson, C. C., & Jones, C. S. (2000). Pediatric sudden cardiac death: What the pediatrician needs to know. *Pediatric Annals, 29*(8), 509–518.

Eugster, E. A., LeMay, D., Zerin, J. M., & Pescovitz, O. H. (2004). Definitive diagnosis in children with congenital hypothyroidism. *Journal of Pediatrics, 144*, 643–647.

Fagerman, L. E., & Farber, L. D. (2007). Intussusception. In N. T. Browne, L. M. Flanigan, C. A. McComiskey, & P. Pieper (Eds.), *Nursing care of the pediatric surgical patient* (2nd ed., pp. 343–348). Boston: Jones & Bartlett Publishers.

Feinstein, S., Keich, R., Becker-Cohen, R., Rinat, C., Schwartz, S. B., & Frishberg, Y. (2005). Is noncompliance among adolescent renal transplant recipients inevitable? *Pediatrics, 115*(4), 969–973.

Feja, K., & Saiman, L. (2005). Tuberculosis in children. *Clinics of Chest Medicine, 26*, 295–312.

Ferguson-Noyes, N. (2005). Bipolar disorder in children. *Advance for Nurse Practitioners, 13*(3), 35–42.

Ferrari, A., Bono, A., Collini, P., Rodolfo, M., & Santinami, M. (2006). What do we know about cutaneous melanoma of childhood? *Contemporary Pediatrics, 23*(9), 42–48.

Fiore, A. E., Wasley, A., & Bell, B. P. (2006). Prevention of hepatitis A through active or passive immunization. *Morbidity and Mortality Weekly Report, 55*(RR07), 1–23.

Fiorino, E. K., & Raffaelli, R. M. (2006). Hemolytic-uremic syndrome. *Pediatrics in Review, 27*(10), 398–399.

Flanigan, L. M. (2007). Biliary atresia and choledochal cyst. In N. T. Browne, L. M. Flanigan, C. A. McComiskey, & P. Pieper (Eds.), *Nursing care of the pediatric surgical patient* (2nd ed., pp. 379–387). Boston: Jones & Bartlett Publishers.

Flume, P. A., O'Sullivan, B. P., Robinson, K. A., Goss, C. H., Mogayzel, P. J., et al. (2007). Cystic fibrosis pulmonary guidelines: Chronic medications for maintenance of lung health. *American Journal of Respiratory and Critical Care Medicine, 176*, 957–969.

Fon, E. W., & Lewin, R. H. (2007). Inhaled corticosteroids for asthma. *Pediatrics in Review, 28*(6), e30–e35.

Fowlkes, A. L., & Fry, A. M. (2006). Respiratory syncytial virus activity—United States, 2005–2006. *Morbidity and Mortality Weekly Report, 55*(47), 1277–1279.

Freeman, J. M., Kossoff, E. H., & Hartman, A. L. (2007). The ketogenic diet: One decade later. *Pediatrics, 119*(3), 535–543.

Froehlich, T. E., Lanphear, B. P., Epstein, J. N., Barbaresi, W. J., Katusic, S. K., & Kahn, R. S. (2007). Prevalence, recognition, and treatment of attention-deficit/hyperactivity disorder in a national sample of US children. *Archives of Pediatric and Adolescent Medicine, 161*, 857–864.

Fu, L. Y., & Moon, R. Y. (2007). Apparent life-threatening events (ALTEs) and the role of home monitors. *Pediatrics in Review, 28*(6), 203–207.

Gabrys, C. A. (2005). Pediatric cardiac transplants: A clinical update. *Journal of Pediatric Nursing, 20*(2), 139–143.

Gallagher, P. G. (2007). Disorders of the red blood cell membrane: Hereditary spherocytosis, elliptocytosis, and related disorders. In M. A. Lichtman, E. Beutler, T. J. Kipps, U. Seligsohn, K. Kaushansky, & J. T. Prchal (Eds.), *Williams hematology* (7th ed.). McGraw Hill's Access Medicine.

Gance-Cleveland, B. (2003). Adaptation to Addison's disease in a child: A case study. *Journal of Pediatric Health Care, 17*(6), 301–310.

Gelfond, D., & Fasano, A. (2006). Celiac disease in the pediatric population. *Pediatric Annals, 35*(4), 275–279.

Ghatan, S. (2006). Surgery for epilepsy. *Pediatric Annals, 35*(5), 386–393.

Giarelli, E., Souders, M., Pinto-Martin, J., Bloch, J., & Levy, S. E. (2005). Intervention pilot for parents of children with autistic spectrum disorder. *Pediatric Nursing, 31,* 389–399.

Gidding, S. S., Dennison, B. A., Birch, L. L., Daniels, S. R., Gilman, M. W., et al. (2005). Dietary recommendations for children and adolescents: A guide for practitioners. Consensus statement from the American Heart Association. *Circulation, 112,* 2061–2075.

Gluck, M. E. (2006). Stress response and binge eating disorder. *Appetite, 46,* 26–30.

Gold, B. D., & Gremse, D. A. (2006). Extinguishing the burn: Case studies in pediatric reflux disease. *Self Study Supplement to Clinician Reviews.*

Goldenring, J. M., & Rosen, D. S. (2004). Getting into adolescent heads: An essential update. *Contemporary Pediatrics, 21*(1), 64–90.

Gottlieb, B. S., & Ilowite, N. T. (2006). Systemic lupus erythematosus in children and adolescents. *Pediatrics in Review, 27*(9), 323–328.

Graham, J. M., Kreutzman, J., Earl, D., Halberg, A., Samayoa, C., & Guo, X. (2005). Deformational brachycephaly in supine-sleeping infants. *Journal of Pediatrics, 146*(2), 253–257.

Grant, E. J. (2004). Burn prevention. *Critical Care Nursing Clinics of North America, 16*, 127–138.

Gray, M., Huether, S. E., & Forshee, B. A. (2006). Structure and function of the renal and urologic systems. In K. L. McCance & S. E. Huether (Eds.), *Pathophysiology: The biologic basis for disease in adults and children* (5th ed., pp. 1301–1335). St. Louis: Elsevier Mosby.

Greydanus, D. E., Matytsina, L., & Gains, M. (2006). Breast disorders in children and adolescents. *Primary Care Clinics of North America, 33*, 455–502.

Grimberg, A., & DeLéon, D. D. (2005). Disorders in growth. In T. M. Moshang (Ed.), *Pediatric endocrinology: The requisites in pediatrics* (pp. 127–167). St. Louis: Elsevier Mosby.

Grimshaw-Mulcahy, L. J. (2006, March). Chlamydia: Diagnosing the hidden STD. *The Clinical Advisor,* 32–41.

Grottkau, B. E., Epps, H. R., & Di Scala, C. (2005). Compartment syndrome in children and adolescents. *Journal of Pediatric Surgery, 40*, 678–682.

Gungor, N., & Arslanian, S. (2004). Progressive beta cell failure in type 2 diabetes mellitus of youth. *Journal of Pediatrics, 144*(5), 656–659.

Gunner, K. B., & Smith, H. D. (2007). Practice guideline for diagnosis and management of migraine headaches in children and adolescents: Part one. *Journal of Pediatric Health Care, 21*(5), 327–332.

Gutierrez, K. (2005). Bone and joint infections in children. *Pediatric Clinics of North America, 52*, 779–794.

Hackman, D. J., Newman, K., & Ford, H. R. (2005). Pediatric surgery. In F. Brunicardi, D. K. Andersen, T. R. Billiar, D. L. Dunn, J. G. Hunter, J. B. Matthews, R. E. Pollock, & S. I. Schwartz (Eds.), *Schwartz's principles of surgery* (8th ed., pp. 1471–1517). New York: The McGraw Hill Companies, Inc.

Hagan, J. G., Shaw, J. S., & Duncan, P. M. (2008). *Bright futures: Guidelines for health supervision of infants, children and adolescents* (3rd ed.). Elk Grove Village, IL: American Academy of Pediatrics.

Halac, I., & Zimmerman, D. (2004). Coordinating care for children with Turner syndrome. *Pediatric Annals, 33*(3), 189–196.

Hansen, R. C. (2003). Atopic dermatitis: Taming the "itch that rashes." *Contemporary Pediatrics, 20*(7), 79–97.

Hardin, D. S., Adams-Huet, B., Brown, D., Chatfield, B., Dyson, M., et al. (2006). Growth hormone treatment improves growth and clinical status in prepubertal children with cystic fibrosis: Results of a multicenter randomized controlled trial. *Journal of Clinical Endocrinology & Metabolism, 91*(12), 4925–4929.

Hart, E. S., Grottkau, B. E., Rebello, G. N., & Albright, M. B. (2005). The newborn foot: Diagnosis and management of common conditions. *Orthopedic Nursing, 24*, 313–321.

Hartford, C. M., Wodowski, K. S., Rao, B. N., Khoury, J. D., Neel, M. D., & Daw, N. C. (2006). Osteosarcoma among children age 5 years or younger. *Journal of Pediatric Hematology and Oncology, 28*, 43–47.

Hay, W. W., Levin, M. J., Sondheimer, J. M., Sondheimer, J. M., Deterding, R. R., & Associate Authors. (2005). *Current pediatric diagnosis and treatment* (17th ed.). New York: Lange Medical Books/McGraw Hill.

Health Resources and Services Administration Office of Special Programs. (2007). National Childhood Vaccine Injury Act vaccine injury table. Retrieved July 3, 2008, from http://www.hrsa.gov/vaccinecompensation/table.htm

Hedrick, H. L., Crombleholme, T. M., Flake, A. W., Nance, M. L., von Allmen, D., Howell, L. J., Johnson, M. P., Wilson, R. D., & Adzick, N. S. (2004). Right congenital diaphragmatic hernia: Prenatal assessment and outcome. *Journal of Pediatric Surgery, 39,* 319–323.

Heeney, M. M., & Ware, R. E. (2008). Hydroxyurea for children with sickle cell disease. *Pediatric Clinics of North America, 55*(2), 483–501.

Henderson, R. A., Mossman, S., Nairn, N., & Cheever, M. A. (2005). Cancer vaccines and immunotherapies: Emerging perspectives. *Vaccine, 23,* 2359–2362.

Henry, S. M. (2004). Discerning differences: Gastroesophageal reflux and gastroesophageal reflux disease infants. *Advances in Neonatal Care, 4,* 235–247.

Hoban, T. F. (2004). Sleep and its disorders in children. *Seminars in Neurology, 24,* 327–340.

Holcomb, S. S. (2005). Managing jaundice in full-term infants. *The Nurse Practitioner, 30*(1), 6–7, 11–12.

Holloway, M., & D'Acunto, K. (2006, June). An update on the ABC's of viral hepatitis. *The Clinical Advisor, 26,* 29–40.

Hon, K. L., Leung, A., Chik, K. W., Chu, C. W., Cheung, K. L., & Fok, T. F. (2005). Critical airway obstruction, superior vena cava syndrome, and spontaneous cardiac arrest in a child with acute leukemia. *Pediatric Emergency Care, 21,* 844–846.

Hornor, G. (2004). Ano-genital warts in children: Sexual abuse or not? *Journal of Pediatric Health Care, 18*(4), 165–170.

Hosalkar, H. S., Horn, B. D., Friedman, J. E., & Dormans, J. P. (2007). The hip. In R. M. Kliegman, R. E. Behrman, H. B. Jenson, & B. F. Stanton (Eds.), *Nelson textbook of pediatrics* (18th ed., pp. 2800–2811). Philadelphia: Saunders Elsevier.

Hoyer, A., & Silberbach, M. (2005). Infective endocarditis. *Pediatrics in Review, 26*(11), 394–399.

Huether, S. E. (2006). Alterations of renal and urinary tract function in children. In K. L. McCance & S. E. Huether (Eds.), *Pathophysiology: The biologic basis for disease in adults and children* (5th ed., pp. 1337–1352). St. Louis: Elsevier Mosby.

Hyams, J. (2005). Inflammatory bowel disease. *Pediatrics in Review, 26*(9), 314–320.

Hyams, J. (2007). Inflammatory bowel disease. In R. M. Kliegman, R. E. Behrman, H. B. Jenson, & B. F. Stanton (Eds.), *Nelson textbook of pediatrics* (18th ed., pp. 1575–1585). Philadelphia: Saunders.

Hyman, P. E., & Danda, C. E. (2004). Understanding and treating childhood bellyaches. *Pediatric Annals, 33,* 97–104.

Jackson, C. S., & Buchman, A. L. (2004). The nutritional management of short bowel syndrome. *Nutritional Clinical Care, 7,* 114–121.

Jaffe, B. M., & Berger, D. H. (2005). The appendix. In F. Brunicardi, D. K. Andersen, T. R. Billiar, D. L. Dunn, J. G. Hunter, J. B. Matthews, R. E. Pollock, & S. I. Schwartz (Eds.), *Schwartz's principles of surgery* (8th ed., pp. 1119–1137). New York: The McGraw Hill Companies, Inc.

James, H. E. (1986). Neurologic evaluation and support in the child with acute brain insult. *Pediatric Annals, 15*(1), 17.

Jankowitz, B. T., & Adelson, P. D. (2006). Pediatric traumatic brain injury: Past, present, and future. *Developmental Neuroscience, 28*, 263–275.

Jellinek, M., Patel, B. P., & Froehle, M. C. (Eds). (2002). *Bright futures in practice: Mental health* (Vol. I). Arlington, VA: National Center for Education in Maternal and Child Health.

Johnson, C. P., Myers, S. M., & the Council on Children with Disabilities. (2007). Identification and evaluation of children with autism spectrum disorders. *Pediatrics 120*, 1183–1215.

Jolliffe, C. J., & Janssen, I. (2006). Distribution of lipoproteins by age and gender in adolescents. *Circulation, 114*, 1056–1062.

Jones, H. (2007). Nurse-administered laser in dermatology. *Nursing Clinics of North America, 42*, 393–406.

Kache, S., & Ferry, R. J. (2005). Diabetes insipidus. In T. M. Moshange (Ed.), *Pediatric endocrinology: The requisites for pediatrics* (pp. 257–267). St. Louis, Elsevier Mosby.

Kaltman, J. R., Madan, N., Vetter, V. L., & Rhodes, L. A. (2006). Arrhythmias and sudden cardiac death. In V. L. Vetter (Ed.), *Pediatric cardiology: The requisites in pediatrics* (pp. 79–96). St. Louis: Elsevier Mosby.

Kaplan, S. L. (2005). Osteomyelitis in children. *Infectious Disease Clinics of North America, 19*, 787–797.

Kasson, B. R. (2007). Necrotizing enterocolitis. In N. T. Browne, L. M. Flanigan, C. A. McComiskey, & P. Pieper (Eds.), *Nursing care of the pediatric surgical patient* (2nd ed., pp. 181–193). Boston: Jones & Bartlett Publishers.

Kavey, R. W., Daniels, S. R., Lauer, R. M., Atkins, D. L., Hayman, L. L., & Taubert, K. (2003). American Heart Association guidelines for primary prevention of atherosclerotic cardiovascular disease beginning in childhood. *Journal of Pediatrics, 142*(4), 368–372.

Kaye. (2006). Newborn screening fact sheets. AAP technical report. *Pediatrics, 118*(3), e934–e963.

Kazak, A. E., Rourke, M. T., Alderfer, M. A., Pai, A., Reilly, A. F., & Meadows, A. T. (2007). Evidence-based assessment, intervention and psychosocial care in pediatric oncology: A blueprint for comprehensive services across treatment. *Journal of Pediatric Psychology, 32*, 1099–1110.

Kelly, D. P., & Aylward, G. P. (2005). Identifying school performance problems in the pediatric office. *Pediatric Annals, 34*, 288–298.

Keri, J. E. (2006). Acne: Improving skin and self-esteem. *Pediatric Annals, 35*(3), 174–179.

Kessman, J. (2006). Hirschsprung disease: Diagnosis and management. *American Family Physician, 74*(8), 1319–1322.

Kirkwood, M. W., Yeates, K. O., & Wilson, P. E. (2006). Pediatric sports-related concussion: A review of the clinical management of an oft-neglected population. *Pediatrics, 117*(4), 1359–1371.

Klar, M. (2007). Hirschsprung disease. In N. T. Browne, L. M. Flanigan, C. A. McComiskey, & P. Pieper (Eds.), *Nursing care of the pediatric surgical patient* (2nd ed., pp. 289–300). Boston: Jones & Bartlett Publishers.

Klein, E. J., Kapoor, D., & Shugerman, R. P. (2004). The diagnosis of intussusception. *Clinical Pediatrics, 43*(4), 343–347.

Klein, G. L., & Herndon, D. N. (2004). Burns. *Pediatrics in Review, 25*(12), 411–416.

Kliegman, R. M., Behrman, R. E., Jenson, H. B., & Stanton, B. F. (2007). *Nelson textbook of pediatrics* (18th ed.). Philadelphia: Saunders Elsevier.

Kliegman, R. M., & Willoughby, R. E. (2005). Prevention of necrotizing enterocolitis with probiotics. *Pediatrics, 115*, 171–172.

Kline, M. W. (2006). Perspectives on the pediatric HIV/AIDS pandemic: Catalyzing access of children to care and treatment. *Pediatrics, 117*, 138–1393.

Knapp, J. M. (2005). Hyperosmolar therapy in the treatment of severe head injury in children: Mannitol and hypertonic saline. *AACN Clinical Issues, 16*(2), 199–211.

Knight, J. R. (1997). Adolescent substance use: Screening, assessment, and intervention. *Contemporary Pediatrics, 14*, 45, 51–56, 61–72.

Kobrynski, L. J. (2006). Combined immune deficiencies in children. *Journal of Infusion Nursing, 29*(4), 213.

Kocher, M. S., Lee, B., Dolan, M., Weinberg, J., & Shulman, S. T. (2006). Pediatric orthopedic infections: Early detection and treatment. *Pediatric Annals, 35*, 112–122.

Kossoff, E. H., & Mankad, D. N. (2006). Medication-overuse headache in children: Is initial preventive therapy necessary? *Journal of Child Neurology, 21*(1), 45–48.

Kowatch, R., Fristad, M., Birmaher, B., Wagner, K. D., Findling, R. L., Hellander, M., & the Child Psychiatric Workgroup on Bipolar Disorder. (2005). Treatment guidelines for children and adolescents with bipolar disorder. *Journal of American Academy of Child and Adolescent Psychiatry, 44*, 236–239.

Krause-Parello, C. A. (2005). Tooth avulsion in the school setting. *Journal of School Nursing, 21*, 279–282.

Kuehn, B. M. (2007). Studies point way to new therapeutic prospects for muscular dystrophy. *JAMA, 298*, 1385–1386.

Kwok, M. Y., Kim, M. K., & Gorelick, M. H. (2004). Evidence-based approach to the diagnosis of appendicitis in children. *Pediatric Emergency Care, 20*, 690–698.

LaFranchi, S. (2007). Disorders of the thyroid gland. In R. M. Kliegman, R. E. Behrman, H. B. Jenson, & B. F. Stanton (Eds.), *Nelson textbook of pediatrics* (18th ed., pp. 2316–2340). Philadelphia: Saunders Elsevier.

Lansford, A. H. (2005). The importance of recognizing a child with bipolar disorder. *Contemporary Pediatrics, 22*(2), 69–78.

Lau, K. K., & Wyatt, R. J. (2005). Glomerulonephritis. *Adolescent Medicine Clinics, 16*(1), 67–85.

Le, P. N., & Chrisant, M. R. K. (2006). Cardiomyopathy. In V. L. Vetter (Ed.), *Pediatric cardiology: The requisites in pediatrics* (pp. 97–109). St. Louis: Elsevier Mosby.

Lee, E. H., & Hui, J. H. (2006). The potential of stem cells in orthopaedic surgery. *Journal of Bone and Joint Surgery, 88*, 841–851.

Legg, V. (2005). Complications of chronic kidney disease. *American Journal of Nursing, 105*(6), 40–49.

Leung, A. K. C., Robson, W. L. M., & Wong, A. L. (2005, February). What's your diagnosis? Bladder exstrophy. *Consultant for Pediatricians*, 77–80.

Levitt, M. A., & Peña, A. (2005). Outcomes from the correction of anorectal malformations. *Current opinion in pediatrics,* 17, 394–401.

Lewis, P., & Glaser, C. A. (2005). Encephalitis. *Pediatrics in Review, 26*(10), 353–362.

Lindsey, T., Watts-Tate, N., Southwood, E., Routhieaux, J., Beatty, J., Calamaras, D., Phillips, M., Lea, G., Brown, E., & DeBaun, M. R. (2005). Chronic blood transfusion therapy practices to treat strokes in children with sickle cell disease. *Journal of the American Academy of Nurse Practitioners, 17*, 277–282.

Linker, C. A. (2008). Hematology. In S. J. McPhee, M. A. Papadakis, & L. M. Tierney, Jr. (Eds.), *Current medical diagnosis and treatment 2008.* McGraw Hill's Access Medicine.

Lipper, G. M. (2007). Isotretinoin and iPLEDGE: Too much regulation or not enough? *Medscape Dermatology.* Retrieved January 31, 2007, from http://www.medscape.com/viewarticle/550255_print

Litmanovitz, I., Dolfin, T., Arnon, S., Regev, R. H., Nemet, D. & Eliakim, A. (2007). Assisted exercise and bone strength in preterm infants. *Calcified Tissue International, 80*, 39–43.

Liu, J., Peterson, A. V., Kealey, K. A., Mann, S. L., Bricker, J. B., & Marek, P. M. (2007). Addressing challenges in adolescent smoking cessation: Design and baseline characteristics of the HS group-randomized trial. *Preventive Medicine, 45*, 215–225.

Loscalzo, M. L., Bondy, C. A., & Biesecker, B. (2006). Issues in prenatal counseling and diagnosis in Turner Syndrome. *International Congress Series, 1298*, 26–29.

Loveland-Cherry, C. J. (2006). Alcohol, children and adolescents. In J. J. Fitzpatrick (Ed.), *Alcohol use, misuse, abuse, and dependence* (pp. 135–177). New York: Springer Publishing.

Luby, J. L., Heffelfinger, A., Koenig-McNaught, A. L., et al. (2004). The Preschool Feelings Checklist: A brief and sensitive screening measure for depression in young children. *Journal of the American Academy of Child and Adolescent Psychiatry, 43,* 708–717.

Lum, G. (2007). Kidney and urinary tract. In W. W. Hay, M. L. Leven, J. M. Sondheimer, & R. R. Deterding (Eds.), *Current pediatric diagnosis and treatment* (18th ed., pp. 684–707). New York: McGraw-Hill.

Lund, C. H., Bauer, K., & Berrios, M. (2007). Gastroschisis: Incidence, complications, and clinical management in the neonatal intensive care unit. *The Journal of Perinatal & Neonatal Nursing, 21*(1), 63–68.

Luxner, K. L. (2003). The complicated prenatal experience. In M. H. Hogan & R. S. Glazebrook (Eds.), *Maternal-newborn nursing.* Upper Saddle River, NJ: Prentice Hall.

Maisels, M. J. (2005). Jaundice in a newborn. *Contemporary Pediatrics,* *22*(5), 34–42, 54.

Mann, G., Attarbaschi, A., Steiner, M., Simonitsch, I., Strobl, H., Urban, C., Meister, B., Haas, O., Dworzak, M., & Gadner, H. (2006). Early and reliable diagnosis of non-Hodgkin lymphoma in childhood and adolescence. *Pediatric Hematology and Oncology, 23,* 167–176.

Manno, C. S., & Larson, P. J. (2005). Transfusion therapy for coagulation factor deficiencies. In R. Hoffman, E. J. Benz, S. J. Shattil, B. Furie, H. J. Cohen, L. E. Silberstein, & P. McGlave (Eds.), *Hematology: Basic principles and practice* (4th ed., pp. 2469–2480). St. Louis: Elsevier.

Manoff, E. M., Banffy, M. B., & Winell, J. J. (2005). Relationship between body mass index and slipped capital femoral epiphysis. *Journal of Pediatric Orthopedics, 25,* 744–746.

Mansfield, R. T. (2007). Severe traumatic brain injury. *Clinical Pediatric Emergency Medicine, 8,* 156–164.

Manworren, R. C. B., & Hynan, L. S. (2003). Clinical validation of FLACC: Preverbal patient pain scale. *Pediatric Nursing, 29*(2), 140–146.

March of Dimes. (2006). Quick reference: Recommended newborn screening tests: 29 disorders. Retrieved December 15, 2007, from http://www.marchofdimes.com/printableArticles/14332_15455.asp

March of Dimes. (2007). Newborn screening overview. Retrieved December 15, 2007, from http://www.marchofdimes.com/peristats/tlanding.aspx?reg=99&top=12&lev=0&slev=1

Marcoux, K. K. (2005). Management of increased intracranial pressure in the critically ill child with an acute neurologic injury. *AACN Clinical Issues, 16*(2), 212–231.

Marin, M., Güris, D., Chaves, S., Schmid, S., & Seward, J. F. (2007). Prevention of varicella: Recommendations of the Advisory Committee on Immunization Practices (ACIP). *Morbidity and Mortality Weekly Report, 56*(RR-4), 1–38.

Marinescu, L. M., & Ilowite, N. T. (2007, July). Update on pediatric rheumatology: Growth spurt in the knowledge base. *Consultant for Pediatricians,* 397–404.

Masharani, U. (2007). Diabetes mellitus and hypoglycemia. In S. J. McPhee, M. A. Papadakis, L. M. Tierney, Jr., R. Gonzales, & R. Zeiger (Eds.), *Current medical diagnosis and treatment 2008.* Retrieved December 20, 2007, from McGraw-Hill's Access Medicine.

McCrory, P., Johnston, K., Meeuwisse, W., Aubry, M., Cantu, R., et al. (2005). Summary and agreement statement of the 2nd international conference on concussion in sport, Prague 2004. *British Journal of Sports Medicine, 39,* 296–204.

McGuinness, T. M., & Pollack, D. (2008). Parental methamphetamine abuse and children. *Journal of Pediatric Health Care, 22*(3), 152–158.

Mehta, S. R., Afenyi-Annan, A., Byrns, P. F., Lottenberg, R. (2006). Opportunities to improve outcomes in sickle cell disease. *American Family Physician, 74*(2), 303–310.

Mercy, N., & Brady-Fryer, B. (2004). Bladder exstrophy: A challenge for nursing care. *Journal of Wound, Ostomy & Continence Nursing, 31*(5), 293–298.

Merkel, S. (2002). Pain assessment in infants and young children: The finger span scale. *American Journal of Nursing, 102*(11), 55–56.

Merkel, S., Voepel-Lewis, T., & Malviya, S. (2002). Pain assessment in infants and young children: The FLACC scale. *American Journal of Nursing, 102*(10), 55–57.

Merritt, L. (2005a). Part 1. Understanding the embryology and genetics of cleft lip and palate. *Advances in Neonatal Care, 5*(2), 64–71.

Merritt, L. (2005b). Part 2. Physical assessment of the infant with cleft lip and/or palate. *Advances in Neonatal Care, 5*(3), 125–134.

Metcalfe, P. D., & Schwarz, R. D. (2004). Bladder exstrophy: Neonatal care and surgical approaches. *Journal of Wound, Ostomy & Continence Nursing, 31*(5), 284–292.

Meyer, R. J., Theodorou, A. A., & Berg, R. A. (2006). Childhood drowning. *Pediatrics in Review, 27*(5), 163–168.

Milana, C., & Chandran, L. (2006). What's new in Kawasaki disease? *Contemporary Pediatrics, 23*(7), 40–47.

Milonovich, L. M. (2007). Meningococcemia: Epidemiology, pathophysiology, and management. *Journal of Pediatric Health Care, 21*(2), 75–80.

Misra, M., & Lee, M. M. (2005). Delayed puberty. In T. M. Moshange (Ed.), *Pediatric endocrinology: The requisites for pediatrics* (pp. 87–101). St. Louis: Elsevier Mosby.

Mitsnefes, M. M. (2006). Hypertension in children and adolescents. *Pediatric Clinics of North America, 53*, 493–512.

Molina, P. E. (2006). Parathyroid gland and Ca^{2+} and Po_4^- regulation. In *Endocrine Physiology* (2nd ed.). Retrieved December 21, 2007, from McGraw-Hill's Access Medicine.

Monroe, J. R. (2005). All that is round is not fungal. *Clinician Reviews, 15*(2), 46–53.

Moore, T. (2005). Bone marrow transplantation. Retrieved September 10, 2007, from http://www.emedicine.com/ped/topic2909.htm

Morcuende, J. A., Dolan, L. A., Dietz, F. R., & Ponseti, I.V. (2004). Radical reduction in the rate of extensive corrective surgery for clubfoot using the Ponseti method. *Pediatrics, 113*, 376–380.

Morgan, K., & McCance, K. L. (2006). Alterations of the reproductive systems. In K. L. McCance & S. E. Huether (Eds.), *Pathophysiology: The biologic basis for disease in adults and children* (5th ed., pp. 771–861). St. Louis: Elsevier Mosby.

Morgan, T. (2007). Turner syndrome: Diagnosis and management. *American Family Physician, 76*(3), 406–410.

Murdock, A. M., & Johnston, S. D. (2005). Diagnostic criteria for coelic disease: Time for change? *European Journal of Gastroenterology and Hepatology, 17*, 41–43.

Murray, D. L. (2003). Infectious diseases. In C. D. Rudolph & A. M. Rudolph (Eds.), *Rudolph's pediatrics* (21st ed., pp. 1102, 1106). New York: McGraw Hill.

Murray, R. B., Zentner, J. P., & Yakimo, R. (2009). *Health promotion strategies through the lifespan* (8th ed.). Upper Saddle River, NJ: Prentice Hall Health.

Nachman, P. H., Jennette, J. C., & Falk, R. J. (2008). Primary glomerular disease. In B. M. Brenner (Ed.), *Brenner & Rector's The Kidney* (8th ed., pp. 987–1066). Philadelphia: Saunders.

National Association of Pediatric Nurse Associates and Practitioners (NAPNAP). (2002). NAPNAP position statement on the pediatric health care home. Retrieved September 25, 2007, from http://www.napnap.org/practice/positions/healthcarehome.html

National Asthma Education and Prevention Program. (2007). *Expert panel report 3: Guidelines for the diagnosis and management of asthma.* Bethesda, MD: National Heart Lung and Blood Institute. Retrieved July 8, 2008, from http://www.nhlbi.nih.gov/guidelines/asthma/asthgdln.htm

National Center for Learning Disabilities. (2004). Learning disability. Retrieved August 15, 2008, from http://www.ldanatl.org/

National Heart, Lung, and Blood Institute. (2004). Blood pressure tables for children and adolescents from the fourth report on the diagnosis, evaluation, and treatment of high blood pressure in children and adolescents. Retrieved June 30, 2008, from http://www.nhlbi.nih.gov/guidelines/hypertension/child_tbl.htm

National Highway Traffic Safety Administration. (2007). Traffic safety. Retrieved June 12, 2007, from http:www.nhtsa.gov

National Institute of Allergy and Infectious Diseases (NIAID). (2004). HIV infection in infants and children. Retrieved September 8, 2007, from http://www.niaid.nih.gov/factsheets/hivchildren.htm

National Maternal and Child Oral Health Resource Center. (2004). Promoting awareness, preventing pain: Facts on early childhood caries (ECC). Retrieved July 12, 2006, from http://www.mchoralhealth.org/PDFs/ECCFactsheet.pdf

National Newborn Screening and Genetics Resource Center. (2006). National newborn screening status report. Retrieved May 22, 2006 from http://genes-r-us.uthscsa.edu/nbsdisorders.pdf

National Sleep Foundation. (2007). Children's sleep habits. Retrieved June 11, 2007, from http://www.sleepfoundation.org

Nehring, W. M. (2004). Down syndrome. In P. L. Allen & J. A. Vessey (Eds.), *Primary care of the child with a chronic condition* (pp. 445–468). St. Louis: Mosby.

Nelson, C. P. (2006). Vesicoureteral reflux. Retrieved May 25, 2007, from http://www.eMedicine.com

Nield, L. S., & Kamat, D. M. (2006). Diaper dermatitis: From "A" to "Pee." *Consultant for Pediatricians*, *5*(6), 373–360.

Nield, L. S., Mangano, L. M., & Kamat, D. (2008). Strabismus: A close-up look. *Consultant for Pediatricians,* January, 17–25.

NINDS—National Institute of Neurological Disorders and Stroke. (2007). NINDS shaken baby syndrome information. Retrieved December 5, 2007, from http://www.ninds.nih.gov/disorders/shakenbaby/shakenbaby.htm?css=print

Ochs, H. D., & Thrasher, A. J. (2006). The Wiskott-Aldrich syndrome. *Journal of Allergy and Immunology, 177*(4), 725–738.

Ogawa, M. T. (2007). Persevering against pediatric pulmonary arterial hypertension. *American Nurse Today, 2*(8), 41–46.

Olsen, E. M. (2006). Failure to thrive: Still a problem of definition. *Clinical Pediatrics, 45,* 1–6.

Olsson, J. (2007). The newborn. In R. M. Kliegman, R. E. Behrman, H. B. Jenson, B. F. Stanton, *Nelson textbook of pediatrics* (18th ed., pp. 41–42). Philadelphia: Saunders Elsevier.

O'Neill, S. G., & Isenberg, D. A. (2006). Immunizing Patients with Systemic Lupus Erythematosus: A Review of Effectiveness and Safety. *Lupus,* 15(11), 778–783.

Orenstein, S., Peters, J., Khan, S., Youssef, N., & Hussain, S. (2007). Congenital anomalies: Esophageal atresia and tracheoesophageal fistula. In R. M. Kliegman, R. E. Behrman, H. B. Jenson, & B. F. Stanton (Eds.), *Nelson textbook of pediatrics* (18th ed., pp. 1543–1544). Philadelphia: Saunders Elsevier.

O'Rourke, D. (2004). The measurement of pain in infants, children and adolescents: From policy to practice. *Physical Therapy, 84*(6), 560–570.

Otitis media with effusion. (2004). Clinical practice guideline. *Pediatrics, 113,* 1412–1429.

Otten, J. J., Hellwig, J. P., & Meyers, L. D. (Eds.). (2006). *Dietary reference intakes: The essential guide to nutrient requirements.* Washington, DC: National Academies Press.

Otten, M. E., & Stoops, M. M. (2007). Splenectomy, cholecystectomy, and Meckel's diverticulum. In N. T. Browne, L. M. Flanigan, C. A. McComiskey, & P. Pieper (Eds.), *Nursing care of the pediatric surgical patient* (2nd ed., pp. 357–375). Boston: Jones & Bartlett Publishers.

Owens, P. L., Thompson, J., Elixhauser, A., & Ryan, K. (2003). Care of children and adolescents in U.S. hospitals. In *HCUP Fact Book No. 4.* Rockville, MD: Agency for Healthcare Research and Quality.

Packman, W., Greenhalgh, J., Chesterman, B., Shaffer, T., Fine, J., Van Zutphen, K., Golan, R., & Amylon, M. D. (2005). Siblings of pediatric cancer patients: The quantitative and qualitative nature of quality of life. *Journal of Psychosocial Oncology, 23,* 87–108.

Palma Sisto, P. A. (2004). Endocrine disorders in the neonate. *Pediatric Clinics of North America, 51*(4), 1141–1168.

Palmer, K., & Burks, W. (2006). Current developments in peanut allergy. *Current Opinion in Allergy and Clinical Immunology, 6,* 202–206.

Panepinto, J. A., & Brousseau, D. C. (2005). Acute idiopathic thrombo-cytopenic purpura of childhood—diagnosis and therapy. *Pediatric Emergency Care, 21*, 691–695.

Pang, S. (2003). Newborn screening for congenital adrenal hyperplasia. *Pediatric Annals, 32*(8), 516–523.

Park, M. K. (2008). *Pediatric cardiology for practitioners* (5th ed.). Philadelphia: Mosby Elsevier.

Parks, J. S., & Felner, E. I. (2007a). Hormones of the hypothalamus and pituitary. In R. M. Kliegman, R. E. Behrman, H. B. Jenson, & B. F. Stanton (Eds.), *Nelson textbook of pediatrics* (18th ed., pp. 2291–2293). Philadelphia: Saunders Elsevier.

Parks, J. S., & Felner, E. I. (2007b). Hypopituitarism. In R. M. Kliegman, R. E. Behrman, H. B. Jenson, & B. F. Stanton (Eds.), *Nelson textbook of pediatrics* (18th ed., pp. 2293–2299). Philadelphia: Saunders Elsevier.

Paskawicz, J. (2005). Latex allergy revisited. *Clinician Reviews 15*(11), 66–75.

Patrick, K., Spear, B., Holt, K., & Sofka, D. (Eds.). (2001). *Bright futures in practice: Physical activity*. Arlington, VA: National Center for Education in Maternal and Child Health.

Pearlman, D. L. (2004). A simple treatment for head lice. Dry-on suffocation based pediculocide. *Pediatrics, 114*, 275–279.

Pellegrino, L. (2007). Cerebral palsy. In M. L. Batshaw, L. Pellegrino, & N. J. Roizen (Eds.), *Children with disabilities* (6th ed., pp. 387–408). Baltimore: Paul H. Brooks Publishing Co.

Pender, N. J., Murdaugh, C. L., & Parsons, M. A. (2006). *Health promotion in nursing practice* (5th ed.). Upper Saddle River, NJ: Prentice Hall.

Peredo-Pinto, H., & Jacobs, N. M. (2008). A 17-month infant with a calf lesion and generalized hypotonia. *Pediatric Annals, 37*(2), 96–98.

Petty, R. E., & Cassidy, J. T. (2005a). Polyarthritis. In J. T. Cassidy, R. E. Petty, R. M. Laxer, & C. B. Lindsley (Eds.), *Textbook of pediatric rheumatology* (5th ed., pp. 261–273). Philadelphia: Elsevier Saunders.

Petty, R. E., & Cassidy, J. T. (2005b). Oligoarthritis. In J. T. Cassidy, R. E. Petty, R. M. Laxer, & C. B. Lindsley (Eds.), *Textbook of pediatric rheumatology* (5th ed., pp. 274–290). Philadelphia: Elsevier Saunders.

Petty, R. E., & Cassidy, J. T. (2005c). Systemic arthritis. In J. T. Cassidy, R. E. Petty, R. M. Laxer, & C. B. Lindsley (Eds.), *Textbook of pediatric rheumatology* (5th ed., pp. 291–303). Philadelphia: Saunders Elsevier.

Petty, R. E., & Laxer, R. M. (2005). Systemic lupus erythematosus. In J. T. Cassidy, R. E. Petty, R. M. Laxer, & C. B. Lindsley (Eds.), *Textbook of pediatric rheumatology* (5th ed., pp. 342–391). Philadelphia: Elsevier Saunders.

Pieper, P. (2007). Pediatric trauma. In N. T. Browne, L. M. Flanigan, C. A. McComiskey, & P. Pieper (Eds.), *Nursing care of the pediatric surgical patient* (2nd ed., pp. 445–464). Boston: Jones & Bartlett Publishers.

Pinyerd, B., & Zipf, W. B. (2005). Puberty—timing is everything. *Journal of Pediatric Nursing, 20*(2), 75–82.

Pitetti, R. D., & Walker, S. (2005). Life-threatening chest injuries in children. *Clinical pediatric emergency medicine, 6*, 16–22.

Platt, A. F., & Eckman, J. (2006, February). Relieving the symptoms of sickle cell disease. *The Clinical Advisor, 54,* 59–62, 67.

Plowfield, L. A. (2007). HIV disease in children 25 years later. *Pediatric Nursing, 33*(3), 274–278, 273.

Potoka, D. A., & Saladino, R. A. (2005). Blunt abdominal trauma in the pediatric patient. *Clinical Pediatric Emergency Medicine, 6,* 23–31.

Prober, C. G. (2007). Central nervous system infections. In R. M. Kliegman, R. E. Behrman, H. B. Jenson, & B. F. Stanton (Eds.), *Nelson textbook of pediatrics* (18th ed., pp. 2512–2524). Philadelphia: Saunders Elsevier.

Pruett, J. R., & Luby, J. L. (2004). Recent advances in prepubertal mood disorders: Phenomenology and treatment. *Current Opinion in Psychiatry, 17,* 31–36.

Quinn, C. T., Rogers, Z. R., & Buchanan, G. R. (2004). Survival of children with sickle cell disease. *Blood, 103*(11), 4023–4027.

Rachmiel, M., Perlman, K., & Daneman, D. (2005). Insulin analogues in children and teens with type 1 diabetes: Advantages and caveats. *Pediatric Clinics of North America, 52,* 1651–1675.

Rafei, K., & Lichtenstein, R. (2006). Airway infectious disease emergencies. *Pediatric Clinics of North America, 53,* 215–242.

Raine, J. E., Donaldson, M. D. C., Gregory, J. W., Savage, M. O., & Hintz, R. L. (2006). Salt and water balance. In J. E. Raine, M. D. C. Donaldson, J. W. Gregory, M. O. Savage, & R. L. Hintz (Eds.), *Practical endocrinology and diabetes in children.*(2nd ed., pp. 147–155). Malden, MA: Blackwell Publishing, Inc.

Raszka, W. V., & Khan, O. (2005). Pyelonephritis. *Pediatrics in Review, 26*(10), 364–369.

Razzaq, S. (2006). Hemolytic uremic syndrome: An emerging health risk. *American Family Physician, 74*(6), 991–996.

Reardon, J. Z. (2007). Environmental tobacco smoke: Respiratory and other health effects. *Clinical Chest Medicine, 28,* 559–573.

Reznik, M., & Ozuah, P. O. (2005). A prudent approach to screening for and treating tuberculosis. *Contemporary Pediatrics, 22*(11), 73–88.

Rezvani, I. (2007). Defects in metabolisim of amino acids. In R. M. Kliegman, R. E. Behrman, H. B. Jenson, & B. F. Stanton (Eds.), *Nelson textbook of pediatrics* (18th ed., pp. 529–532). Philadelphia: Saunders Elsevier.

Rheingold, S. R., & Lange, B. J. (2006). In P. A. Pizzo & D. G. Poplack (Eds.), *Principles and practice of pediatric oncology* (5th ed., pp. 1202–1230). Philadelphia: Lippincott Williams & Wilkins.

Richardson, M. (2007). Microcytic anemia. *Pediatrics in Review, 28*(1), 5–14.

Ringdahl, E., & Teague, L. (2006). Testicular torsion. *American Family Physician, 74*(10), 1739–1743.

Riviello, J. J., Ashwal, S., Hirtz, D., Glauser, T., Ballaban-Gil, K., et al. (2006). Practice parameter: Diagnostic assessment of the child with status epilepticus (an evidence-based review). *Neurology, 67,* 1542–1550.

Rivkees, S. A., & Dinauer, C. (2007). An optimal treatment for pediatric Graves' disease is Radioiodine. *The Journal of Clinical Endocrinology & Metabolism, 92*(3), 797–800.

Roach, J. P., & Bruny, J. L. (2008). Advances in the treatment and understanding of biliary atresia. *Current Opinion in Pediatrics, 20,* 315–319.

Roberts, P. F., Waller, T. A., Brinker, T. M., Riffe, I., Sayre, J. W., & Bratton, R. L. (2007). Henoch-Schönlein purpura: A review article. *Southern Medical Journal, 100*(8), 821–824.

Robertson, J., & Shilkofski, N. (Eds.). (2005). *The Harriet Lane handbook* (17th ed.). Philadelphia: Elsevier Mosby.

Robinson, R. F., Nahata, M. C., Mahan, J. D., & Batisky, D. L. (2003). Management of nephrotic syndrome in children. *Pharmacotherapy, 23*(8), 1021–1036.

Rosenbaum, P., Paneth, N., Leviton, A., Goldstein, M., Bax, M., et al. (2007). A report: The definition and classification of cerebral palsy, April 2006. *Developmental Medicine and Child Neurology, 49,* 8–14.

Rouse, B., & Azen, C. (2004). Effect of high maternal blood phenylalanine on offspring congenital anomalies and developmental outcome at ages 4 and 6 years: The importance of strict dietary control preconception and throughout pregnancy. *Journal of Pediatrics, 144,* 235–239.

Ruth, E. M., Landolt, M. A., Neuhaus, T. J., & Kemper, M. J. (2004). Health-related quality of life and psychosocial adjustment in steroid-sensitive nephrotic syndrome. *Journal of Pediatrics, 145*(6), 778–783.

Ruth, E. M., Kemper, M. J., Leumann, E. P., Laube, G. F., & Neuhaus, T. J. (2005). Children with steroid-sensitive nephrotic syndrome come of age: Long-term outcome. *Journal of Pediatrics, 14* (2), 202–207.

Sampson, H. A. & Leung, D. Y. M. (2007). Anaphylaxis. In, R. M. Kliegman, R. E. Behrman, H. B. Jenson, & B. F. Stanton, *Nelson textbook of pediatrics* (18th ed., pp. 983–985). Philadelphia: Saunders Elsevier.

Saulsbury, F. T. (2007). Clinical update: Henoch-Schönlein purpura. *The Lancet, 369,* 976–978.

Saunthararajah, Y., Vichinsky, E. P., Embury, S. H. (2005). Sickle cell disease. In R. Hoffman, E. J. Benz, S. J. Shattil, B. Furie, H. J. Cohen, L. E. Silberstein, & P. McGlave (Eds.), Hematology: Basic principles and practice (4th ed., pp. 605–644). St. Louis: Elsevier.

Saxena, A. K. (2006). Abdominal trauma. Retrieved October 13, 2007, from http://www.emedicine.com/ped/topic3045.htm

Schiller, C., & Allen, P. J. (2005). Follow-up of infants prenatally exposed to cocaine. *Pediatric Nursing, 31*(5), 427–436.

Schultz, K. A., Ness, K. K., Whitton, J., Recklitis, C., Zebrack, B., Robison, L. L., Zeltzer, L., & Mertens, A. C. (2007). Behavioral and social outcomes in adolescent survivors of childhood cancer: A report from the childhood cancer survivor study. *Journal of Clinical Oncology, 25,* 3649–3656.

Schwaderer, A. L., & Schwartz, G. J. (2004). Back to basics: Acidosis and alkalosis. *Pediatric Review, 25,* 350–357.

Sciscione, P., & Krause-Parello, C. A. (2007). No-nit policies in schools: Time for a change. *Journal of School Nursing, 23*(1), 13–20.

Sectish, T. C., & Prober, C. G. (2007). Pneumonia. In R. M. Kliegman, R. E. Behrman, H. B. Jenson, & B. F. Stanton (Eds.), *Nelson textbook of pediatrics* (18th ed., pp. 1795–1800). Philadelphia: Saunders Elsevier.

Sepa, A., Wahlberg, J., Vaarala, O., Frodi, A., & Ludvigsson, J. (2005). Psychological stress may induce diabetes-related autoimmunity in infancy. *Diabetes Care, 28*(2), 290–295.

Shaw, N. M. (2003). Assessment and management of the hematologic system. In C. Kenner & J. W. Lott (Eds.), *Comprehensive neonatal nursing: A physiologic perspective* (3rd ed., pp. 586–602). St. Louis, MO: Saunders.

Sheffer, A. L., Feldweg, A., & Castells, M. (2006). Anaphylaxis. In S. T. Holgate, M. K. Church, & L. M. Lichtenstein (Eds.), *Allergy* (3rd ed., pp. 167–178). Philadelphia: Mosby Elsevier.

Shelov, S. P. (Ed.). (2004). *The American Academy of Pediatrics: Caring for your baby and young child: Birth to age 5* (4th ed.). New York: Bantam Books.

Shetty, K. (2006). Oral lesions commonly associated with pediatric HIV infection—presentation, management, and review of the literature. *General Dentistry, 54,* 284–287.

Shipman, S., Helfand, M., Nygren, P., & Bougatsos, C. (2006). Screening for developmental dysplasia of the hip. Evidence synthesis 42. *Agency for Healthcare Research and Quality*, 1–98.

Shuler, P., Huebscher, R., Miller, H., & Rauckhorst, L. (2004). Genitourinary concerns. In R. Huebscher & P. A. Shuler (Eds.), *Natural, alternative and complementary health care practices* (pp. 567–658). St. Louis: Mosby.

Shy, R. (2007). Tinea corporis and tinea capitis. *Pediatrics in Review*, *28*(5), 164–174.

Silbermintz, A., & Markowitz, J. (2006). Inflammatory bowel disease. *Pediatric Annals*, *35*(4), 269–274.

Silverstein, J., Klingensmith, G., Copeland, K., Plotnick, L., Kaufman, F., Laffel, L., et al. (2005). Care of children and adolescents with type 1 diabetes. *Diabetes Care, 28*(1), 186–212.

Simon, E., Flaschker, N., Schadewaldt, P., Langenbeck, U., & Wendel, U. (2006). Variant maple syrup urine disease (MSUD)—The entire spectrum. *Journal of Inherited Metabolic Disease, 29*, 716–724.

Simons, E., Weiss, C. C., Furlong, T. J., & Sicherer, S. H. (2005). Impact of ingredient labeling practices on food allergic consumers. *Annals of Allergy, Asthma and Immunology*, *95*(5), 426–428.

Singh, J., & Arrieta, A. C. (2004). Management of meningococcemia. *The Indian Journal of Pediatrics, 71*(10), 909–913.

Sladden, M. J., & Johnston, G. A. (2005, May 21). Clinical review: More common skin infections in children. *British Medical Journal*, *330*, 1194–1198.

Small M. J., & Copel, J. A. (2004, February). Ultrasound Clinics: Practical guidelines for diagnosing and treating fetal hydronephrosis. *Contemporary OB/GYN, 49*(2), 59–60, 64, 66.

Smoot, L. C., Boothby, L. A., & Gillett, R. C. (2007). Clinical assessment and treatment of ADHD in children. *International Journal of Clinical Practice, 61*, 1730–1738.

Soldin, S. J., Brugnara, C., & Wong, E. C. (2005). *Pediatric reference ranges* (5th ed.). Washington, DC: AACC Press.

Spinazze, S., & Schrijvers, D. (2006). Metabolic emergencies. *Critical Reviews in Oncology/Hematology, 58*, 79–89.

Starke, J. R. (2007). New concepts in childhood tuberculosis. *Current Opinion in Pediatrics, 19*(3), 306–313.

Steadman, B., & Ellsworth, P. (2006). To circ or not to circ: Indications, risks, and alternatives to circumcision in the pediatric population with phimosis. *Urologic Nursing, 26*(3), 181–194.

Stevenson, K. L. (2004). Chiari type II malformation: Past, present, future. *Neurosurgical Focus, 16*(2), E5.

Stichweh, D., Arce, E., & Pascual, V. (2004). Update on pediatric systemic lupus erythematosus. *Current Opinion in Rheumatology, 16*, 577–587.

Stoll, B. J. (2007a). Metabolic disturbances. In R. M. Kliegman, R. E. Behrman, H. B. Jenson, & B. F. Stanton (Eds.), *Nelson textbook of pediatrics* (18th ed., pp. 777–782). Philadelphia: Elsevier Saunders.

Stoll, B. J. (2007b). The umbilicus. In R. M. Kliegman, R. E. Behrman, H. B. Jenson, & B. F. Stanton (Eds.), *Nelson textbook of pediatrics* (18th ed., pp. 775–777). Philadelphia: Saunders Elsevier.

Strausbaugh, S. D., & Davis, P. B. (2007). Cystic fibrosis: A review of epidemiology and pathobiology. *Clinics of Chest Medicine, 28*, 279–288.

Suwandhi, E., Ton, M. N., & Schwarz, S. S. (2006). Gastroesophageal reflux in infancy and childhood. *Pediatric Annals, 35*(4), 259–266.

Tamburrini, S., Brunetti, A., Brown, M., Sirlin C., & Casola, G. (2007). Acute appendicitis: Diagnostic value of nonenhanced CT with selective use of contrast in routine clinical settings.*European Radiology, 17*, 2055–2061.

Tezcan, I., Ersoy, F., Sanal, O., Turul, T., Uckan, D., Balci, S., Hicsonmez, G., Prieur, M., Caillat-Zucmann, S., Le Deist, F., & Basile, G. S. (2005). Long-term survival in severe combined immune deficiency: The role of persistent maternal engraftment. *The Journal of Pediatrics, 146*, 137–140.

Theos, A., & Korf, B. R. (2006). Pathophysiology of neurofibromatosis type 1. *Annals of Internal Medicine, 144*(11), 842–849.

Thomas, J. A., & Van Hove, J. L. K. (2007). Inborn errors of metabolism. In W. W. Hay, M. J. Levin, J. M. Sondheimer, & R. R. Deterding (Eds.), *Current pediatric diagnosis and treatment* (18th ed.). Access Medicine: McGraw-Hill Companies.

Tofte, S. (2007). Atopic dermatitis. *Nursing Clinics of North America, 42*, 407–419.

Towbin, J. A., Lowe, A. M., Colan, S. D., Sleeper, L. A., Orav, E. J., et al. (2006). Incidence, causes, and outcomes of dilated cardiomyopathy in children. *Journal of the American Medical Association, 296*(15), 1867–1876.

Trigg, M. E. (2004). Hematopoietic stem cells. *Pediatrics, 13*, 1051–1057.

Twombly, R. (2007). Childhood cancer survivor study doubles to examine late effects of new treatments. *News – Journal National Cancer Institute, 99*, 1574–1576.

Tyler, C., & Edman, J. C. (2004). Down syndrome, Turner syndrome, and Klinefelter syndrome: Primary care throughout the life span. *Primary Care Clinics for Office Practitioners, 31*, 627–648.

Ummpierrez, G. E. (2006). Ketosis-prone type 2 diabetes. *Diabetes Care, 29*(12), 2755–2757.

U.S. Department of Health and Human Services. (2006). *Healthy people 2010: Midcourse review*. Washington, DC: Author.

U.S. Department of Health and Human Services. (2008a). Guidelines for the use of antiretroviral agents in pediatric HIV infection. Retrieved April 20, 2008, from http://aidsinfo.nih.gov/contentfiles/PediatricGuidelines.pdf

U.S. Department of Health and Human Services. (2008b). Pediatric antiretroviral drug information. Retrieved April 20, 2008, from http://aidsinfo.nih.gov/contentfiles/PediatricGL_SupI.pdf

Utterson, E. C., Shepherd, R. W., Sokol, R. J., Bucuvalas, J., Magee, J. C., McDiarmid, S. V., & Anand, R. (2005). Biliary atresia: Clinical profiles, risk factors, and outcomes of 755 patients listed for liver transplantation. *The Journal of Pediatrics, 147*(2), 180–185.

Vaira, D., Gatta, L., Ricci, C., Tampieri, A., Cavina, M., & Bernabucci V. (2005). Symposium on peptic acid disease. Peptic ulcer and *Helicobacter pylori*: Update on testing and treatment. *Postgraduate Medicine, 117*(6), 17–22, 46.

Vajnar, J. (2007). A common cause of vomiting in infancy. *Journal of the American Academy of Physician Assistants, 20*(1), 58–59.

Van Riper, M. (2007). Families of children with Down syndrome: Responding to "a change of plans" with resilience. *Journal of Pediatric Nursing, 22*, 116–127.

Vegunta, R. K., Ali, A., Wallace, L. J., Switzer, D. M., & Pearl, X. X. (2004). Laparoscopic appendectomy in children: Technically feasible and safe in all stages of acute appendicitis. *The American Surgeon, 70*, 198–202.

Vetter, V. L. (2006). Kawasaki disease. In V. L. Vetter (Ed.), *Pediatric cardiology: The requisites in pediatrics* (pp. 131–144). St. Louis: Elsevier Mosby.

Viera, A. J. (2002). Hyperparathyroidism. *Clinics in Family Practice, 4*(3), 627–638.

Visner, G. A., & Goldfarb, S. B. (2007). Posttransplant monitoring of pediatric lung transplant recipients. *Current Opinion in Pediatrics, 19*(3), 321–326.

Voepel-Lewis, T., Malviya, S., & Tait, A. R. (2005). Validity of parent ratings as proxy measures of pain in children with cognitive impairment. *Pain Management Nursing, 6*(4), 168–174.

Vogt, B. A., & Avner, E. D. (2007a). Conditions particularly associated with proteinuria. In R. M. Kliegman, R. E. Behrman, H. B. Jenson, & B. F. Stanton (Eds.), *Nelson textbook of pediatrics* (18th ed., pp. 2188–2195). Philadelphia: Saunders Elsevier.

Vogt, B. A., & Avner, E. D. (2007b). Toxic neuropathies: Renal failure. In R. M. Kliegman, R. E. Behrman, H. B. Jenson, & B. F. Stanton (Eds.), *Nelson textbook of pediatrics* (18th ed., pp. 2204–2219). Philadelphia: Saunders Elsevier.

Volkmar, F. R., Wiesner, L. A., & Westphal, A. (2006). Healthcare issues for children on the autism spectrum. *Current Opinions in Psychiatry, 19*, 361–366.

Walle, J. V., Mauel, R., Raes, A., Vanderkerckhove, K., & Donckerwolcke, R. (2004). ARF in children with minimal change nephrotic syndrome may be related to functional changes of the glomerular basement membrane. *American Journal of Kidney Diseases, 43*(3), 399–404.

Walsh, M. C., Szefler, S., Davis, J., Allen, M., Van Martin, L., et al. (2006). Summary proceedings from the bronchopulmonary dysplasia group. *Pediatrics, 117*(3), S52–S56.

Wang, J., Wiley, J. M., Luddy, R., Greenberg, J., Feuerstein, M., & Bussel, J. B. (2005). Chornic immune thrombocytopenic purpura in children: Assessment of Rituximab treatment. *The Journal of Pediatrics, 146*, 217–221.

Warady, B. A., & Chada, V. (2007). Chronic kidney disease in children: the global perspective. *Pediatric Nephrology, 22* (12), 1999–2009.

Wathen, J. E., MacKenzie, T., & Bothner, J. P. (2004). Usefulness of the serum electrolyte panel in the management of pediatric dehydration treated with intravenously administered fluids. *Pediatrics, 114*, 1227–1234.

Weerasooriya, V. S., White, F., & Shepherd. R. W. (2004). Hepatic fibrosis and survival in biliary atresia. *The Journal of Pediatrics, 144*(1), 123–125.

Weinstein, S. L., & Gaillard, W. D. (2007). Epilepsy. In M. L. Barshaw, L. Pellegrino, & N. J. Roizen, (Eds.), *Children with disabilities* (6th ed., pp. 439–460). Baltimore: Paul H. Brooks Publishing Co.

Weston, S., Halbert, A., Richmond, P., & Prescott, S. L. (2005). Effects of probiotics on atopic dermatitis: A randomized controlled trial. *Archives of Disease in Childhood, 90*, 892–897.

White, P. C. (2007). Disorders of the adrenal glands. In R. M. Kliegman, R. E. Behrman, H. B. Jenson, & B. F. Stanton, *Nelson textbook of pediatrics* (18th ed., pp. 2349–2374). Philadelphia: Saunders Elsevier.

Willis, M. H. W., Merkel, S. I., Voepel-Lewis, T., & Malviya, S. (2003). FLACC behavioral pain assessment scale: A comparison with the child's self-report. *Pediatric Nursing, 29*(3), 195–198.

Wilne, S., Collier, J., Kennedy, C., Koller, K., Grundy, R., & Walker, D. (2007). Presentation of childhood CNS tumors: A systematic review and meta-analysis. *The Lancet Oncology, 8*, 685–695.

Wilne, S. H., Ferris, R. C., Nathwani, A., & Kennedy, C. R. (2006). The presenting features of brain tumors: A review of 200 cases. *Archive of Diseases in Children, 91*, 502–506.

Wilson, B. A., Shannon, M. T., & Shields, K. M. (2009). *Nurses' drug guide 2009*. Upper Saddle River, NJ: Pearson Prentice Hall.

Wilson, W., Taubert, K. A., Gewitz, M., Lockhart, P. B., Baddour, L. M., et al. (2007). Prevention of infective endocarditis: Guidelines from the American Heart Association Rheumatic Fever, Endocarditis, and Kawasaki Disease Committee, Council on Cardiovascular Disease in the Young, and the Council on Clinical Cardiology, Council on Cardiovascular Surgery and Anesthesia, and the Quality of Care and Outcomes Research Interdisciplinary Working Group. *Circulation, 116*, 1736–1754.

Wolraich, M. L., Wibbelsman, C. J., Brown, T. E., Evans, S. W., Gotlieb, E. M., Knight, J. R., Ross, C., Shubiner, H. H., Wender, E. H., & Wilens, T. (2005). Attention-deficit/hyperactivity disorder among adolescents: A review of the diagnosis, treatment, and clinical implications. *Pediatrics, 115,* 1734–1746.

Wong, D. L., & Baker, C. M. (1988). Pain in children: Comparison of assessment scales. *Pediatric Nursing, 14,* 9–16.

Woods, C. R. (2007). Neisseria meningitidis. In R. M. Kliegman, R. E. Behrman, H. B. Jenson, & B. F. Stanton (Eds.), *Nelson textbook of pediatrics* (18th ed., pp. 1164–1169). Philadelphia: Saunders Elsevier.

World Health Organization. (1996). *Basic document* (36th ed.). Geneva, Switzerland: Author.

Wyllie, R. (2007). Pyloric stenosis and congenital anomalies of the stomach. In R. M. Kliegman, R.E. Behrman, H. B. Jenson, & B. F. Stanton (Eds.), *Nelson textbook of pediatrics* (18th ed., pp. 1555–1558). Philadelphia: Saunders Elsevier.

Yaeger, D., McCallum, J., Lewis, K., Soslow, L., Shah, U., Potsic, W., Stolle, C., & Krantz, I. D. (2006). Outcomes of clinical examination and genetic testing of 500 individuals with hearing loss evaluated through a genetics of hearing loss clinic. *American Journal of Medical Genetics, 140,* 827–836.

Yazdy, M. M., Honein, M. A., & Xing, J. (2007). Reduction in orofacial clefts following folic acid fortification of the U.S. grain supply. *Birth Defects Research (Part A), 79*(1), 16–23.

Yazigi, N., & Balistreri, W. F. (2007). Viral hepatitis. In R. M. Kliegman, R. E. Behrman, H. B. Jenson, & B. F. Stanton (Eds.), *Nelson textbook of pediatrics* (18th ed., pp. 1680–1690). Philadelphia: Saunders Elsevier.

Young, N. S., Calado, R. T., & Scheinberg, P. (2006). Current concepts in pathophsiology and treatment of aplastic anemia. *Blood, 108*(8), 2509–2519.

Zaenglein, A. L., & Thiboutot, D. M. (2006). Expert committee recommendations for acne management. *Pediatrics, 118*(3), 1188–1199.

Zelnik, N., Pacht, A., Obeid, R., & Lerner, A. (2004). Range of neurological disorders in patients with celiac disease. *Pediatrics, 113,* 1672–1677.

Zimmerman, B. T. (2007). Abdominal wall defects. In N. T. Browne, L. M. Flanigan, C. A. McComiskey, & P. Pieper (Eds.), *Nursing care of the pediatric surgical patient* (2nd ed., pp. 261–271). Boston: Jones & Bartlett Publishers.

INDEX